WOMEN'S HEALTH
98/99
First Edition

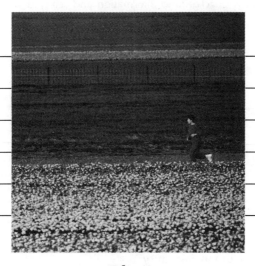

Editors

Maureen Edwards
Montgomery College

Dr. Maureen Edwards is coordinator of the Health Education Program at Montgomery College in Rockville, Maryland, and a faculty research assistant in the Department of Health Education at the University of Maryland, College Park. A private consultant in health behavior, including pain management, weight control, and smoking cessation, her areas of specialization are stress management and gerontology. During her tenure at the University of Maryland Health Center, Dr. Edwards served as coordinator of the Stress Management Education Program. In addition, Dr. Edwards has served as a stress management consultant to a number of government and private agencies.
Dr. Edwards holds a doctorate in health education from the University of Maryland. She also is certified as a health education specialist.

Nora L. Howley
Montgomery College

Nora Howley is an adjunct faculty member in the Health Education Program at Montgomery College in Rockville, Maryland, where she teaches Women's Health, among other courses. In addition, she is a private consultant in health education, working in the areas of women's health, worker health education, and needs assessment and evaluation issues.
Ms. Howley is the former Health Educator for the Association of Occupational and Environmental Clinics, where she developed health education programs for health professionals and community members. She also developed field placement programs in occupational health for medical students and undergraduate health education students. Presently, she is a consultant to the American Federation of Teachers' Breast and Cervical Cancer Education Project.
Ms. Howley has a master's degree in health education from the University of Maryland. She is also a certified health education specialist.

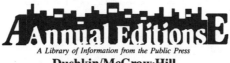

Annual Editions
A Library of Information from the Public Press
Dushkin/McGraw·Hill
Sluice Dock, Guilford, Connecticut 06437

Visit us on the Internet—http://www.dushkin.com/

The Annual Editions Series

ANNUAL EDITIONS, including GLOBAL STUDIES, consist of over 70 volumes designed to provide the reader with convenient, low-cost access to a wide range of current, carefully selected articles from some of the most important magazines, newspapers, and journals published today. ANNUAL EDITIONS are updated on an annual basis through a continuous monitoring of over 300 periodical sources. All ANNUAL EDITIONS have a number of features that are designed to make them particularly useful, including topic guides, annotated tables of contents, unit overviews, and indexes. For the teacher using ANNUAL EDITIONS in the classroom, an Instructor's Resource Guide with test questions is available for each volume. GLOBAL STUDIES titles provide comprehensive background information and selected world press articles on the regions and countries of the world.

VOLUMES AVAILABLE

ANNUAL EDITIONS
Abnormal Psychology
Accounting
Adolescent Psychology
Aging
American Foreign Policy
American Government
American History, Pre-Civil War
American History, Post-Civil War
American Public Policy
Anthropology
Archaeology
Astronomy
Biopsychology
Business Ethics
Child Growth and Development
Comparative Politics
Computers in Education
Computers in Society
Criminal Justice
Criminology
Developing World
Deviant Behavior
Drugs, Society, and Behavior
Dying, Death, and Bereavement
Early Childhood Education

Economics
Educating Exceptional Children
Education
Educational Psychology
Environment
Geography
Geology
Global Issues
Health
Human Development
Human Resources
Human Sexuality
International Business
Macroeconomics
Management
Marketing
Marriage and Family
Mass Media
Microeconomics
Multicultural Education
Nutrition
Personal Growth and Behavior
Physical Anthropology
Psychology
Public Administration
Race and Ethnic Relations

Social Problems
Social Psychology
Sociology
State and Local Government
Teaching English as a Second
    Language
Urban Society
Violence and Terrorism
Western Civilization,
    Pre-Reformation
Western Civilization,
    Post-Reformation
Women's Health
World History, Pre-Modern
World History, Modern
World Politics

GLOBAL STUDIES
Africa
China
India and South Asia
Japan and the Pacific Rim
Latin America
Middle East
Russia, the Eurasian Republics,
    and Central/Eastern Europe
Western Europe

Cataloging in Publication Data
Main entry under title: Annual editions: Women's health, 1998/99.
    1. Women—Health and hygiene. I. Edwards, Maureen, *comp.* II. Howley, Nora L., *comp.* III. Title:
Women's health.
ISBN 0-07-012568-6   613.042'44'05

First Edition

Cover image © 1996 PhotoDisc, Inc.

Printed in the United States of America

Printed on Recycled Paper

Editors/Advisory Board

Members of the Advisory Board are instrumental in the final selection of articles for each edition of ANNUAL EDITIONS. Their review of articles for content, level, currentness, and appropriateness provides critical direction to the editor and staff. We think that you will find their careful consideration well reflected in this volume.

Editors

Maureen Edwards
Montgomery College

Nora L. Howley
Montgomery College

ADVISORY BOARD

Staff

To the Reader

In publishing ANNUAL EDITIONS we recognize the enormous role played by the magazines, newspapers, and journals of the *public press* in providing current, first-rate educational information in a broad spectrum of interest areas. Many of these articles are appropriate for students, researchers, and professionals seeking accurate, current material to help bridge the gap between principles and theories and the real world. These articles, however, become more useful for study when those of lasting value are carefully *collected, organized, indexed,* and *reproduced* in a *low-cost format,* which provides easy and permanent access when the material is needed. That is the role played by ANNUAL EDITIONS. Under the direction of each volume's *academic editor,* who is an expert in the subject area, and with the guidance of an *Advisory Board,* each year we seek to provide in each ANNUAL EDITION a current, well-balanced, carefully selected collection of the best of the public press for your study and enjoyment. We think that you will find this volume useful, and we hope that you will take a moment to let us know what you think.

In this first edition of *Annual Editions: Women's Health 98/99,* we have tried to address the most current issues in women's health, which is no easy task. After a long period of neglect and lack of interest from the medical community, the past 20 years have seen increased interest in this field. The National Institutes of Health have targeted women's health with large research initiatives such as *The Women's Health Initiative; The Nurses' Health Study;* and the *Study of Women's Health across the Nation.* Because of this heightened level of interest, large quantities of new information, at times contradictory, are now available. In preparing this volume, we have sifted through a diverse range of publications. Our goals are both to provide factual information and to challenge the reader to think critically about some of the more controversial issues in the field.

Not every issue is clear cut. Consensus does not always exist, and we have tried to represent multiple viewpoints. It is not surprising that after the years of neglect of women's health, there are now differences of opinion. It is our hope that this set of readings can be a supplement to the existing women's health texts. We recognize that we are not able to address every area, but we have tried to survey many of the issues in the public consciousness.

Women's health is more than reproductive health issues. Women's health is nutrition, mental health, fitness, chronic disease, and so on. We have attempted to touch as many of those areas as possible, without neglecting the reproductive arena. Women are not monocultural. We have tried to address some of the issues from the perspective of nonwhite women. Most of the articles selected come from nonprofessional literature, which we hope will make the health information more easily accessible. We have also included articles from health newsletters and journals that provide current information from the research in a timely manner.

The book is divided into eight units that correspond to major areas of health, such as nutrition and fitness and psychological health, or that address key topics, such as violence, chronic diseases, and reproductive health. The first chapter, Women and Health, is designed to explore issues of how women participate in the health care system, including managed care and alternative medicine. This chapter is intended to provide an overview of the status of women's health and the leading issues.

To facilitate the use of this volume by teachers and students of women's health, we have included a number of features. Because so many health issues cut across chapter headings, the *topic guide* provides a cross-reference for finding information on topics in all the locations where it is addressed. This allows the student to see the interaction of the different areas of health. The *table of contents* also includes abstracts, in which we have tried to summarize the key points of each article. Instructors may find this useful in choosing readings to assign. Each unit begins with an overview, providing background information on the area as well as more detailed information on how articles were chosen. We have also included *challenge questions* to help students focus their reading.

We will be updating *Annual Editions: Women's Health* annually. It is our goal that this collection should be useful and effective for those teaching and learning. We welcome your advice, suggestions, and comments. Please complete and return the postage-paid *article rating form* on the last page of the book. Thank you.

Maureen Edwards

Nora L. Howley
Editors

Contents

UNIT 1

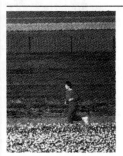

Women and Health

The six articles in this section consider the way women are treated in today's health care system.

UNIT 2

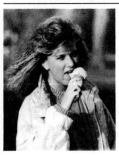

Nutrition and Fitness

Eight selections in this unit look at the current popularity of dieting and the need for a healthful fitness program.

The concepts in bold italics are developed in the article. For further expansion please refer to the Topic Guide and the Index.

v

UNIT 3

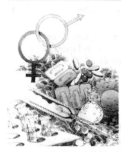

Gynecological and Sexual Health

In this section, nine articles consider the importance of periodic physical examinations, the latest data on birth control, and the abortion debate.

UNIT 4

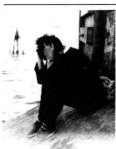

Psychological Health

Seven selections in this section look at how stress, depression, eating disorders, and children impact on a woman's psychological health.

The concepts in bold italics are developed in the article. For further expansion please refer to the Topic Guide and the Index.

vii

UNIT 5

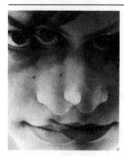

Chronic Diseases

How heart disease, cancer, and other chronic diseases affect women are addressed in the eleven articles in this section.

The concepts in bold italics are developed in the article. For further expansion please refer to the Topic Guide and the Index.

viii

UNIT 6

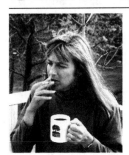

Substance Abuse: New Trends for Women

In this unit, seven articles look at the latest on women's abuse of tobacco, alcohol, and drugs.

The concepts in bold italics are developed in the article. For further expansion please refer to the Topic Guide and the Index.

UNIT 7

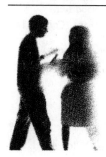

Violence in Women's Lives

Five selections in this section
discuss violence and women,
particularly domestic
violence and rape.

x

The concepts in bold italics are developed in the article. For further expansion please refer to the Topic Guide and the Index.

UNIT 8

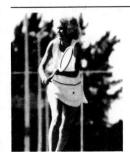

Special Issues for Older Women

The six selections in this section consider health challenges that older women face.

The concepts in bold italics are developed in the article. For further expansion please refer to the Topic Guide and the Index.

Topic Guide

This topic guide suggests how the selections in this book relate to topics of concern to students and professionals involved with women's health. It can be used to locate articles that are related to each other for reading and research. The guide is arranged alphabetically according to topics. Articles may, of course, treat subjects that do not appear in the topic guide. In turn, entries in the topic guide do not necessarily constitute a comprehensive listing of all the contents of each selection. **In addition, relevant Web sites, which are annotated on the next two pages, are noted in bold italics under the topic articles.**

TOPIC AREA	TREATED IN	TOPIC AREA	TREATED IN
Abortion	22. National Abortion Debate 23. Psychological Aftereffects of Abortion *(6, 14, 15)*	**Diet**	7. Say Good-Bye to Dieting 8. Confessions 10. Diet Pills 12. Who *Isn't* on a Diet? 13. Diet Fix 14. Weighty Matters in Women's Health 31. Mending the Female Heart 34. Redesigning Women: Breast Cancer 37. Silent Epidemic 55. Who Age Better—Men or Women? *(10, 11, 12, 13, 16, 18, 19, 27, 28, 29)*
Addictions	42. What Does Being Female Have to Do with It? 43. Facts about Women and Smoking 44. Up in Smoke 45. Smoker's Tale 47. Alcohol and Health: Mixed Messages 48. Way Out West and Under the Influence *(16, 17, 22, 23, 24)*		
		Eating Disorders	11. Dying to Win 12. Who *Isn't* on a Diet? 14. Weighty Matters in Women's Health 28. Treating Eating Disorders 44. Up in Smoke *(11, 12, 13, 16)*
Aging	13. Diet Fix 30. New Rite of Passage 39. When Arthritis Strikes 54. Our Mothers, Ourselves 55. Who Age Better, Men or Women? 56. Hormone Therapy 57. Silent Sabotage 58. Mammography Muddle *(9, 10, 11, 12, 14, 18, 19, 27, 28, 29)*	**Estrogen**	16. Politically Incorrect Surgery 20. Endometriosis: The Hidden Epidemic 32. Heart Disease in Women: Special Symptoms 33. Consensus: No Long-Term Link 34. Redesigning Women: Breast Cancer 55. Who Age Better—Men or Women? 56. Hormone Therapy 57. Silent Sabotage *(14, 15, 18, 21, 27, 28, 29)*
Arthritis	38. Living with Lupus 39. When Arthritis Strikes *(2, 9, 10, 27, 28, 29)*		
Cancer	13. Diet Fix 15. Smart Pap 16. Politically Incorrect Surgery 33. Consensus: No Long-Term Link 34. Redesigning Women: Breast Cancer 35. Cancer Nobody Talks About 36. Mole Patrol 56. Hormone Therapy 58. Mammography Muddle 59. Options for Hysterectomy *(1, 4, 9, 19, 20, 21, 27, 28, 29)*	**Ethics**	5. Fitting into Our Genes 8. Confessions 22. National Abortion Debate 23. Psychological Aftereffects of Abortion 45. Smoker's Tale 49. Female Genital Mutilation 52. "I Was Raped" *(5, 6, 10, 14, 15, 22, 25, 26)*
		Exercise	7. Say Good-Bye to Dieting 9. Rebel against a Sedentary Life 26. Stressed Out—and Sick from It 30. New Rite of Passage 34. Redesigning Women: Breast Cancer 37. Silent Epidemic 55. Who Age Better—Men or Women? *(4, 6, 10, 11, 12, 13, 16)*
Contraception	17. Prevent Sexually Transmitted Diseases 18. Condom Report 19. Rethinking Birth Control 22. National Abortion Debate 33. Consensus: No Long-Term Link *(4, 6, 10, 14)*		
Depression	9. Rebel against a Sedentary Life 16. Politically Incorrect Surgery 27. Depression Way beyond the Blues 40. Running on Empty 44. Up in Smoke 52. "I Was Raped" *(1, 6, 10, 14, 16, 17, 27, 28, 29)*	**Gynecology**	15. Smart Pap 16. Politically Incorrect Surgery 17. Prevent Sexually Transmitted Diseases 20. Endometriosis: The Hidden Epidemic 21. Overcoming Infertility 59. Options for Hysterectomy *(5, 6, 14, 15, 19, 21)*
Diabetes	9. Rebel against a Sedentary Life 14. Weighty Matters in Women's Health 37. Silent Epidemic *(2, 3, 4, 9, 19, 21, 27, 28, 29)*	**Health Care System**	1. Women's Health Studies 2. Women *Are* Different 3. Work with Me, Doctor *(5, 6, 7)*

TOPIC AREA	TREATED IN	TOPIC AREA	TREATED IN
Heart Disease	9. Rebel against a Sedentary Life 13. Diet Fix 14. Weighty Matters in Women's Health 26. Stressed Out—and Sick from It 31. Mending the Female Heart 32. Heart Disease in Women: Special Symptoms 40. Running on Empty 47. Alcohol and Health: Mixed Messages 56. Hormone Therapy *(9, 10, 18, 21, 22, 27, 28, 29)*	**Reproduction**	19. Rethinking Birth Control 20. Endometriosis: The Hidden Epidemic 21. Overcoming Infertility 22. National Abortion Debate 23. Psychological Aftereffects of Abortion 33. Consensus: No Long-Term Link 59. Options for Hysterectomy *(6, 14, 15, 16)*
Infertility	16. Politically Incorrect Surgery 20. Endometriosis: The Hidden Epidemic 21. Overcoming Infertility 19. Rethinking Birth Control *(10, 14, 15, 22)*	**Self-Image**	11. Dying to Win 12. Who *Isn't* on a Diet? 14. Weighty Matters in Women's Health 16. Politically Incorrect Surgery 23. Psychological Aftereffects of Abortion 28. Treating Eating Disorders 29. Childless by Choice 30. New Rite of Passage 43. Facts about Women and Smoking 44. Up in Smoke 46. Cigars, Women, and Cancer 52. "I Was Raped" 53. Dangerous Men 55. Who Age Better—Men or Women? *(10, 11, 12, 13, 16, 17, 25, 28, 29)*
Menopause	16. Politically Incorrect Surgery 30. New Rite of Passage 55. Who Age Better—Men or Women? 56. Hormone Therapy 57. Silent Sabotage *(9, 10, 14, 15, 16, 27, 28, 29)*		
Menstruation	13. Diet Fix 20. Endometriosis: The Hidden Epidemic *(6, 11, 12, 14, 15)*	**Sexually Transmitted Diseases**	17. Prevent Sexually Transmitted Diseases 18. Condom Report 19. Rethinking Birth Control *(6, 14, 15)*
Minority Women	4. Forgotten Women 14. Weighty Matters in Women's Health 24. How Real Women Keep Stress at Bay 37. Silent Epidemic 38. Living with Lupus 52. "I Was Raped" *(10, 14, 15, 16, 19, 25, 26)*	**Smoking**	43. Facts about Women and Smoking 44. Up in Smoke 45. Smoker's Tale 46. Cigars, Women, and Cancer *(22, 23, 24)*
Obesity	8. Confessions 10. Diet Pills 12. Who *Isn't* on a Diet? 14. Weighty Matters in Women's Health 37. Silent Epidemic 40. Running on Empty *(12, 13, 16, 17, 23)*	**Stress**	13. Diet Fix 21. Overcoming Infertility 24. How Real Women Keep Stress at Bay 25. Myth of the Miserable Working Woman 26. Stressed Out—and Sick from It 44. Up in Smoke *(16, 17, 22, 23, 24)*
Osteoporosis	13. Diet Fix 55. Who Age Better—Men or Women? 56. Hormone Therapy 57. Silent Sabotage *(9, 12, 13, 27, 28, 29)*	**Treatment**	16. Politically Incorrect Surgery 20. Endometriosis: The Hidden Epidemic 21. Overcoming Infertility 27. Depression Way beyond the Blues 28. Treating Eating Disorders 31. Mending the Female Heart 41. What to Do for Urinary Tract and Vaginal Infections 59. Options for Hysterectomy *(4, 5, 14, 15, 16, 18, 19, 20, 24, 29)*
Pregnancy	20. Endometriosis: The Hidden Epidemic 21. Overcoming Infertility 22. National Abortion Debate 37. Silent Epidemic *(5, 6, 10, 11, 13, 14, 15)*		
		Violence	50. Domestic Violence 51. Women's Killer Is Likely to Be Her Partner 52. "I Was Raped" 53. Dangerous Men *(25, 26)*
Prevention	4. Forgotten Women 15. Smart Pap 31. Mending the Female Heart 58. Mammography Muddle *(5, 6, 7, 10, 14, 15, 19, 24)*	**Weight Management**	10. Diet Pills 12. Who *Isn't* on a Diet? 14. Weighty Matters in Women's Health 40. Running on Empty 44. Up in Smoke *(6, 11, 12, 13, 14, 16)*

Selected World Wide Web Sites for Annual Editions: Women's Health

All of these Web sites are hot-linked through the *Annual Editions* home page: *http://www.dushkin.com/annualeditions* (just click on a book). In addition, these sites are referenced by number and appear where relevant in the Topic Guide on the previous two pages.

Some Web sites are continually changing their structure and content, so the information listed may not always be available.

General Health Sites

1. Healthfinder: Gateway Consumer Health and Human Services Information Web Site—*http://www.healthfinder.gov/*—Healthfinder can lead you to selected online publications, clearinghouses, databases, Web sites, and support and self-help groups, as well as to the government agencies and not-for-profit organizations that produce reliable information for the public.

2. National Institutes of Health: Health Information Index—*http://www.nih.gov/health*—This index will help you identify the NIH's role and responsibility in all areas of medical research. Links also to a collection of NIH publications and a list of information clearinghouses with their phone numbers. From here you can also access Internet Grateful Med v2.3 for free access to the Medline and PubMed data bases.

3. NIH: Consumer Health Information—*http://www.nih.gov/health/ consumer/conicd.htm*—The publications of the agencies of the National Institutes of Health are listed at this site and can be accessed online.

4. Starting Point: Health—*http://www.stpt.com/health/health.html*—Search engine to excellent resources on health and fitness. Click on Women's Health for complete menu of links to relevant sites.

Women and Health

5. American Medical Women's Association—*http://www.amwa-doc. org/*—The home page of the AMWA, an organization of over 13,000 female physicians and medical students dedicated to the care of the woman patient and serving as a unique voice for women's health. Changing articles on a host of health topics can be found here and links to other sites.

6. Guide To Women's Health Issues—*http://www.coil.com/~tsegal/ womens_health.html*—This guide is an effective launching site for gender issues in health care, and includes a Table of Contents and Emotional, Physical, and Sexual Health Issues, which can be accessed by topic. Abstracts help you decide whether or not to read further. Includes bibliographical materials and links to the Argus Clearinghouse.

7. National Women's Health Information Center—*http://www. 4woman.org/*—This brand-new site is still under construction but worth a visit. It will also contain the resources of the U.S. Public Health Service's Office on Women's Health and the Defense Women's Health Information Center.

8. Program on Women's Health—*http://www.cmwf.org/wmhealth. html*—This is the Commonwealth Fund's site for its program on women's health. Table of Contents leads to Overview of Program, Work in Progress, and Completed Initiatives.

9. Women's Health Initiative—*http://odp.od.nih.gov/whi/*—The WHI is one of the largest preventive studies of its kind in the United States. It focuses on the major causes of death, disability, and frailty in postmenopausal women, with a goal of reducing coronary heart disease, breast and colorectal cancer, and osteoporotic-fractures among this study group.

10. WWW Virtual Library for Women—*http://www.nwrc.org/vlwomen. htm*—Interactive, peer-reviewed guide to information on the health and environment of women across the life cycle. Links primarily to pages with content rather than simply referring to other links. Categories are specific to female adolescents, older women, African American women, Latinas, Asian women, Native American women, lesbians, homeless women, women with HIV/AIDS, and women with disabilities.

Nutrition and Fitness

11. FitnessLink: The Health and Fitness Source—*http://www.fitnesslink. com/*—An excellent resource for fitness information, which includes the following indexes: Nutritional Information and Mind/Body Connection, each of which is useful to a discussion of women's health.

12. Food and Nutrition Information Center—*http://www.nal.usda.gov/ fnic*—Run by the Agriculture Network Information Center, this Web site contains a Search Engine plus Publications and Databases, and links to information produced by other USDA agencies, as well as an Index of Food and Nutrition Internet Resources.

13. Mayo Clinic Diet & Nutrition Resource Center—*http://www.mayo. ivi.com/mayo/common/htm/dietpage.htm*—At this site find many new diet and nutrition articles, plus a Virtual Cookbook: Send your recipes and have them altered for health; Ask the Mayo Dietician; Quizzes that test nutrition knowledge; Reference Articles; and Links to Other Organizations.

Gynecological and Sexual Health

14. A Forum for Women's Health—*http://www.womenshealth.org/*—Internet resource for women's health information hosts a collection of information, advice, and suggestions to help women deal with their health concerns. Organized under Ask a Woman Doctor; Subjects (such as Reproductive, Social/Psychological, and Wellness); Lifecycle (containing Girl's Reproduction, Midlife, Mature); What's New; Search the Forum; and Links. Helpful place to deal with birth control and pregnancy issues.

15. Women's Health Interactive—*http://www.womens-health.com/*—This interactive learning environment facilitates the exchange of information among participants and motivates individual proactive response. Featured are The Infertility Center, The Gynecological Health Center, and comprehensive health resources. Special services include Bleeding Assessment Diary and Infertility Insurance Advisor. Interactive sites are Assessment of Pregnancy Factors, Assessment of Gynecological Factors, Symptoms, and Cardiovascular Health Assessment.

Psychological Health

16. Mental Health Net: QuickFind Results—*http://www.cmhc.com/mhn/*—Link to many articles on women and stress by using the search engine at this site. Then explore this comprehensive guide to mental health online, which contains information on depression, substance abuse, eating disorders, and much more. You can also take a Self-Help Quiz.

17. National Women's Resource Center—*http://www.nwrc.org/*—Site contains bibliographic databases with current citations to literature related to women's substance abuse and mental illness.

Chronic Diseases

18. Heartinfo Search Directory Index: Women's Health—*http://www.heartinfo.org/wmhd.htm*—Links interesting articles about heart disease and other chronic diseases of women to other sites that discuss women's health.

19. Mayo Clinic's Women's Health Resource Center—*http://www.mayo.ivi.com/mayo/common/htm/womenpg.htm*—In addition to Ask the Mayo Physician and a comprehensive collection of articles covering women's health issues, and articles for the Mayo Clinic's own Women's Health Resource Newsletter, click on Cancer Center, Heart Center, Pregnancy and Child Health Center, and Diet and Nutrition Center for additional information and links.

20. NCI's CancerNet Cancer Information for Patients—*http://wwwicic.nci.nih.gov/patient.htm*—A wide range of accurate, credible cancer information is at this site, from peer-review statements from PDQ (Physicians Data Inquiry) covering latest cases, to cancer fact sheets and other publications. All have been reviewed by oncology experts and are based on results of current research. Some examples: Prototype Breast Cancer Resource and Information for Ethnic/Racial Groups. Glossary and global resources.

21. Search Health and Human Services—*http://www.hhs.gov/search/*—At SEARCH enter "articles-about-cancer-in-women" and a list of 50 articles will appear at this search site of the Department of Health and Human Services. Go to *http:www.hhs.gov/* also and explore What's New. Use the Search feature to initiate your own quest.

Substance Abuse: New Trends for Women

22. National Clearinghouse for Alcohol and Drug Information—*http://www.health.org/women.htm*—Material from many sources about alcohol, tobacco, and other drugs can be accessed at this clearinghouse. Bibliographies are also available. Click on Making the Link: Alcohol, Tobacco, and Other Drugs & Women's Health for: Women's Health, Sex under the Influence, Pregnancy and Parenthood, and Alcohol, Tobacco, and Other Drugs

23. NWRC: Documents—*http://www.nwrc.org/document.htm*—In addition to several online reports at this site, there is a list of bibliog-

raphies, including these subjects: Gender Specific Treatment, Substance Abuse: Risk and Resilience in Adolescents, Women and Life Stress, Treatment Barriers for Substance-Abusing Women, Fetal Alcohol Effect.

24. NWRC: Gender Specific Substance Abuse Treatment—*http://www.nwrc.org/respkg.htm*—At this site, read a complete publication on the Web, "Gender-Specific Substance Abuse Treatment," prepared for the National Women's Resource Center for the Prevention and treatment of Alcohol, Tobacco, and Other Drug Abuse and Mental Illness, which was a current project of the National Association for Families and Addiction Research and Education. It is a thoroughly researched work, complete with table of contents, tables, and a bibliography.

Violence in Women's Lives

25. Domestic Violence—*http://www.s-t.com/projects/DomVio/domviohome.HTML*—The main page of this site leads to 60 articles that explore domestic violence—its causes, victims, and some solutions. There is also a special help file and a guide to resources on the Internet.

26. The WWW Virtual Library for Women—*http://www.nwrc.org/vlwomen.htm#v*—Under Violence at this site there is a list of organizations that deal with the subject of domestice violence, battered women, and abuse.

Special Issues for Older Women

27. National Institute on Aging—*http://www.nih.gov/nia/*—The main page of the NIA leads to What's New, NIA Research, Health Information, and Related Sites, many of which concern the health problems of older women.

28. National Survey for Women's Health—*http://www.cmwf.org/whhilite.html*—Survey results of major health problems that affect older women are included in this study.

29. WWW Virtual Library for Women—*http://www.nwrc.org/vlwomen.htm#h*—Scroll to Aging for a list of resources that concern menopause, breast cancer in older women, issues of hormone replacement therapy, and links to some general sites on aging.

We highly recommend that you review our Web site for expanded information and our other product lines. We are continually updating and adding links to our Web site in order to offer you the most usable and useful information that will support and expand the value of your *Annual Editions*. You can reach us at: *http://www.dushkin.com/annualeditions/*.

Women and Health

The purpose of this first unit is to provide an introduction to some of the issues facing women in the changing health care environment. The existence of women's health as a discipline of study is the result of a long history of advice and activism that has pushed the particular issues of women out of the background and into the light.

After many years of neglect by the medical establishment, women's health has been discovered. The studies described in the article "Women's Health Studies" are a response both to the realization that "one size does not fit all" in health care and to years of advocacy and pressure from women. The process of investigating what is unique about women's health will provide the basis for women's health courses for years to come. Gaye Feldman, in "Women *Are* Different," investigates the health differences between men and women and feels that medical training needs to change to incorporate them, which would be beneficial to both women and men.

Next, the *Women's Health Advocate Newsletter* further urges women to become alert health care consumers in order to obtain the best possible care for themselves.

While women as a whole have been neglected by the health system, minority women have received a double dose. Even as things start to improve, minority women are still the "Forgotten Women." Lisa Collier Cool demonstrates that minority women, whatever their insurance status, do not get as many screenings, may receive less aggressive care, or may not be told of new treatment options. Historically, they have been neglected by the research trials both as women and as minorities. The implications of this for women's health are also discussed.

As health care becomes ever more complicated, and perceived by many to be highly impersonal, two parallel and seemingly contradictory trends in medicine are seen. These are the availability of increasingly high-tech tests and treatments, such as genetic testing, and the increased interest in "low-tech" methods of healing, such as herbal medicines. "Fitting into Our Genes" looks at the impact on women of the increased ability to test for genetic risk factors, the presence of which does not guarantee that a disease state will follow. What are the implications of knowing that one carries a "defective" gene—for screening, prevention, and even insurance coverage?

In response to the perceived impersonalness of much of allopathic medicine, many people are developing an increasing number of alternatives. However, there is much confusion about what is safe and effective, and scientific testing has only recently begun. The irony, of course, is

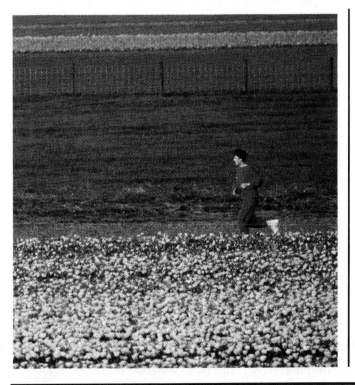

that the cultural emphasis on medical treatment leads many women to the doctor's office, even when it is not needed. Women are more likely than men to be consumers of health care services. In "Give Your Body Time to Heal," the author uses her own experiences to make the potentially controversial proposition that sometimes the best treatment is no treatment.

In reading this section, we hope that you will see the common thread that unites these articles. As health care in the United States changes and evolves, women are faced with a myriad of questions and challenges. The primary challenge is how to receive appropriate care in a system which is only just beginning to learn what works for women.

Looking Ahead: Challenge Questions

What are some of the reasons why minority women may receive substandard care? How can this be changed?

Genetic testing raises many questions regarding privacy, ethics, and effectiveness. What are some of the pros and cons of genetic testing for diseases like breast cancer?

What are some of the consequences of the neglect of women in research studies?

Women's Health Studies

The gender gap in medical research is closing. It has been since 1990, when the Office of Research on Women's Health was established at the National Institutes of Health to address the underrepresentation of women in medical studies. Since then, women in such investigations have increased not only in number, but also in diversity. Postmenopausal women, once all but ignored in scientific investigations, have become the focus of several new projects, and efforts to include African-American, Asian, and Hispanic women have expanded. These studies should provide information to guide us in reducing our risks of heart disease, cancer, osteoporosis, and other degenerative diseases. They generally take one of two forms — observational or interventional investigations.

Observational studies are designed to reveal possible associations between physical characteristics or health habits and disease. They usually include large numbers of people who are followed for several years. The participants may answer periodic questionnaires and may also be tracked through hospital records, tumor registries or death records.

Interventional studies are designed to determine the effects of specific treatments, diets, or health practices. Controlled trials are considered the gold standard of interventional studies. In these investigations, participants are randomly assigned to groups and each group follows a certain treatment, with at least one of the groups receiving a placebo or no treatment at all. At the end of the study, the results in each of the groups are compared.

The following studies are the first major investigations to deal exclusively with health issues of women at mid-life and beyond.

• *The Women's Health Initiative.* The largest study of women to date, the WHI includes both observational and interventional components. Researchers at 40 centers around the country are studying 160,000 healthy, postmenopausal women who were between the ages of 50 and 79 when they enrolled.

In the Observational Study, 100,000 women will undergo a physical examination upon entry and again after 3 years. Every year, the participants will complete questionnaires on their health habits.

The remaining 60,000 women are being enrolled in one or more of three controlled trials — the Dietary Modification (DM) Study, the Hormone Replacement Therapy (HRT) Study, or the Calcium and Vitamin D Supplementation (CaD) Study. The DM is designed to determine whether a low-fat diet reduces the risk of breast and colorectal cancer. The CaD study will test the effects of taking calcium and vitamin D supplements on osteoporosis risk.

The HRT Study should help to determine whether postmenopausal hormone supplementation actually lowers the risk of heart disease and osteoporosis and increases the risk of breast cancer, as some observational studies have indicated. It may also help to resolve the question of estrogen's effect on mental acuity and on the risk of developing Alzheimer's disease: women over age 65 will take annual examinations to test memory and reasoning. To enroll in this study, call 1-800-54-WOMEN.

• *The Nurses' Health Study.* This ongoing observational study, conducted by researchers at Brigham and Women's Hospital, Harvard Medical School, and Harvard School of Public Health, was inaugurated in 1976, when 120,000 women between the ages of 30 and 55 were enrolled. They are asked to fill out extensive questionnaires about their health and lifestyles every two years. By changing the questions asked, the researchers are able to examine the relationship between different lifestyle factors and medical outcomes. The more than 100 reports emanating from this study have provided the foundation for additional research into women's health risks. These reports have, among other things, indicated that there are health benefits in regular exercise, diets high in fruits and vegetables, and maintaining a lean body mass. They have suggested that oral contraceptive use does not increase the risk of cardiovascular disease, that postmenopausal replacement therapy with estrogen alone is linked with an increased risk of endometrial cancer, that drinking alcohol increases the risk of breast cancer, that the risk of gallstones rises with obesity, that suntanning increases the likelihood of melanoma, and that aspirin, estrogen, and exercise may reduce the risk of colon cancer.

The participants in the Nurses' Study are now between 50 and 75. Not only have their answers changed with age — more have suffered heart attacks, osteoporosis or cancer — but the questions have, too. The next round of inquiry is designed to obtain information on the psychosocial factors, such as stress, anxiety, social isolation and mood changes, that may influence health and longevity.

• *Study of Women's Health Across the Nation* (SWAN). This observational investigation, sponsored by the National Institute on Aging, is underway at seven medical centers in the United States. Researchers are selecting 3,200 women between the ages of 42 and 52, whom they will track for about five years. The project will focus on the physical and psychological differences among African-American, Hispanic, Asian-American, and Caucasian women during menopause.

The researchers will look at body composition, bone density, hormone levels, cardiovascular function, and menstrual bleeding. They will also consider psychosocial influences, such as sexuality, interpersonal relationships, commitment toward work, social values, and attitudes toward aging. Lifestyle factors — diet, exercise, smoking, and alcohol consumption — will also be included.

Women *Are* Different

Sex is only the beginning. From heart to brain to bowel, women are not the same as men, and this may change medicine forever.

Gayle Feldman

Linda is 36 years old, on the go all day, and can hardly spare the time for her annual physical. She knows what the doctor will tell her: Lose weight, quit smoking, work out. Fat chance, given her schedule. In fact, she would like to put off the physical, but she's been feeling so tired and short of breath lately. On top of that, the past couple of weeks she's been sick to her stomach. She can't figure out why—she hasn't changed her diet or routine, and she's on the Pill, for goodness' sale, so she can't be pregnant. She'd better get the physical over with and find out what's going on.

What's going on, the doctor tells her, is that Linda has heart disease; in fact she's already had a mild heart attack. It's a complete shock. Like most women, Linda thinks heart disease is something that happens to men. Her image of a heart attack is a man clutching his chest or doubling over in life-stopping pain. The truth is, heart disease is the number-one killer of women, too; it kills more women than all cancers, AIDS, domestic violence and osteoporosis combined.

Most women are like Linda, not only completely unaware that heart disease could happen to them, but also that its symptoms and risk factors are often very different in women and in men. Their ignorance isn't surprising since heart disease—along with almost every other disease or condition outside the reproductive area—was until recently studied almost exclusively in men, and the results extrapolated, undifferentiated, to women.

But ignorance is not bliss; it's dangerous. Women are not simply pint-size men with different sexual plumbing. Now a new medical frontier is opening up, one that researchers are calling gender-based medicine. It is not only saying vive la différence but is aggressively setting out to learn from that difference and to make up for the years of neglect. It's looking at the biological specifics in areas that range from heart disease to pain management to how our bodies metabolize drugs.

Government and business are paying attention. Procter & Gamble is investing more than $2.5 million over the next few years to help establish the Partnership for Women's Health at Columbia University, located at Columbia–Presbyterian Medical Center in New York City, precisely to study gender-based medicine. Drug industry surveys show that more products are being developed specifically for women. And the Women's Health Initiative (WHI), the largest-ever prevention study

funded by the U.S. government, is, among other things, researching how female hormones and lifestyles affect the development over time of heart disease, osteoporosis and other conditions in women.

Researchers know that women are far more prone to certain diseases or conditions than men. For example, we are:

- Twice as likely to suffer from major depression, anxiety disorders and phobias.
- Fifteen times more likely to have autoimmune or thyroid diseases.
- Three times more prone to rheumatoid arthritis and irritable bowel syndrome.
- Far more likely to suffer from migraine headaches.

The challenge that gender-based medicine has set for itself is to find out what causes the disproportion in women, and how treatment options might eventually be tailored more specifically—and more successfully—to help them.

Women's hearts are smaller, they weigh 50 to 100 grams less, and they beat more often and more quickly than men's.

Think about Linda's situation: A doctor grounded in gender-based medicine would recognize that her fatigue, shortness of breath and nausea were common heart disease symptoms in women. This doctor would know the best tests for coronary disease in women and would recognize that Linda is putting herself at risk for major heart problems by the very fact that she smokes while taking birth-control pills, which can cause the development of life-threatening blood clots. Smoking while on the Pill is something no woman over age 35 should ever do. A gender-based approach would recognize the heart benefits of hormone-replacement therapy after menopause for a woman like Linda.

Unfortunately, though, many primary-care physicians aren't yet looking at patients through a gender-specific lens. Astonishingly, a 1995 Galllup survey for the American Medical Women's Association (AMWA) found that one out of three of the 300 primary-care doctors surveyed didn't know that heart disease is the number-one cause of death in American women; two out of three didn't know risk factors for women are different; and nine out of 10 thought that male and female symptoms were the same. All the more reason for women to be educated participants in their own care.

Estrogen and oral contraceptives can have a significant impact on how drugs are metabolized.

One of the easiest ways to begin to appreciate what gender-based medicine is about is to look more closely into the female heart. Women's hearts are smaller, they weigh 50 to 100 grams less, and they beat more often and more quickly than men's. Our arteries also tend to be smaller, so it takes less fatty plaque to block them. When these arteries do become blocked and bypass operations, balloon angioplasty or other procedures are necessary to open or circumvent them, it can be trickier and riskier for heart surgeons to use on their female patients the standard instruments that have been designed to go into bigger male arteries. Sometimes they have to use surgical instruments that were designed for use on children; on other occasions, they just can't operate on certain arteries.

Statistically, our 36-year-old friend Linda was unlucky, since most premenopausal women are—to a large degree—protected against heart disease by their own estrogen. Once a woman enters menopause, heart problems can mushroom. One in nine women ages 45 to 64 has some cardiovascular disease, and the statistics skyrocket to one in three after age 65. Of course, until modern medical advancements like antibiotics extended women's life spans from an average of 48 years in 1900 to 79 years today, chronic illnesses such as heart disease, stroke and late-onset diabetes were hardly a problem at all: Women tended to die of infectious diseases or during childbirth; many never reached menopause. That is one of the reasons why the study of these diseases in women has lagged.

Although we know that estrogen protects the cardiovascular system, we still don't completely understand how. Traditionally, doctors thought that the hormone's beneficial effect was to help maintain a high level of high-density lipoproteins (HDLs, or "good cholesterol") and a low level of low-density lipoproteins (LDLs, or "bad cholesterol"). Now it has become clear that LDL levels are a better predictor of heart disease risk for men; HDL and triglyceride levels (triglycerides are another kind of fat, not found in cholesterol) are a better predictor for women, according to Debra R. Judelson, M.D., the Beverly Hills cardiologist who is the current president of AMWA. Linda's HDL level was found to be low and her triglyceride level was very high.

A unique benefit of estrogen that we do know is that it preserves the normal dilating response of blood vessels during stress. "You preserve the dilating response even in damaged blood vessels, an effect that is totally different between men and women," Dr. Judelson says.

Women often have very distinctive cardiovascular disease symptoms. According to Elizabeth Ross, M.D., author of *Healing the Female Heart,* the pain that a man with heart disease in danger of a heart attack feels tends to be severe and sudden. A woman may feel that, too, or, like Linda, may only feel

What We'll Learn in the Year 2006

Ten years from now we will have answers to some of our gender-based women's health questions, courtesy of the Women's Health Initiative (WHI), an unprecedented 15-year, 40-site, $628 million study of 164,500 postmenopausal women from 50 to 79 years old that was begun in 1991.

The largest part of this study is "observational," with 100,000 women participating. They will have periodic physical exams and respond to annual surveys about their health, focusing on heart disease, cancer and osteoporosis. Lifestyle, attitude, diet and medications will be taken into account.

The other 64,500 women will each be

in one or more of three clinical trials:
• 27,500 will be involved in a randomized HRT trial. No previous randomized trials of estrogen have gone on longer than three years, so up till now doctors have essentially been dispensing HRT in the dark. This study should finally tell us about its real benefits and risks.
• 48,000 will be studied to see if a low-fat, high-fiber, high-fruit-and-vegetable diet lowers breast and colon cancer rates.
• 45,000 women from the two previous groups will also be tracked to see the effects of calcium and vitamin D supplements on osteoporosis and colon cancer risk.

In 1995, another project, the $25

million, five-year Study of Women's Health Across the Nation (SWAN), involving women ages 42 to 52, was begun. It is studying 3,200 women for alterations in body composition, bone density and cardiovascular function; risk factors for cardiovascular disease and arthritis; the endocrine system; and sexuality. Lifestyle and psychological factors will also be taken into account, and a special feature of the study is that it was designed to include a large proportion of African Americans, Hispanics and Asian Americans.

We'll have to wait for an equivalent study of younger women. —*G.F.*

Shaking Up the Medical Establishment

Throughout history, a woman's unique ability to bear children has largely determined society's attitude toward her, and medicine was no exception. Inspired by feminism, groups such as the Boston Women's Health Collective—authors of the pathbreaking book *Our Bodies, Ourselves*—began in the 1970s to look at women's health in a new way. Only during the past decade have the medical and political establishments started to catch up.

Pressure to shift the focus to gender-specific aspects of women's health has been coming from grassroots advocacy and the efforts of female scientists who have worked to change the agenda. One of them, gynecologist Florence Haseltine, Ph.D., M.D., arrived at the National Institutes of Health to direct the Center for Population Research in 1985. Once there, she became angry about the unfairness of excluding women from government-funded clinical trials.

From 1977 to 1993, women were officially barred from early drug trials overseen by the FDA, partly in response to the tragic birth defects of children whose pregnant mothers had taken thalidomide and DES. The FDA feared the possible side effects of experimental drugs on fetuses or on future pregnancies, as well as legal liability issues. Women were also excluded to ensure a "homogeneous" testing population, and because of the extra "complications" in cost, timing and "unreliability" of dealing with people who have menstrual cycles.

So, for example, during the 1980s, when 25,000 men were studied to see if aspirin worked as a preventive measure for heart disease, not one woman was included. Even earlier, estrogen was tested to see if it helped prevent heart disease—in men only. Dr. Haseltine also discovered that in the NIH there were fewer gynecologists than veterinarians. So in 1988, with psychiatrist Susan J. Blumenthal, M.D. (now deputy assistant secretary for women's health at the Department of Health and Human Services, or HHS), she cofounded the Society for the Advancement of Women's Health Research.

To be fair, the government hadn't been completely unaware of the need for change. A Public Health Service report in 1985 clearly stated that "biomedical and behavioral research should be expanded to ensure an emphasis on conditions and diseases unique to, or more prevalent in, women," and in 1986 the NIH issued a policy statement advising that women be included in clinical trials. But those good intentions had not been carried out. So Haseltine, Dr. Blumenthal and others turned to the Congressional Caucus for Women's Issues for help.

The caucus requested that the Government Accounting Office (GAO) determine the extent to which women had been left out of federally funded research. The GAO findings, issued in a June 1990 report, were scathing.

The reaction was swift. Within two months, the NIH instructed its staff that beginning the following February, no grant applications for studies would be accepted unless women were adequately represented; soon thereafter, the organization established the Office for Research on Women's Health. In fall 1990, Bernadine Healy, M.D., became the first female head of the NIH. That September, the NIH conference in Hunt Valley, Maryland, issued the watershed "Hunt Valley report," setting its priorities for women's health research. Finally, in 1993, it was mandated that women be included in clinical trials. A year later, President Clinton named Blumenthal to the first senior level post at HHS exclusively devoted to women's health. —*G.F.*

---

nausea, pain in the arm or shoulder or jaw, extreme fatigue or shortness of breath. Or, she might only suffer from swelling in the ankles or lower legs.

Women have the ability to fight off viruses better than men do because they have higher immunoglobulin levels.

Thanks to her estrogen, a woman tends to get heart disease, on average, 10 years later than a man, and yet she is twice as likely to die after a heart attack. How can that be? First many women are so completely unaware of their risk that they don't realize their bodies are giving them warning signs. Second, many primary-care physicians are unaware of women's more subtle symptoms. Third, Dr. Ross emphasizes, the traditional gold-standard exercise stress test "is not as accurate in women as it is in men, because women's physiology of response to exercise may be different." Some doctors still don't realize that heart disease can be diagnosed more accurately in women by two other tests (a nuclear stress test or a stress echo-cardiogram). So by the time many women are diagnosed, they are far sicker than men.

Knowing already that heart disease was a factor in her life, Linda's physician wasn't surprised to find some evidence of mild diabetes when her blood test results came back from the lab. Diabetes is a stronger cardiovascular risk factor in women than in men, and as our population ages, its prevalence is greatly increasing, even more so in the African American population. Obesity and a sedentary lifestyle are the two biggest predictors of diabetes risk. Ross reminds us that "one third of American women past the age of 30 are obese, and too many subscribe to the concept that dieting makes you healthy. But unless you also begin to exercise regularly, dieting will accomplish nothing useful in the long term."

Then, of course, there's smoking. Quite simply, it cancels out the beneficial effects of estrogen. According to Judelson, "smoking makes a man get a heart attack seven years earlier than usual, but a woman 19 years earlier than usual."

In fact, one of the major goals of gender-specific medicine is to determine how much lifestyle factors (regular exercise, eating a low-fat diet and not smoking, for example) can affect a woman's health. Researchers already know that how a woman treats her body when she's young affects what happens after menopause. Yet findings also show that too many young women are ignorant about that relationship or feel immune to it.

A 1993 survey by the Commonwealth Fund's Commission on Women's Health found that nearly one out of three women never exercised, and one out of four smoked. In addition, tobacco seems to slow lung function and growth in adolescent girls more than in boys. Since cigarette manufacturers recognized the profits to be made in targeting advertising to women decades ago, preventive medicine has a lot of catching up to do to tailor antismoking campaigns specifically to young girls.

And, of course, the whole debate over whether women should take hormone replacement therapy (HRT) after they have reached menopause is connected to their risk of cardiovascular disease. The higher their risk, the more they should consider HRT. Hormone replacement also looms large in any discussion of osteoporosis.

The next time you're in a crowd, notice all the senior citizens whose shoulders and backs are stooped and bent. Most of them are women, not men. That's because older women are the main victims of the disentegrating bone disease osteoporosis. In fact, two out of five women now alive will have had an osteoporosis-related fracture by the age of 70, according to Marianne J. Legato, M.D., the Columbia University professor who is directing the Partnership for Women's Health. The loss of estrogen after menopause is the most obvious factor in female osteoporosis, so why should younger women pay attention to a disease of middle and old age? Simple: because how we treat our bodies when we're young affects development of the disease after menopause. The osteoporosis that younger women should be concerned about is Type 1, which affects women six times more often than men and is associated with estrogen decline. (Type 2 affects women twice as often as men, but isn't really a factor until after age 70.)

Osteoporosis is the loss of bone mass or density, which leads to fragility and unexpected fractures. Throughout our lives, our bones are constantly being rebuilt, with new bone matter replacing the bone mass we lose. But around age 30, bone loss begins very subtly to exceed bone formation in both men and women. Once a woman reaches menopause—and for eight to 10 years immediately afterward—the hormonal changes cause increased breakdown of bone. During that decade, as much as 5 percent of bone mass can be lost in a single year.

Building Better Bones

So it's essential to build maximum bone mass when young and lead a lifestyle that will help maintain as much of it as possible later on. But women's bones are at a disadvantage from a very early age. Since most women have smaller frames and are less physically active as teenagers, they have less bone density than men do. If a teenager does not eat well or diets a lot, she will have a calcium deficiency and never build optimum mass. Similarly, if a woman is an exercise fanatic and begins to have irregular periods (or none at all), her body isn't producing enough estrogen. She'll pay the price later on.

Obviously, estrogen deficiency is not the only factor in the disease, since not every postmenopausal woman has osteoporosis. All women require a certain amount of calcium, but many don't get it through their diet. Although researchers agree that calcium supplements can be a beneficial preventive measure, according to the Commonwealth Fund survey, four out of five women ages 18 to 44 (and three out of five women 45 and older) do not take them.

Smoking, caffeine, too much alcohol and lack of weight-bearing physical exercise throughout adulthood make a woman susceptible to the disease. So too, does the abuse of thyroid medications, which some women misguidedly use to speed up their metabolisms to lose weight.

Thyroid disorders predispose women to osteoporosis, and they are much more a woman's problem than a man's. One in eight women develops some thyroid problem during her lifetime; one in 20 does so after having a baby. That's why during the past few years some doctors have started to advocate the TSH (thyroid stimulating hormone) test as part of a regular physical exam.

Drugs for Women Only?

The drugs men and women take may affect them differently solely because of gender, and the instructions that come with them may one day contain dosage variations for sex, weight, age and other factors. Freda Lewis-Hall, M.D., who heads the Lilly Center for Women's Health in Indianapolis, says that drug companies will have to address two major questions when developing new medications: first, whether there are differences in their effectiveness or in adverse side effects in men and women; and, second, whether the effectiveness of the medicine varies during a woman's menstrual cycle.

Think of the changes the menstrual cycle imposes on women's bodies; indeed, consider the multiplicity of hormonal changes throughout a woman's life and the effects they can have. Judelson describes a scenario that is all too familiar to every woman: "When I'm premenstrual, my GI tract slows down, my stomach takes forever to empty, and my belly bloats—doesn't that affect medication absorption?"

Remember, standard dosages of most medications until very recently were designed for and tested on men. According to a 1993 research report by the Food and Drug Administration's Working Group on Women in Clinical Trials, the popular painkillers acetaminophen, aspirin and lidocaine take longer to be eliminated from a woman's body. Does that mean women need different dosages or need to time them differently for optimum

2. Women *Are* Different

effect? We don't know. Seventy percent of psychotropic drugs are prescribed to women, yet basic studies of them were done primarily on male rats.

We have only limited knowledge about how oral contraceptives lessen some of the gender differential effects for drug metabolism and heighten others; we know even less about how HRT enters into the equation. The tranquilizer Valium, for example, takes longer to clear a woman's body than a man's, but only until menopause. What happens if a menopausal woman is on both Valium and HRT? As yet, nobody knows.

Migraine headaches occur in up to 17 percent of women in the U.S., compared with up to 6 percent of men.

Then, too, consider not only the variations of the monthly cycle, but also the fact that women's circadian rhythms are different from men's. There may be certain times of day when a woman's body would do a quicker, better job of absorbing a drug and circulating it throughout her system, and it may be very different from the timing that works best in a man. We need to find out.

One thing we do know is that our higher body-fat content and lower body-water volume contribute to higher blood-alcohol concentrations. Women produce less of a liver enzyme—alcohol dehydrogenase—that breaks down alcohol. This is why a woman who drinks a smaller amount of an alcoholic beverage than does a man of the same size will nevertheless get more intoxicated.

Then there are drugs that have been tested and abandoned in men-only clinical trials, but if given a chance might work beautifully in women. Take, for example, the recent discovery by a team of researchers at the University of California San Francisco regarding a group of painkilling drugs called kappa-opioids. These drugs do not have the significant side effects of the more familiar mu-opioids—morphine, codeine, etc.—and had originally been developed as an alternative to them. In men-only tests, their effectiveness had been disappointing.

The team at San Francisco decided to try them out again, this time on a group of 48 young men and women who were having impacted wisdom teeth removed. The kappa-opioids worked very well for the women in the group—so well that the leader of this National Institutes of Health (NIH)–funded project, Jon D. Levine, M.D. Ph.D., recommended that their use for women with moderate to severe pain be reevaluated. Further, Dr. Levine stated, "our studies provide evidence that biologically, women and men do not obtain pain relief in the same way. It may be that the brain circuitry regulating pain relief differs between the sexes."

There's much to find out about gender differentiation in brain function. Some experts, like Dr. Legato, speculate that it may reveal the most fascinating gender specificity of all. Sex differences have already been recognized in cognition as well as in epilepsy, Alzheimer's disease and sleep disorders.

While research is crucial, it must be accompanied by new attitudes in the medical profession. AMWA believes doctors must fundamentally change the way they think about women. The organization has developed an education program for practicing physicians, the Advanced Curriculum in Women's Health, to help them do so. "Instead of grouping information by organ systems, it's much more suitable to look at life phases and consider how to prevent illness and maintain health in each phase," says Lila Wallis, M.D., clinical professor of medicine at Cornell University Medical College, head of the team that designed the course. The five life phases are adolescence (12 to 20 years old); young adulthood (from 20 to 45); perimenopause (45 to 60); postmenopausal, "mature" (60 to 85); and "advanced" (85-plus).

Changes also must be made in the way future doctors are trained. In 1994, doctors at Philadelphia's Allegheny University of the Health Sciences joined with AMWA to create *Women's Health in the Curriculum,* a resource guide for medical school professors and health care educators. But experts say that curriculum shifts will only occur if gender-specific questions become part of the licensing exams that every aspiring physician must take. Florence Haseltine, Ph.D., M.D., director of the Center for Population Research at the NIH, doesn't see "real changes happening for another 10 years."

The research establishment needs to rethink the way it conducts medical studies and reports results. Experts like Vivian W. Pinn, M.D., director of the Office of Research on Women's Health at the NIH, are concerned that medical journal articles don't routinely address gender differences in studies. Hormonal variations are not typically taken into account; rarely does a study report whether the subjects were pre- or post-menopausal, or taking HRT.

Dr. Haseltine believes medical students will be the agents of change, actively seeking out gender-specific information in their courses, as will the pharmaceutical industry, which sees the profit potential in new, differentiated products for the two sexes. In the end, gender-specific women's health also implies gender-specific men's health. Learning more about the special characteristics of women will inevitably produce corresponding action for men. That can only be good for both.

GAYLE FELDMAN, the author of *You Don't Have to Be Your Mother,* is a writer living in New York City. She last wrote for SELF about genetic testing for breast cancer (October 1996).

13

This is the first of a two-part* story on how to get better care, whether you're covered

under traditional insurance or are in a managed care plan.

Work with Me, Doctor: How to Get Better Care

It's the best of times and the worst of times to be a patient. The advances of the last 50 years have been breathtaking, and never has so much medical information been available directly to health care consumers.

What's more, the doctor-patient relationship has undergone a subtle shift in the last 10 to 15 years. Paternalism is out; partnerships are in. Many doctors today are more attuned to patient advocacy issues, and patient satisfaction is a topic that appears more and more often in physician publications, says Mike Donio, director of projects at the People's Medical Society.

However, this shift in power is occurring simultaneously with a profound shift in the way medicine is practiced. Increasingly, managed care—HMOs, PPOs, and other corporate-influenced arrangements—is the name of the game.

As a result, the doctor-patient relationship often includes a third party—and many third parties carry a big stick. In some HMOs, doctors who would like to spend more time listening to their patients and providing them with more information simply can't. Thus, any advice on how to form a "health care partnership" with your doctor is, by necessity, general and subject to adaptation to individual circumstances.

Ten Steps to Better Care
In the best of all worlds—and under the ideal insurance plan—here are some steps you can take to help forge

a satisfying doctor-patient relationship. (Most of these approaches will work well under any type of provider relationship, although next month's issue of *WHA* will carry tips on navigating the world of managed care.)

1 Schedule an interview. If you have a choice in physicians, get recommendations. Find out from the office staff whether the doctor is accepting new patients. If so, ask for other basic information, such as the doctor's specialization, training, fees, and office hours.

Then arrange for a get-acquainted interview. (If the doctor refuses, go on to the next physician on your list.) Be aware that some physicians charge for a get-acquainted visit; others don't.

This first-time interview may take about 10 to 15 minutes. Ideally, it should be conducted in person, although it can be done over the phone. Either way, this is the time to ask about things that are important to you, such as wellness and screening strategies and attitudes toward vitamins or alternative treatments.

Evaluate your "gut level" response—did the doctor seem harried? distracted? irritated or offended by your questions? Or did he or she make good eye contact, listen, and take your concerns seriously? Were things explained in terms you could understand? Will you feel comfortable in revealing important information to him or her? Most importantly, do you feel that this is someone you can work with?

2 Come prepared. Before your first medical visit to any new doctor, gather all relevant information about all major illnesses and treatments. List current medications and any problems you've had with particular drugs. Bring copies of relevant test results—mammograms or other x-rays, for example. Include your family medical history—first- or second-degree relatives who've had heart disease, cancer, diabetes, or other chronic diseases.

3 Jot it down. Before an appointment, make a list of any questions or concerns. A written list is more time-efficient, and it can keep you from forgetting to ask something important. Keep a notebook handy for taking notes.

If you're facing a complex medical procedure, consider taking along a family member or friend to help you remember important details.

You might also ask the doctor if you can tape record a lengthy or complicated discussion. If your doctor's initial reaction to this request is a negative one, point out that you don't want to miss or forget something.

4 Be observant. You are the only person who can describe how you feel. When you have a problem, keep track of your symptoms and write down anything that might be helpful.

For instance, if you're experiencing pain, when does it occur? How long does it last? What does it feel like—jabbing, squeezing, or a dull ache? The more specific you can be, the better.

5 **Tell the truth.** Be honest about eating, exercise, smoking, drinking, and other habits. Holding back information because you're embarrassed—or you're trying to avoid conflict—could jeopardize your health.

The same is true when a treatment is prescribed. For instance, if you aren't taking your medication or you haven't consistently altered your eating habits, let your doctor know. It isn't easy to admit to noncompliance, but being evasive can lead to diagnostic confusion and perhaps to a more complicated or invasive treatment than you actually need.

And if a doctor wants you to do something you suspect might be a problem—such as waking up in the middle of the night to take a pill—be honest about your concerns. There may be an alternative.

6 **Do your homework.** Find out all you can about your particular medical condition or the drug you're taking. The purpose isn't to diagnose your own illness but to learn what questions to ask and help you negotiate with your doctor.

7 **Don't be afraid to ask.** If you don't understand a medical phrase, or something is unclear, say so. Above all, don't leave your doctor's office until you're clear about your diagnosis and any treatment or follow-up plan.

8 **Speak up.** If you run into a problem—if, for instance, you don't feel as if your doctor is spending enough time with you or taking your problem seriously—you need to speak up and make your feelings known.

An assertive, straightforward expression of your feelings usually can bring an end to the bothersome behavior. For example, if the doctor regularly conducts post-examination discussions while you're still on the table in a paper gown, you might say,

Assertiveness Helps Your Health

What's an ounce of assertiveness worth? Your health, perhaps. Consider the following:

Tufts University researchers conducted four separate trials in which patients with a chronic illness—hypertension, ulcers, diabetes, or breast cancer—were assigned to one of two groups.

In each trial, patients in the first group were given general information about their particular disease and the importance of self-monitoring and self-care.

Those in the second were given this basic information plus training in assertiveness and communication techniques. These patients also were shown their own medical records and given information on treatment strategies; their training

session took place immediately before a scheduled office visit.

Six to eight weeks later, researchers assessed each patient's health status, measuring it subjectively (via the patient's own assessment) and objectively (through medical tests).

The findings: In all four trials, patients who had had the assertiveness training were in better health.

Similar research has supported these findings. What's the underlying connection between good health and assertiveness? It may be feelings of self-confidence or a sense of control. Over the years, numerous studies have suggested that a sense of control over one's situation—be it a job or a health condition—lowers stress and boosts mental and physical well-being.

"I feel uncomfortable when our discussions take place in the examining room; I'd like to get dressed first."

If you find it hard to express yourself during an office visit, Donio suggests writing the physician a letter or calling later and asking for a brief appointment to discuss your concerns. If your physician responds negatively or continually ignores your wishes, it's time to find a new doctor.

9 **Don't be intimidated.** Even the most involved patients have been known to fall into the trap of letting themselves be intimidated by a doctor's perceived prestige or expertise.

It's important to remember two things: First, behind the starched white persona is a human being. Secondly, you're paying for his or her services.

10 **Consider a second opinion.** If you're facing an invasive procedure, are told you have a life-threatening illness, or are uncomfortable with—or uncertain about—the diagnosis or recommended treatment, tell your doctor that you'd like to get a second opinion.

If your doctor balks at the request, find another physician. For one thing, such consultations are common. More importantly, it's your right—and your duty to yourself—to ask for and receive the kind of medical care you need.

*See *Women's Health Advocate,* May 1997 for the second part "Managing Managed Care." **Ed.**

Resources:
Related stories published previously in *WHA* include: How to find medical information (July 1995); how to keep your own medical history (December 1995); and older women's health care rights (October 1996).

People's Medical Society. Write 462 Walnut St., Allentown, Pa. 18102, or call (800) 624-8773.

Forgotten Women: How Minorities Are Underserved by Our Health Care System

LISA COLLIER COOL

Imagine living in a place where going to a doctor involves a difficult or even dangerous trek to a distant, over-crowded clinic where you wait hours for a few minutes

of questionable medical care—a place where preventive treatment is so lacking that breast tumors sometimes protrude through the skin before they are diagnosed.

You might expect these conditions in a third world country, but actually they're faced every day by minority women in some parts of the U.S. Statistics show that "an African-American woman born in Harlem today has less chance of surviving to age 65 than a woman from Bangladesh, one of the poorest nations on earth," says Colin McCord, M.D., associate director of surgery at Harlem Hospital in New York City.

Although you may think that poverty is to blame, the truth is that even affluent minority women—whether black, Hispanic, Asian-American or Native American—fare poorly in our medical system. "An African-American woman who earns triple what a Euro-American female earns still has a greater chance of mortality from disease like breast cancer," says Faye Gary, Ed.D., distinguished service professor at the College of Nursing of the University of Florida in Gainesville.

What makes this all the more shocking is that even as progress has been made in women's health as a whole, the health disparities between black and white women have remained. Mortality from heart disease and cancer has fallen among white women, yet is unchanged in blacks. At every age, "African-American, Native American, Hispanic and Asian-American women suffer from poorer health and greater risk of premature death," says Dr. Gary.

Deadly Discrimination Socioeconomic factors explain only some of these inequities. While it's true that black women have triple the rate of poverty of white women and are slightly less likely to be insured, research reveals that they're also the victims of subtle but potentially fatal

YOUR HERITAGE, YOUR HEALTH

Here's how your background may affect your disease risk. (Except where noted, individual groups are compared to U.S. women as a whole.)

Native American women:
◆ are 10 times likelier to suffer from diabetes.
◆ have 12 times the odds of dying from alcohol-related causes before age 34.
◆ are much likelier to live more than half an hour away from the nearest health facility.

Hispanic women:
◆ are 60% likelier to say their health is fair or poor.
◆ have a greater risk of obesity.
◆ have the greatest rate of severe depression.

Black women:
◆ have quadruple the high blood pressure risk of whites in young adulthood and a higher rate of serious complications, including stroke, later in life.
◆ have the highest death rate from colon cancer.

Asian-American/Pacific Island women:
◆ are least likely to be satisfied with their health care.
◆ have the highest rate of stomach cancer.
◆ are at greater risk for the genetic disorders alpha- and beta-thalassemia, which cause retardation, as well as for hepatitis B.

medical bias. A recent study at Boston University found that at every income level, black women over age 64 are only half as likely as whites to have a mammogram ordered for them by a doctor, even if they see a primary-care physician just as often. Mammography rates are even lower for Native American women. The result is that black and Native American women have a 30% higher risk of dying of breast cancer, despite the fact that the disease is much less common in these groups than in whites.

The same pattern of prejudice prevails in hospital care: A study at Beth Israel Hospital in Boston found that doctors order 1½ times as much surgery and other high-tech treatment for whites as for equally ill blacks. It's not just costly procedures these patients are shortchanged on, either: 20% of Latinas and 65% of Korean Americans have never had a Pap smear, yet lab costs start at $16.

Even in the emergency room, your race or ethnicity can have more impact on your care than your condition, says Jane Delgado, Ph.D., president and CEO of the National Coalition of Hispanic Health and Human Services Organizations in Washington. "A study of people treated for a broken leg showed that the single greatest predictor of who got painkillers was whether they were Hispanic," she says. "The doctors often withheld painkillers from Hispanic patients even though Hispanic and non-Hispanic patients rated their pain as equally severe." This reminds Dr. Gary of the segregated care she received growing up in the South in the '50s. "My parents had to drive 100 miles to take me to the only white dentist who would see black people," she recalls. "I remember feeling grateful when he yanked out my teeth at his kitchen table, because I wasn't allowed into his office."

Deep-Rooted Stereotypes Not only are minorities' medical needs dangerously neglected, but doctor prejudice can also result in substandard care for those who get treated, says Claudia R. Baquet, M.D., associate dean for policy and planning at University of Maryland School of Medicine in Baltimore. "In focus groups," she says, "minority women say that doctors assume they have multiple partners or start having sex at an early age. Racial and ethnic stereotyping is still rampant and a barrier to quality care."

Minority women are doubly disadvantaged because they may be subjected to sexism in addition to racial bias, notes Aida Giachello, Ph.D., director of the Midwest Latino Health Research, Training and Policy Center at the University of Illinois in Chicago. Many Latinas report that doctors dismiss their complaints. "The stereotype is that Latinas overuse the health system," says Dr. Giachello. "But when we did a focus group with these women, the reality was that they had to go to their doctors over and over with the same symptoms, because the physicians would say it was stress while the real problem went undiagnosed, sometimes causing serious complications."

Equally damaging are the assumptions physicians may make if they judge a patient's ethnicity based on her skin color or surname. "If a Native American woman from the Southwest has a Latino last name, a doctor may misclassify her and not test for gallbladder disease, which is epidemic in that population," says Dr. Baquet. Others question the medical value of determining ethnicity at all. "Asking someone what race she considers herself to be doesn't tell you what her genetics are," points out Olivia Carter-Pokras, Ph.D., an epidemiologist and public health analyst at the Office of Minority Health in Washington. "Even sickle-cell anemia, thought of as a 'black' disorder, also appears in white people of Mediterranean origin."

Research Bias More serious still is the situation in clinical trials, where scientists develop the medicine of the future by testing new drugs, diagnostic techniques and other treatments. Despite laws mandating the inclusion of women and minorities in trials sponsored by the National Institutes of Health, many doctors don't seem to have gotten the message, reports Dr. Carter-Pokras, who says she constantly sees unconscious or even overt prejudice on the part of researchers. "A doctor may decide to recruit from her own clinic, never stopping to think that since her patients are 80% white, she needs to be aggressive about finding minority cases," she says. Investigators often try to recruit Spanish speakers with no

---

Equal Opportunity Health Resources

To lobby for better care for minority women, or to get more information about minority women's health risks, contact the following:

- **Minority Health Consortium**, in Richmond, VA (804-355-4502), offers free women's health pamphlets and referrals to other resources.
- **National Black Women's Health Project** in Washington (202-835-0117) provides free information on subjects of special interest to black women.
- **National Coalition of Hispanic Health and Human Services Organization** in Washington (202-387-5000; http://www.cossmho.org) offers a free catalog listing bilingual literature, videos and hot lines.
- **Office of Minority Health Resource Center** (800-444-6472; http://www.omhrc.gov) provides customized database searches and referrals.

translators or bilingual materials. Not only do such attitudes reduce minority women's access to state-of-the-art care, but also underrepresentation in studies ensures that the second-class medical care will continue for decades to come.

Increasing the number of women of color participating in medical studies is important, but Dr. Gary feels it doesn't go far enough. "There also needs to be better representation of ethnic groups among the people who do the studies," she says. Despite doctors' best intentions, subtle biases and cultural differences can still interfere with good research.

Constructive Changes The outrage from women of color is finally starting to be heard on Capitol Hill. To determine how to end these inequities, 740 experts convened in Washington last January for the nation's first minority women's health conference, sponsored by the U.S. Public Health Service's Office on Women's Health. The agency is developing a culturally sensitive women's health curriculum for medical and nursing schools, and it has started programs to recruit more minority women into health careers and as participants in clinical trials.

Other federal agencies are creating their own initiatives. The Centers for Disease Control and Prevention is funding studies of chronic disease that affect women of color disproportionately (see "Your Heritage, Your Health"). But it's still up to women to help alert doctors to the potential for bias in diagnosis and treatment and to become more attuned to how our racial or ethnic background may affect our health. Each of these efforts shares the same crucial goal: to create a healthier tomorrow for *all* women.

Award-winning journalist Lisa Collier Cool lives in Pelham, NY.

fitting into our genes

News about breast cancer genes is being discovered so fast that our laws and ethics are having trouble keeping up.

Leslie Schwartz

Eve Gold (not her real name) was worried about her daughters. Her mother and both grandmothers had all died of breast cancer. Then the 71-year-old Los Angeles psychologist learned that 1 percent of 400 European Jewish women tested carried a mutated BRCA1, one of two known breast cancer genes. So Eve, who is of Ashkenazi (European) Jewish descent, decided to take a simple blood test she'd read about that could detect the presence of inherited breast cancer genes.

t his year, 182,000 American women will develop breast cancer, according to the American Cancer Society. Researchers believe that as many as 5 percent of these women carry a mutated form of the genes BRCA1 and BRCA2 (named for BReast CAncer).

Everyone, regardless of gender, inherits two BRCA1 and two BRCA2 genes, one of each from each parent. In some cases, one of the genes is mutated. The normal genes actually work to prevent the growth of breast cancer and other cancers, while the mutated genes do not. "In hereditary breast cancer," explains Jeffrey Holt, M.D., associate professor of cell biology at Vanderbilt University in Nashville, Tenn., "there's a mutation in one of the genes that doesn't allow the cells to suppress tumor growth."

Will Gene Research Lead to Treatment?

BRCA1 was discovered by a team of researchers at the University of Utah in 1994. A year later, BRCA2 was found simultaneously by researchers from the Institute of Cancer Research in London and researchers from the University of Utah. The researchers have shown that for women in families with a high incidence of breast and ovarian cancer, the BRCA1 mutation has been linked to an 85 to 90 percent lifetime risk of getting breast cancer and a 50 percent lifetime risk of ovarian cancer. In addition, there may be a connection between the BRCA1 mutation and an increase in colon cancer for both men and women, as well as an increase in prostate cancer for men.

Less is known about BRCA 2, but because it has a similar structure and function to the BRCA1 mutation, researchers believe that its mutation in the body also could lead to an 85 to 90 percent lifetime risk of getting breast cancer. Unlike the BRCA1 mutation, the BRCA2 mutation doesn't seem to increase a woman's risk of developing ovarian cancer; and initial studies indicate that it is associated with an increased risk of male breast cancer.

Though these discoveries may seem ominous, the real implications could be very encouraging. Experts say that if research continues at the meteoric pace it has since the discovery of BRCA1, drugs to combat some types of breast and ovarian cancers may soon exist.

In fact, a study done in March by Holt and Roy Jensen, M.D., assistant professor of pathology and cell biology at Vanderbilt, looks promising. Researchers injected nonhereditary human breast cancer cells into the abdomens of mice. After tumors grew, the mice were injected with healthy BRCA1 genes.

"We found that if you give the [tumor] healthy BRCA1, it doesn't grow like a cancer," says Holt. "This suggests that BRCA1 slows down breast and ovarian cancer growth." In addition, this could be true for some types of both hereditary and nonhereditary cancer, since the cells injected into the mice were from nonhereditary cancer sources.

Jenson says there are reasons to be even more hopeful. Most other cancer genes do their damage within the nucleus of the cell. But BRCA1 is secreted outside the cell, which makes it easier for pharmaceutical companies to develop drugs that can interfere with cell action.

An effective drug remedy for breast and ovarian cancers — though perhaps at least 10 years away — could eliminate the need for radiation or chemotherapy and their painful effects.

The Genetic-Testing Gamble

Equally as important, a successful drug treatment may one day curb a current debate about the availability of testing for the genes. Though genetic-testing firms now make testing for a mutated BRCA1 available to

From *Shape*, October 1996, pp. 35, 39. Reprinted by permission of *Shape*, published by *Shape* Magazine, Inc., Woodland Hills, CA 91367.

19

everyone, some feel the test should be restricted to the realm of research.

Francis S. Collins, M.D., Ph.D., director for the National Center for Human Genome Research, is one example. His chief concern is that there is no cure for breast cancer now. Treatment is costly, he says, and women who test positive for the gene could be dropped from their health insurance. "It's tragic," he says.

that your employer or insurer won't try to evade the law by citing "other" reasons for firing or dropping you.

Collins also warns that no test for BRCA1 is definitive. More than 100 mutations can appear on any BRCA1 gene, not all of which cause cancer, so risk for false positives abounds. Likewise, the potential for false negatives arises since not all mutations will necessarily be picked up in the screening.

are more prevalent.) The most important thing to remember about the test, however, is that even if you do find you have a genetic predisposition, it does not guarantee that you'll get breast or ovarian cancer. But, as Knell says, the result may help you take more aggressive preventive steps.

Eve Gold paid $475 for the test at a private testing center. It took 12 weeks

A drug remedy for breast and ovarian cancers—though perhaps at least 10 years away—could eliminate the need for radiation and chemotherapy.

His concern is a valid one. If you submit a claim to your insurance company for payment for the test, the fact that you took the test and the results may become available to future medical and life insurance companies. Even if you pay for the test yourself and then report the results to your physician, that information may become part of your medical record, to which insurance companies also have access.

As yet, there is no national policy established to address genetic testing and patient's rights. "This is ethically unjust," says Collins. "You just don't get to pick your genes." Though 15 states have enacted legislation designed to protect against abuses of privacy and discrimination related to insurance and genetic testing, there's no guarantee

On the other hand, says Ellen Knell, Ph.D., director of medical genetics at the Los Angeles Oncologic Institute, restricting testing to a research setting does women a grave disservice. "All women have a right to information that will allow them to maximize their health and longevity," she says. Women who test positive, says Knell, are more likely to do breast self-exams and get regular mammograms.

If you do decide to take the BRCA1 test, you'll be required to undergo counseling before and after the test to discuss all the medical, legal and ethical implications involved. (Counselors also will explain that in smaller population groups, such as Ashkenazi Jewish women, the gene pool is limited. Therefore, BRCA 1 or 2 mutations

for the results to come in. When they were negative, she was surprised. "Of course it doesn't mean I'm cancer-proof. It just means I don't have a built-in mutation [that was detected]," says Gold. "I took the test partly to see if I'd beaten the odds. But mostly I wanted to tell my daughters so that they could make choices for their future."

To take the BRCA1 test, contact the National Society of Genetic Counselors at (610) 872-7608, 233 Canterbury Drive, Wallingford, PA 19086-6617, for a list of counselors near you who specialize in cancer-risk assessment and breast cancer gene testing.

Leslie Schwartz *is a writer in Los Angeles.*

It's only natural: When you hurt, you want a diagnosis and treatment—right away. But slow down. When it comes to your everyday medical care, the best doctors do the least.

GIVE YOUR BODY TIME TO HEAL

By Ann Japenga

IN THE SPRING OF 1987 I was living a Nike ad. Brimming with vitality, I routinely jetted off—reporter's notebook in hand—to kayak in ocean storms or go helicopter skiing in the Sierras. To wind down at the end of an eventful day, I'd swim laps or run along Santa Monica beach, six blocks from my house. Then I began suffering "swoops," as a friend called them, periods when for weeks at a time the color drained from my face and my body felt like it was made of clay. Once the swoops came on, I couldn't even muster the energy to stroll down to the pier for gelato.

My mother, a pediatrician, came to my house one day, laid my arm on the kitchen counter, and drew some blood. She tucked the vial into her cracked black bag. A few days later the results came back. Mononucleosis.

I was relieved. At the time I had a sunny view of medicine. A test would lead to a diagnosis; a diagnosis, to treatment; a treatment, to wellness. And now I had a diagnosis, a disease.

There was only one problem: I didn't get well. Long after the mono virus should have run its course I was still shuttling from one time-consuming doctor's visit to another, feeling irritated because I had skydiving appointments to keep.

The doctors opined that I might just be overworked or depressed, or that I might qualify for a new malady—chronic fatigue syndrome—which was untreatable anyway. I became obsessed with finding a physician who could give me a more concrete explanation. More than once I had blood drawn and checked for every disease you can name. When still no answer came, I named my sickness "the voodoo bug" and cursed the profession too incompetent to cure it.

Of course, I wasn't the only one who spent at least part of his or her thirties demanding answers from doctors. Sickness seemed a rite of passage, judging from my equally vigorous friends and coworkers' susceptibility to fatigue, chronic viruses, insomnia, infertility, depression, bad backs, and bum knees.

My peers shared the belief that tests would lead to a treatment and therefore a cure. Unwittingly, all of us had been indoctrinated by a cultural phenomenon known as medicalization. This is the tendency to see bona fide illness behind every discomfort, coupled with an inordinate belief in the ability of doctors to relieve the pain.

Medicalization has been in ascendancy for much of my lifetime, prompted by the apparent ease with which Marcus Welby and Ben Casey cured illness, researchers' announcements of high-tech "breakthroughs," and ferocious marketing of everything medical—doctors, tests, drugs, cures. By the mid-1980s there were few symptoms left that might not warrant a doctor's visit. Tired? A blood test should find something. Stomachache? Could be an ulcer or cancer; see a specialist. Backache? Time for an MRI.

But during the year my voodoo bug took hold, medicalization began to come under scrutiny. In 1986 an article published by University of Oklahoma researchers James Mold and Howard Stein in the *New England Journal of Medicine*

Docs Through the Decades
How They Lost Our Trust

WHY DO WE EXPECT so much from doctors, then suspect the worst when they don't diagnose and cure our ailments fast? Look back at the medicine depicted on television since the 1960s. For two decades these shows—which the American Medical Association screened until the late 1970s—glorified physicians and trumpeted their healing power. But no longer, says Joseph Turow, a communications professor at the University of Pennsylvania and the author of *Playing Doctor: Television, Storytelling, and Medical Power*. "The doctors have been knocked off their pedestal."—*Kathleen Moloney*

DR. KILDARE
1961–1966
Richard Chamberlain stars as part superhero, part eagle scout. (He described Kildare as "good, high-minded, loyal, kind, warm-hearted, friendly, sincere, and chaste.") "If I suffered from a deadly disease," Kildare says to a recalcitrant alcoholic, "I'd do everything in my power to help the doctors who were helping me." Though little actual treatment is shown—most action takes place in the hospital's break room and cafeteria—the patients always get better.

BEN CASEY
1961–1966
Vince Edwards stars as a brooding neurosurgeon at County General. The show is low-tech, offering only vague shots of equipment while most clinical scenes take place in a shadowy room with a bed and a table. Casey is brusque and powerful. "If you don't want medical help, you've taken leave of your senses, woman," he barks. "I'm a neurosurgeon. My job is to identify, isolate, and cure."

MARCUS WELBY, M.D.
1969–1976
Robert Young ("Father Knows Best") stars as a beloved family physician. Welby gives injections on screen—a TV-doc first—and spends hours counseling patients on autism, abortion, impotence, addiction, menopause, and homosexuality. (He has trouble believing that a gay patient doesn't actually like girls.) He makes house calls, rarely uses medical terms, and almost always—with the help of a crack specialist—heals the patient.

MEDICAL CENTER
1969–1976
Chad Everett stars as Joe Gannon, a young yet seasoned physician-turned-department-chief beset by personal and professional crises. Often hurried and abrupt, Gannon tosses off terms like aortic stenosis and mastectomy. He operates on screen and is cagey with his back-talking, eccentric patients. Still, hardly anyone dies.

ER
1994–present
In a seething emergency room, the staff—with Anthony Edwards as Dr. Mark Greene and George Clooney as Dr. Douglas Ross—practices harsh, snap-judgment medicine. ("Two-day-old male infant, full-term, vaginal delivery, found cyanotic in his crib. Resp 50, heart rate 160.") Yet for all the techy talk and shiny equipment, the doctors struggle. "We work 36 hours on, 18 off, which is 90 hours a week, 52 weeks a year," says Dr. Peter Benton (Eriq LaSalle). "For that we are paid $23,739 before taxes—and we make our own coffee."

ST. ELSEWHERE
1982–1988
At Boston's fictional St. Elegius Hospital, actors Ed Begley, Jr., Denzel Washington, and countless others mark a shift by playing up medicine's seedy side. Patients die as often as they live, doctors are mugged in the ER, blood and jokes flow, and the screen fills with people in hospital greens darting amid gadgets. One doctor gets AIDS, another becomes a rapist, a third kills himself.

CHICAGO HOPE
1994–present
In a large city hospital, Hector Elizondo (Dr. Phillip Watters), Mandy Patinkin (Dr. Jeffrey Geiger), and Adam Arkin (Dr. Aaron Shutt) wallow in ethical and personal dilemmas. This show flaunts what the old shows hid: profiteering, gore, and death. ("That bowel stinks like a cesspool. I'll never operate on anybody with a stinking bowel. Air freshener!") Doctors display heroism, then rush off to gouge a colleague. "Sometimes it feels like we spend all our time saving people we don't know," says a surgeon. "People who are ignorant and racist."

was one of the first to point out that in the rush for diagnosis patients often just frighten themselves and make their symptoms worse.

The authors told of a 59-year-old patient admitted to a hospital to have a hernia repaired. While awaiting surgery, the patient complained of mild chest pain, so doctors began a battery of tests, which increased his agitation and pain. The patient ended up in the coronary care unit with a catheter in his heart and an IV dripping nitroglycerin into a vein. The original operation had been forgotten entirely, and as it turned out, there was nothing wrong with his heart.

"The chain of events seemed to be fueled by both the patient's anxiety and the 'anxiety' of the health care system," wrote the authors. They coined a new phrase to describe how events had gotten out of hand: *clinical cascade*. And the catalyst in most of these cases, said the authors, was a medical test.

Not long after, a panel of experts released the nation's first-ever evaluation of medical tests, from Pap smears to electrocardiograms, and the results confirmed Mold and Stein's warning. Of 169 tests, only nine actually reduced the incidence of disease—and many tended to lead to faulty diagnosis, launching patients into treatments they didn't need.

In one study, 80 percent of subjects whose hearts registered "abnormal" on a treadmill stress test actually had no heart problems. In another, scans employed to test for bulging disks as the source of back pain found them in nearly half of people whose backs were perfectly fine. Yet doctors were using both tests to recommend surgery. This was alarming: People with nothing more serious than passing chest or back pain were being marched off to get their hearts repaired or spines fixed as a matter of course.

You may think you'd never let yourself fall headlong into such a tangle of unnecessary treatment. But every cascade starts with something as simple as an aching wrist, a jabbing pain, a touch of malaise. It might all start with a voodoo bug.

MY MALADY HUNG AROUND for several years. I never suffered a classic clinical cascade, but I did experience an emotional one familiar to researchers of patient-physician interaction: My visits to the doctor's office increased my worry that something was really wrong with me. The anxiety made me focus on my symptoms so much that they seemed worse. And every failed attempt to elicit relief left me resentful of money and time wasted. This made me sicker; resentment is hardly a healing emotion.

Despite my frustration, I began to notice that the swoops would run their course. If I rested and spent time with jovial friends, the bad days went away sooner. I found that no matter what the doctors did or didn't do I'd eventually be able to dust the sand off my Boogie board and hit the beach again.

I was learning something about patience, not just in health but in life. Stormy weather, broken hearts, houseguests—nothing ever seemed to go away as fast as I wanted it to. But I had to admit that it all got better over time.

Many of my friends were experiencing similar medical revelations: the bad knee that repaired itself with rest, the depression that lifted without antidepressant drugs. In fact, the majority of all complaints people bring to their doctors do resolve spontaneously, according to Arnold Relman, a former editor in chief of the *New England Journal of Medicine.* "Life is one vast collection of little aches and pains, and the vast majority of aches and pains and worries get better on their own," he says.

By my mid-thirties I was starting to believe a little less that medicine had all the answers and a little more that my body could heal on its own. But clearly I had more to learn.

Five years after the voodoo bout I skidded on wet leaves and fell on my arm, bruising the ulnar nerve. Day and night the nerve dispatched urgent messages from my elbow to my little finger. The pain kept me from swimming and typing my assignments—actually, I never could type, but now I couldn't even peck.

Once again, outrage at being deprived of my activities sent me into a flurry of consultations. This brings me to the humbling low point of my tale: the day I allowed a doctor to plunge spikes into my arm and electrify my flesh.

These were nothing so inoffensive as acupuncture needles, mind you; they felt more like crochet needles. I tried to hold still while the physician zapped electricity back and forth between the needles. My muscles contracted and my arm jerked like a marlin on a line. When it was over, the doctor announced: "They say this is the worst test in medicine."

The worst test has value for some: It can determine if a nerve is, in effect, dying. If that proves to be the problem, sometimes it can be corrected surgically. But my doctor said that even if my test revealed serious damage he wasn't optimistic he could repair it.

The episode forced me to acknowledge my own role. By demanding answers even when there was no good treatment, I was letting myself in for an excruciating test and, if I'd pushed harder, surgery that would undoubtedly have led only to complications and more intervention.

As it was, I could have saved myself a lot of misery by waiting. In a few months the bruised nerve began to heal and my hunt-and-peck was fully restored.

WHILE I WAS HAVING that lesson jabbed home, medical experts started to look beyond tests, to the treatments at the end of any clinical cascade. Most procedures developed out of tradition, and recipients weren't tested to see how they fared. The cost crisis finally prompted a review of these practices. The results again gave the lie to our blind faith in medicine.

Researchers found the usual therapies for lower back pain—ultrasound, nerve stimulation, bed rest, and surgery—to be of little use. (Chiropractic, by contrast, did help.) Among men with early-stage prostate cancer, those who underwent surgery or radiation got no better results than those who were sent home untreated. Ailment by ailment, researchers advised backing off from medical care. Because often, they learned, the most effective treatment was to do nothing.

It wasn't just big-ticket items that flunked. Antibiotics for colds? They only make it harder to treat a real virus later. Common procedures to ease vascular leg pain? Three in four patients get relief just by walking more.

In an ideal world these findings along would make us think twice before rushing to the doctor. But for years we've been conditioned to believe that our health is precarious. Human nature being what it is, it'll take more than a bunch of studies to persuade us of the reverse, that we are basically durable. This conviction can only come from a shift inside ourselves.

My own worldview has been tested recently. In ten-year commemoration of the voodoo bug, I've developed a new mystery ailment involving a persistent ache in the neighborhood of my right kidney. A CAT scan revealed nothing. When the doctor suggested more tests, I flashed back to all the dead-end doctor visits I'd endured over the years and decided then and there to invoke what I'd learned. I'm trying to have faith in my powers of regeneration, though that doesn't come easily.

To counteract my tendency to backslide, I'm trying yoga, an age-old method for getting reacquainted with the body's inherent well-being. I've tacked a poster of 908 positions on my bedroom wall, and I spend a few minutes each evening settling into new poses. You might wonder if I'm missing the boat here. While I'm busy coaxing my toe to my ear in the pigeon pose, might I be neglecting a potentially life-threatening problem?

That's conceivable. In the past decade I've witnessed not just the slow wonder of healing but out-of-control illness as well. My brother ignored a stomachache and would have died from a ruptured appendix if he hadn't been rushed to surgery. An editor friend was too busy with work to attend to a suspicious mole; during the time I spent writing this article, she died, at age 40, of melanoma.

Yes, it's always possible that the voodoo ache could be something dire. If the

ARE YOU AND YOUR DOCTOR GOOD PARTNERS?

THE BEST WAY TO avoid the cycle of overtreatment—where every symptom seems to require a drug or a test—is to cultivate a good relationship with your doctor. You need to be comfortable asking questions, weighing alternatives, and taking your time. Basically, you need someone who is willing to consider you a partner in your medical care. Here's a short quiz to help you determine whether your doctor fits the bill, followed by some tips on how to nudge him or her in that direction. Circle true or false for each of these statements.

My doctor never makes me feel that I'm imposing by asking lots of questions.
TRUE or FALSE

At the end of an appointment, my doctor always asks me if I have any additional questions or concerns.
TRUE or FALSE

If I ask ahead of time for a longer appointment, my doctor will usually give it to me.
TRUE or FALSE

My doctor always explains why she's giving me a particular test.
TRUE or FALSE

My doctor explains things without using medical jargon, in words I can understand.
TRUE or FALSE

If she doesn't, I can ask her to rephrase the explanation until I understand it.
TRUE or FALSE

I can reach my doctor or a nurse for advice by phone.
TRUE or FALSE

My doctor always asks what prescription or over-the-counter medicines I'm taking.
TRUE or FALSE

My doctor discusses the possible side effects of any drug she prescribes.
TRUE or FALSE

I feel calm and comforted after interacting with my doctor.
TRUE or FALSE

My doctor presents several approaches to treating a problem, in a manner that helps me decide what to do.
TRUE or FALSE

When an insurer creates difficulties, my doctor will stand up for my rights.
TRUE or FALSE

When I'm unhappy with my doctor for any reason, I feel comfortable enough to tell her.
TRUE or FALSE

.... Total number of trues

SEVEN OR MORE TRUES
You and your physician have an enviable partnership. You talk easily about your concerns, and it sounds as though the two of you can work together to solve any problems that arise.

SIX OR FEWER TRUES
You and your doctor need to treat a nagging ailment: your relationship. But if you had at least three trues, the prognosis is good, as long as you're willing to make an effort and approach the process with an open mind.

Getting the Kind of Care You Want

Be friendly. Even the best physicians may find themselves constrained in this era of cost-cutting and abbreviated office visits. But being busy doesn't necessarily mean a person will be unsympathetic, and sometimes all it takes to get the ball rolling is a little natural, human contact. Start by broaching your concerns the same way you would with a friend. Explain what you want—more time, more information, more compassion—and see how your doctor reacts. He or she may be perfectly willing and able to accommodate your needs.

Put it in black and white. If your doctor needs help in the communication department, write down your questions ahead of time and bring the list to each appointment, suggests Boston internist Timothy McCall, author of *Examining Your Doctor: A Patient's Guide to Avoiding Harmful Medical Care*. If you're prepared, you won't get flustered and forget what you wanted to say.

Request a longer appointment. If you'd like to have a more open-ended discussion—say you're thinking about whether to go on hormone replacement therapy or you want to consider a new treatment for your chronic headaches—ask for more time when scheduling your next appointment. Feeling rushed is frustrating and may compel you to make decisions before you're ready.

Do your homework. The more informed you are about your condition, the better you can evaluate your treatment options. Doctors aren't always up on the latest remedies for every ailment. So do some research at the library or on the Internet, then share what you learned at your next appointment.

Consider switching. If you've tried everything you can think of to improve the relationship but you're still not happy, you may want to shop around for a different doctor. In the end, you have to trust your instincts. Despite the hassle involved, you may be better off starting fresh with someone new.

This brings me to the humbling low point of my tale: the day I allowed a doctor to plunge spikes into my arm and electrify my flesh.

symptoms change or get worse, I'll jump back on the medical hamster wheel. But I'm letting go of the idea that another test is the breakwater standing between me and mortality. Gilbert Welch, a Vermont physician and researcher, says: "The public really overestimates the ability of the medical profession to significantly change the course of events in many situations."

The work of my thirties was to relinquish the childhood notion that there's always someone who can protect me, someone out there—a parent, teacher, or doctor—with the answer. The work of my forties, I imagine, will be to invite doctors back into the equation in a more realistic light. But if I no longer expect physicians to supply me with diagnoses and cures on demand, what do I expect them to do?

I expect them to behave a little more like my mother. Although she's retired now, she really was a prototype of the postmedicalization doc. At dinnertime when I was small, she was often summoned to the phone to talk to a worried parent about a sick child. My siblings and I listened in as her voice dipped an octave and she murmured, "That's normal. Normal. Nothing to worry about."

She was slow to prescribe drugs and tests, quick to reassure. Most important, her tone conveyed: This is a question worth asking, a concern worth interrupting my dinner for. No matter how many times the parent phoned back in the subsequent hours, days, or weeks, she always had time for him or her.

After all, these were her patients, and one meaning of the word *patient* is having the ability to persevere in trying circumstances. To bear discomfort graciously. To wait.

Ann Japenga has been a contributing editor since 1992.

Nutrition and Fitness

The United States has a national obsession with thinness, which is particularly focused on women. Until very recently the hot look for female fashion models was an emaciated thinness, achievable only by those on drugs or with severe eating disorders. At the same time, as a country we are heavier than ever. We also suffer from a variety of chronic diseases (which will be discussed in more detail in a later unit) that are caused by or influenced by our nutritional and fitness behavior.

Our decision to pair these issues is based on the belief that, as we look at the role of each in women's health, they cannot be separated. We also note that the new generation of diet pills provides yet another "quick fix," which may have unintended consequences.

As Laura Fraser points out in "Say Good-Bye to Dieting," the thinness many women strive for can, in fact, cause ill health. The focus on "dieting" as opposed to healthy eating leads many women to choose behaviors that are both physically and psychologically dangerous. Exercise can help to provide the balance between a need to feel good and to eat a well-balanced diet.

In "Who *Isn't* on a Diet?" Michelle Stacy discusses the historical changes which have led us to a point where "normal" for American women means to be concerned about food and weight. In fact, it could be argued that most American women demonstrate some level of disordered thinking about food.

African American women have special issues regarding food, weight, and exercise. Eric Houston, in "Weighty Matters in Women's Health," notes that 50 percent of

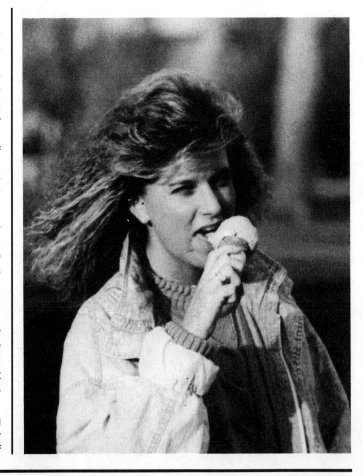

African American women are obese, placing them at greater risk for many chronic diseases. This rate is higher than that for white women (33.5 percent). Houston examines the reasons for this, including heredity, lack of physical activity, eating habits that favor high-fat foods, as well as socioeconomic factors. However, Houston also notes that African American women may have different cultural views about weight and attractiveness, that is, they may see larger bodies as more attractive. This view has allowed African American women to avoid many of the eating disorders more common in white women, but it may place them at risk in the area of weight.

The irony is that despite our national obsession with fat, we are more obese than ever—and more confused. In "The Diet Fix," Elizabeth Somer takes the current nutrition recommendations and summarizes them in an easily usable form. In addition, she looks at the seven major health concerns of women and provides specific nutritional recommendations for each.

Exercise also plays a critical role in psychological health. In her article "Rebel against a Sedentary Life," Katherine Griffin describes a 92-year-old woman who maintains her health through regular daily activity. Griffin also notes the role that our culture plays in making us more sedentary. For those who cannot or will not participate in regular formal exercise, it is critical to find ways to incorporate activity into our lives. While the view has been that exercise must be regular and intense to provide benefits, new research now shows that activity at the level of a 30-minute brisk walk can provide health benefits.

This activity does not have to be all at once; it can be broken out over the course of the day.

The highly medicalized state of our culture and the desire for quick fixes has led many women to seek a pill that will provide a quick-fix weight loss. "Diet Pills" examines the newest generation of pills designed to promote weight loss. While many people see these drugs as a panacea, the *Women's Health Advocate Newsletter* points out that they can have serious consequences and that all of the side effects are not yet known. It notes that for these drugs to be effective they must be combined with changes in eating and exercise behaviors.

Looking Ahead: Challenge Questions

What are the factors that influence women's view of their bodies? What role does culture play in these factors?

Many people seek out quick fixes for health problems. How does this view impact on long-term weight and health status?

Nutritional information can be very confusing. Summarize the current recommendations in a form which can be easily understood and implemented.

Exercise (or activity) has a number of physical and psychological benefits. What are these, and how can they be integrated into your lifestyle?

The image of the "ideal" woman has changed over time. Describe some of the past views of the ideal woman and how they compare with the present view. Is any one of them more realistic?

For years women have been driven by their desire to be thin. Now research shows you don't need to lose weight to be healthy. And you sure don't need to be skinny to look great.

SAY GOOD-BYE TO DIETING

By Laura Fraser

AST SUMMER I went to the beach with a friend who, at age 42, looks lean and carefree in a bikini. Lying in the sand beside her, I wondered: What would it be like not to have to think about sucking in your stomach? Not to have to wrap a towel around your waist to hide your chubby thighs? Not to feel embarrassed during that awful moment when you drop the cloth and head for the water? I envied her, and like so many other women who have avoided two-piece swimsuits all of their lives, I wished for the zillionth time that I was thin.

Later that day my friend, who is an art teacher, commented that when I merged from the ocean after my swim, waves lapping at my ankles, I looked like a figure from a 16th century painting. "A venus," she said. With my smallish waist, slightly rounded tummy, ample hips, and fleshy thighs, I do have some traits in common with Titan's famous *Lying Venus*. But I don't have her lusciously confident gaze, and frankly, I don't even like being compared to her.

"Great," I told my friend. "But we're living at the end of the 20th century." And with this body, that's not always easy.

A blanket of fat was once a sign of prosperity and sexuality, but over the past century or two our culture has turned its back on the plump female physique. Chubbiness stopped being a badge of status as soon as everyone had plenty to eat. And when women started to demand roles other than mother and housekeeper, they shunned the maternal shape that symbolized former constraints. Thinness came to represent everything modern, disciplined, and healthy. If Titian were painting the ideal female today, he would hardly need to color in between the lines.

Most of us realize that the ideal put forward in ads and magazines is unattainable. But that doesn't stop us from wanting to be runway thin ourselves. And too often losing weight becomes so important we lose our marbles instead.

Like many otherwise sensible women, I'm astonished at the stupid things I tried over the years to shed a few pounds: 500-calorie-a-day diets, fat-free junk food binges, fruit juice fasts, even bulimia. Fortunately, I'm older now, and the years have brought not only some reason to my chaotic eating habits and a weariness with the whole topic of weight, but also an acknowledgment that women in their mid-thirties aren't meant to have prepubescent-looking bodies.

So I stopped dieting. But even so, I often felt the sting of shame about my size.

Famous Dieters

Who Lost—and Who Won

YOU AND ME, WE PUT ON A FEW POUNDS and sigh as we struggle to fasten our pants. Celebrities gain weight and there's a national lynching. When actress Alicia Silverstone (*Batman and Robin*) appeared at the 1996 Oscars a bit chunkier than her *Clueless* size, the tabloids proclaimed: FATGIRL. Alicia took her personal trainer and slunk away, not to be seen again until she lost those extra pounds.

But if we delight in guffawing at overweight celebrities, we've also been eager to snap up their diet books to learn how they went from whale to wisp in 30 short days. For years this was our mistake; stars were wedded to the strict calorie counting we now know is a prescription for disaster. But some notables are learning. Here we grade the decade's celebrity diet books by the quality of the advice. Just as researchers have discovered that the only smart way to "diet" is to eat sensibly, exercise, and learn to accept your body as it is, thankfully, so have Oprah and a few others. —*Danelle Morton is a writer at People.*

Elizabeth Taylor
Grade: D+

BOOK: *Elizabeth Takes Off,* 1987
PRE-DIET WEIGHT: 180 +
DESIRED WEIGHT: 122
PLAN: 1,000 calories a day for 14 days, with some swimming or walking

A good way to drop pounds quickly but an impossible way to live. Liz soon regained most of what she'd lost and returned to covering up all of the mirrors in her house except the hand mirror—her standard denial strategy when she thinks she's overweight.

Victoria Principal
Grade: D

BOOK: *The Diet Principal,* 1987
PRE-DIET WEIGHT: 140
DESIRED WEIGHT: 105
PLAN: As little as 800 calories a day for 30 days

Having just lost a coveted part because she wasn't rail thin, Principal cut her calories to this unhealthy level—a bad idea for anyone, even a work-starved Hollywood actress. Also troublesome is her ban on fatty or sugary foods you love; allow yourself a nibble, she says, and you'll lose control.

Oprah Winfrey
PART I
Grade: F

"The Oprah Winfrey Show," 1988
PRE-DIET WEIGHT: 211
DESIRED WEIGHT: 140
PLAN: Four months on Optifast liquid protein with minimal exercise

It seemed like a triumph. But in retrospect, hauling a little red wagon filled with 76 pounds of beef fat on stage to let people see exactly how much weight you lost makes you a caricature of a yo-yo dieter. Two years later she was back over 200.

Jane Fonda
Grade: C +

BOOK: *Jane Fonda's New Workout & Weight-Loss Program,* 1986
PRE-DIET WEIGHT: 125
DESIRED WEIGHT: 125
PLAN: 1,200 calories a day on a high-protein, high-carbo diet with an hour of aerobic and floor exercise

For years Jane's big problem was eating too *little*. Why? As a plump child she saw her older sister had written: "June is busting out all over." She misread it as: "Jane is busting out all over." This plan is still too strict with calories, but it helped her drop the illusion that she was overweight.

Susan Powter
Grade: B

BOOK: *Stop the Insanity!* 1993
PRE-DIET WEIGHT: 260

DESIRED WEIGHT: 127
PLAN: About 2,300 calories a day (mainly carbohydrate and vegetables) along with abundant exercise

The buzz-cut infomercial queen lets you eat all you want of some healthy foods, and it's a delight to come across a dozen pages of her and an overweight woman demonstrating exercises. But her ban on sweets is insupportable; in her nutritional worldview, one cookie equals *20 cups* of rice.

Angela Lansbury
Grade: B-

BOOK: *Angela Lansbury's Positive Moves,* 1990
PRE-DIET WEIGHT: 165
DESIRED WEIGHT: 150
PLAN: Low-fat, high-fiber eating plus walks and gardening

She was prompted to eat better when she discovered that the "Murder, She Wrote" wardrobe guy bought her clothes at the plus-size shop. Egad! "Don't count calories" is good advice. But she advocates a lifetime of tiny portions—which you halve during an initial period of weight loss.

Oprah Winfrey
PART II
Grade: A

BOOK: *Make The Connection* (with Bob Greene), 1996
HEALTHY WEIGHT: 150
PLAN: Eat a balanced, low-fat diet full of fruits and vegetables; commit to exercising five times a week; and let your body settle at its ideal weight.

Oprah's unrestricted-portion, whole-food recommendations deserve applause, as do the daily 45-minute walks or bike rides. Not bad for someone who once broke a diet by eating defrosted, two-year-old hot dog buns slathered with pancake syrup.

And year after year, experts' proclamations reminded me anew that, at 5 foot 6 and about 155, if I didn't lose 20 pounds, I was endangering my health.

But recently that view changed. First, researchers revisited long-ignored findings that dieters are vulnerable to depression and rarely keep off lost weight. Then, last year, studies found that being overweight is not as risky as we once thought. For many women, in fact, it isn't risky *at all*.

These are two heady notions: Diets are bad for us. We don't need to lose weight to be healthy. From them has sprung an alternative to dieting that every woman should consider.

WHY DOES DIETING seldom work? University of Toronto psychologists Janet Polivy and Peter Herman were the first to show that people on diets binge more often than normal eaters. In one study the researchers gave dieters and nondieters milk shakes before a snack. The nondieters did what makes sense: They ate less after the drink. But the dieters did the opposite, eating much more. The reason, Polivy and Herman decided, is that people on diets don't eat according to whether they feel hungry or full but according to their sense of whether they're being "good" or "bad." When they're bad (the milk shake), they figure they've blown their diets and, like a coil wound too tight, tend to spring apart—losing control and binging. Such episodes intensify dieters' anxieties about their weight and spawn new vows to do "better." This cycle is familiar to anyone who has ever tried to lose weight, but researchers now say we should give ourselves a break: It's the diet, not the dieter, that's to blame.

The problem with limiting food is that the body reacts as if it's being starved. Neurotransmitters in the brain start clamoring for food, producing cravings. Metabolic rate slows so the body can survive the apparent famine. And then the mind starts a rebellion. "It's the deprivation effect," says Polivy. "If you're told you can't have something, then that's what you want. You want it so much, in fact, that you become preoccupied with food at the expense of emotional stability." Many obesity researchers now agree. "Clearly the psychological consequences of dieting are horrible," says John Foreyt, a psychologist at Baylor University.

Nevertheless, few medical experts have challenged the practice of treating overweight people with diets. Drastic measures were necessary, doctors said, for patients with this serious health problem. The so-called healthy weight tables developed years ago by the life insurance industry told physicians which patients should lose pounds. And the message that weight kills kept getting confirmed by new, similar studies.

Then, in 1986, gerontologist Reubin Andres looked at the data behind the tables and wasn't impressed. The studies making connections between obesity and death made no allowance for whether the subjects smoked or were ill. They also ignored many elderly people's need for extra pounds to fend off osteoporosis. Other researchers went further, showing that a person's weight alone—without regard to body shape, blood pressure, cholesterol levels, and fitness—was essentially useless as a predictor of health.

Last year, when Cornell University nutrition professor David Levitsky and his colleagues analyzed 19 studies of weight and mortality, they found that only people at the extremes of weight died younger than the general population. Levitsky's conclusion: If they don't have other health problems, even the most overweight people have no additional risk of dying early. "Nobody ever dies of obesity itself," he says.

Then Steven Blair, an epidemiologist at the Cooper Institute for Aerobics Research, reviewed the health of 25,000 men and found that once he accounted for how much exercise they got, their weight had no bearing on their life span. Blair and Levitsky are quick to say that all people—fat or not—must exercise and eat well to cut their risk. But they also point out that it does no good to tell anyone except those who are excessively fat—50 to 100 pounds heavier than average—to lose weight.

Make no mistake, there's still heated debate over whether they're right. But more and more experts agree with Andres. "Extreme obesity is dangerous," he says, "but I don't think we're doing a service to the rest of the American public to create massive anxieties about weight."

THAT IS comforting news, but how many of us are neurotic about our weight because we want to live longer? If Satan offered us slenderness in exchange for five years off our lives, many of us would take the deal.

In this culture it's easy to get stuck disliking our bodies and believing we

One day when I was feeling depressed, I asked an old friend the question men dread most: "Do you think I'm fatter?"

should deprive or punish ourselves to look better. Sometimes, when I stand in front of the mirror and acknowledge that I will never pass for svelte (not even dressed all in black), I still get depressed. But with researchers now debunking diets, things are clearer to me. I realize that my obsession with weight made me lose touch with myself. It may be easier to face a weight-loss program than to tackle the vague project of learning to listen to, and respect, your body. Over many years I have learned to eat when I feel hungry rather than when a diet plan says I can.

Think of this approach, which experts call internal regulation, as nature's feeding plan. Left to themselves, children will choose a variety of foods and stop eating when they've had enough, according to research by Penn State psychologist Leann Birch. By adulthood physical signals have often been drowned out, usually by judgments from a parent or a diet identifying "good" and "bad" foods. The way back to normal eating, psychologists say, is to stop listening to anyone's advice about weight or food. What it meant for me was to quit tracking how many calories I'd eaten in a day or burned at the

ARE YOU HUNG UP ABOUT YOUR WEIGHT?

EAT WHEN YOU'RE hungry, stop when you're full, and choose foods that are good for you. Oh, and while you're at it, learn to love your body, whatever its shape or size. If only it were so simple. But experts say that until we learn to respect our natural hunger signals and to accept the way we look, we'll never be able to kick the dieting habit. To find out how close you are to that healthy goal, pick up a pencil and circle true or false for each of the following statements.

My life would be better if only I could lose some weight.

T R U E o r F A L S E

I often eat when I am upset, depressed, anxious, or angry as a way of feeling better.

T R U E o r F A L S E

I tend to overeat in social situations.

T R U E o r F A L S E

I avoid mirrors.

T R U E o r F A L S E

I keep eating even when I'm full.

T R U E o r F A L S E

If I ate whenever I wanted to, I would get very fat.

T R U E o r F A L S E

I choose clothes that hide the size of my body.

T R U E o r F A L S E

I often feel guilty after I eat.

T R U E o r F A L S E

I'm afraid to have even a taste of dessert because I might lose control and eat too much.

T R U E o r F A L S E

I have tried many diets.

T R U E o r F A L S E

I prefer to make love in the dark because I'm embarrassed about my body.

T R U E o r F A L S E

I eat even when I don't feel hungry.

T R U E o r F A L S E

I compare my body unfavorably with those of others.

T R U E o r F A L S E

I eat normally when I'm with friends; when I'm by myself I tend to pig out.

T R U E o r F A L S E

I think about food nearly all the time.

T R U E o r F A L S E

I'm embarrassed about the fact that I like to eat.

T R U E o r F A L S E

.... Total number of trues

FIVE OR FEWER TRUE

Congratulations. You're in tune with your hunger, and you've resisted the pressures—cultural or otherwise—that make so many women dissatisfied with their bodies.

SIX OR MORE TRUE

You probably realize that your relationship with food and your view of your body are somewhat troubled. Try to ease up on yourself and take steps to relearn a more natural way of eating.

Making Peace With Your Body

Make mealtimes sacred. Rather than reading or working while you eat, focus on the food; chew slowly and savor each mouthful. Also, pause periodically to see if you're still hungry. It takes roughly 20 minutes from the time you start eating before your stomach lets your mind know you've had enough.

Don't deprive yourself. It's better to eat one or two cookies than to swear off sweets entirely, say experts. Deprivation only makes people unhappy, which in turn makes them much more likely to overindulge.

Get moving. The evidence is overwhelming. Not only does exercise help you stay healthy and live longer, it also makes your body look better. A combination of aerobic exercise and weight training will tone you up—and help you go down a size or two in clothes—even if you don't lose any weight.

Accentuate the positive. Play up the parts of your body you *do* like. Get a great haircut, wear a low-cut dress, find a sweater in a color that flatters your complexion. And console yourself with the fact that almost all women, thin or not, are unhappy with some parts of their bodies.

Know thyself. Figure out whether your concerns about weight could be substituting for other unmet needs. Too many women try to eat their way out of anxiety, boredom, or loneliness, and their bodies—and minds—are paying the price. If that sounds like you, reach out to your friends, rethink your job, figure out what's missing in your life and how you can work on getting it. If necessary, seek professional help.

FOR MORE INFORMATION
Overcoming Overeating (Fawcett Columbine Trade Paperbacks, 1989, $11) and *When Women Stop Hating Their Bodies* (Fawcett Columbine, 1996, $23), by Carol Munter and Jane Hirschmann, are both invaluable resources for women dealing with weight and body-image issues.

gym, give up weighing myself, and start trusting myself to make what are actually pleasurable choices about what to eat and when to exercise.

The irony about my to-hell-with-diets attitude is that I've developed habits obesity doctors would love all their patients to have. For exercise I choose only activities I enjoy, and I've reached the point where I feel restless if I don't have a chance to get sweaty every day. With bingeing no longer a part of my life, I've discovered I'm not that fond of junk food. I gravitate toward fruits, vegetables, and pasta; occasionally I eat a few cookies but never the whole bag. I check in with myself: Do I really want the rest of this angel hair, or should I ask the waiter to pack it up for lunch tomorrow?

Through it all, my weight has stayed more or less the same (without a scale all I can say is my size 12 jeans still fit). That weight is about 20 pounds lighter than it was when I was bingeing and 20 pounds heavier than what some doctors might say it should be, but it seems to be the weight my body likes. And I feel good.

One day a few years ago when I was feeling depressed, I asked an old college friend the question men dread most: "Do you think I'm fatter?"

Brave and foolish man, he answered me honestly. "You're definitely heavier," he said. "But you're much sexier because you look like you live in your body." And I suppose that's true. I feel like I carry myself with a confidence that makes fewer concessions to my weight.

I've discovered nothing magical, of course. I've just had to learn the hard way what some women know intuitively from the start. Your body is all you've got. Accept it. Yet even if you can start to live more cheerfully and rebelliously with a less-than-ideal figure, you may not feel fabulous in a bikini. I don't.

But does anyone in this culture feel completely comfortable in her body? I take perverse pleasure in knowing that even those people who are genetically slender would probably change something about their bodies if they could. Maybe they wish they didn't have knobby knees and scrawny arms. Maybe, just maybe, they wish they were blessed with a few more curves, like me.

Contributing editor Laura Fraser is the author of Losing It: America's Obsession With Weight and the Industry That Feeds on It.

CONFESSIONS OF A FORMER WOMEN'S MAGAZINE WRITER

Marilynn Larkin

Ms. Larkin is a freelance writer in New York City. In 1985, she received a first-place award for consumer journalism from the National Press Club. Her most recent work is *What You Can Do About Anemia* [Dell Publishing, 1993].

Writing about "hot" nutrition topics still has impact. During the decade or so that I wrote for women's magazines, I received much positive feedback from readers.

In 1989, at the height of oat bran's popularity as a panacea to lower cholesterol, the president and chief operating officer of a leading cereal manufacturer estimated that sales of oat-bran cereals would grow to nearly $600 million annually. I wrote five oat-bran stories that year for various women's magazines. A year later, when a study called oat bran's health-promoting properties into question, sales plummeted 50 percent within a week; at that point, I couldn't give away an article on oat bran.

I also covered other "hot" nutrition topics. But although they appeared on the nutrition page, these articles tended to be either "food-of-the-month" stories (the grapefruit diet, carrot power) or quasi-entertainment pieces that positioned foods as medicine: to fight cancer, strengthen the immune system, lower blood pressure, cut cholesterol, stave off heart attacks, prevent osteoporosis, reduce stress, or improve your sex life.

Earning a living this way was quick, easy, and—for a while at least—fun. I readily recycled material from publication to publication, since all were prone to hopping on the same bandwagons. And editors who saw my work in one magazine often asked me to "do a story like this for *our* audience." It never dawned on me that I might be misleading the public by promoting "food-as-magic-bullet" mythology. I labored under the illusion that by carefully executing assignments according to the editors' parameters, I was informing the public and being a good writer.

What I was really doing was helping to sell magazines by presenting a lopsided point of view: the world according to women's magazine editors. Their world (and my assignments) was shaped primarily by two considerations: providing a "nice environment" for advertisers and making sure readers were not challenged by anything more than simple tips for healthy living.

(The word *healthful* does not exist in women's magazine stylesheets.)

Elizabeth Whelan, Sc.D., M.P.H., president of the American Council on Science and Health, thinks women's magazines are shirking responsibility by focusing on trivia and ignoring the devastating effects of cigarette smoking. In a recent op-ed piece in *The New York Times,* she said, "What advice do the magazines offer on how to stay healthy? Here is a sampling: Eat lots of broccoli to ward off cancer . . . take vitamins E and C and beta-carotene; eat garlic to fight colds and flu . . . and eat active-culture yogurt to live longer."

Conflicting views are seldom presented in women's magazines. After all, the "logic" goes, readers might become confused if they actually have to weigh more than one side of a story. Instead, editors usually decide in advance what readers should think, infantilizing readers in the process. This condescending philosophy was a major reason why I decided to get out of the whole business and into writing for physicians. Today, more than two years after making the transition, I savor the fact that I am writing for grown-ups.

How Articles Evolve

One reason why trivial and/or incorrect nutrition advice appear so often is the desire to please the magazines' lifeline: advertisers. Most marketing executives view women's magazines as "products" or "vehicles" that are part of a "marketing package" for their wares. That's where the "nice environment" comes in. Before agreeing to buy space, advertisers want to know what kinds of articles will appear in the magazine—and, particularly, what copy will appear near the ad. "Negative" stories—topics that may upset readers or otherwise interfere with a "feel-good" atmosphere—are routinely rejected. Unfortunately, this means that manuscripts that tell the truth (for example, that the link between specific foods and specific health effects is largely hype) seldom get published.

"Women's magazines are controlled by advertisers in ways that other magazines aren't," *Ms.* co-founder Gloria Steinem told a gathering of writers from the American Society of Journalists and Authors in 1991. She described how women's magazines began as catalogs, with short stories woven in between the ads. The link between advertising and editorial has remained, she said, creating a situation wherein "85 percent of women's magazine copy is really 'unmarked advertorial.'" A few months later, co-founder Patricia Carbine talked about "Advertising and Editorial—The Uneasy Coexistence" to a group of advertising, marketing, and public relations professionals attending a forum on business ethics. "Advertisers are insisting on concessions from women's service magazines that they wouldn't insist on from *Time* or *Newsweek*," she said. According to Ms. Carbine, declining circulation has put even greater pressure on women's publications to continually cross the line between advertising and editorial. Examples include presenting a certain number of recipes that use soup as an ingredient to satisfy a soup advertiser, or refusing to run results of "taste tests" that could offend an advertiser whose product appears at the bottom of the heap.

When I wrote regular nutrition columns for women's magazines, my topics were determined in most cases by advertisements already commissioned or those the publication hoped to bring in. "[A major cereal manufacturer] is advertising in September. Why don't you do a fiber story for that issue?" one editor suggested. "We'd love to get an ad from [a leading manufacturer of lowfat dairy products]. We want you to do a story on foods that are low in fat and high in calcium," said another.

Michael Hoyt, associate editor of *Columbia Journalism Review*, has expressed concern about the blurred boundaries between advertising and editorial content. In the March/April 1990 issue, in an article called "When The Walls Come Tumbling Down," he stated:

> From a reader's perspective this confluence of advertising and editorial is confusing: Where does the sales pitch end? Where does the editor take over?…Magazines of all stripes are suddenly competing to give advertisers something extra—"value added" in ad-world lingo—in return for their business. Many of these extras are perfectly legitimate and have little or nothing to do with editorial content; others fall into a gray and foggy area; still others involve the selling of pieces of editorial integrity, from slivers to chunks to truckloads.

When it comes to nutrition information, the "confusion" Hoyt alludes to is rampant. In a recent interview (*not* for a women's magazine), Richard Rivlin, M.D., of New York Hospital told me: "The public is enormously confused. They need a better understanding of the role nutrition plays with respect to disease. We haven't been doing a very good job of putting things in perspective." Writing in the *Journal of the American Medical Association*, Dr. Rivlin stressed that it is more realistic to think that good nutrition can help delay the onset or reduce the effects of such illnesses as heart disease, stroke, cancer, and diabetes—not that nutrition can prevent or eliminate these disorders entirely. He added that proper nutrition won't do much to protect an individual who continues to smoke cigarettes, drinks excessively, or leads a sedentary lifestyle.

But that type of moderate message seldom makes its way into magazines where "food as medicine" themes are regarded as an essential editorial ingredient. During my tenure as a health and nutrition writer, I wrote everything from the "diet that can save your life" to the "fertility diet" and the "brain power diet." I also wrote about diets to calm your kids, boost their I.Q., and keep them from becoming overweight adults.

The Ingredients of a "Good" Nutrition Article

The other force that drives the editorial content of women's magazines is the desire to grab attention to boost sales. The quickest, surest way to sell article ideas to a women's magazine is to come up with a great cover line. Once I learned this secret, getting assignments was a snap. Whereas some writers labored long and hard over query letters, I would think up titles and bullet them on a page, fleshing out the "story" with one or two sentences. Examples include: "16 Great Food Finds," "20 Hunger-Fighting Foods," "6 Myths That Keep You Fat," and "What Your Snacks Say About You." At least 75% of the topics I proposed in this way ended up as assignments.

Of course, the process also worked in reverse. Editors would call me and say, "We want such-and-such story (naming a provocative headline). You figure out what to put in the article." Although all this smacks of deception, I did have scruples. Despite the jazzy-sounding titles, in most instances I merely repackaged basic nutrition advice into my articles, slipping in qualifiers ("there's no proof as yet") for spurious speculations and liberally peppering my articles with "may" and "they speculate." Does this excuse me? Not really. What astounds me in retrospect is how many "experts" were willing to go along with this charade.

Another essential ingredient in good articles is the voice of authority. As a women's magazine writer, I needed "experts" to validate my editor's point of view. Many "experts" who regularly appear in women's magazines are willing to trade scientific credibility for the opportunity to have their name in print. Some would give me quotes even when the premise of a story made little sense. For example, one women's magazine editor asked me to do a feature article called "Ten Foods to Make You Prettier." I balked, saying that unless an "expert" would corroborate that such a story could include some substance, I wouldn't do it. I was given the name of an "authority" at the school of public health of a major university. *She* convinced *me* it could be done and provided me with additional sources. I not only wrote the article but recycled it to other women's publications under such titles as "Eat Your Way to Perfect Skin" and "Beauty Is More Than Skin Deep."

Some "experts" I had quoted once were only too pleased to appear in subsequent articles—but not just the spin-offs. In some cases, they "trusted me" to put quotes in their mouths without even doing another interview or clearing the information with them. At one point, I had a psychiatrist, a psychologist, several nutritionists, an eating disorder specialist, and a dietitian that I could pull out of my hat (by making up quotes based on past interviews) whenever an editor wanted a particular viewpoint point substantiated. In other words, I had "instant sources."

I won't speculate on the reasons why people with M.D.s and Ph.D.s (the ones most coveted as sources by women's magazines), who presumably know better, permit themselves to be used in that way. The fact is, many do. Of course, not all have been manipulated. But I'll bet that most are not challenged, either by the writer who interviews them or by others who are quoted.

"Hiring" of Writers

A little-publicized, unethical practice that is more common than writers would like to admit can directly affect what "expert" information gets into a women's magazine and what doesn't. On several occasions, people from public relations agencies representing weight-loss centers and other clients have called me with a proposition. They would "hire" me to write a nutrition story that quoted their client if I would "place" it in a women's magazine. (I was never asked to place a piece in a more "reputable" type of magazine. I guess it was assumed that only women's magazines, and their writers, could be bought.) For an unscrupulous writer, this is an opportunity to be paid twice for the same article. I have consistently refused such work, telling callers that if their client's views were appropriate for something I am writing, they would be used without charge.

In another typical women's magazine scenario, the writer is required to skip attribution altogether—the rationale being that "we want the magazine to be the authority." The result of this abuse of power is that the magazine gives itself a free hand to say whatever it wants, merely by having the writer pepper the article with convenient phrases such as "experts agree," "scientists have found," and "experts say." What experts? The writer and editor, of course.

Style over Substance

Another practice that makes it easier for writers to write for women's magazines than for many other publications—and that has the potential of leaving readers seriously misinformed—is lack of fact-checking. Although some women's magazines call sources to check quotes for accuracy and require writers to provide backup material for statistics, many (I would venture to guess most) don't. I wrote weekly nutrition columns for one women's magazine that preferred to be the authority (in other words, no experts were to be quoted). In more than a year and a half, no one on the magazine's staff ever asked where I got my information. Each column was composed of an article that provided a good headline, a Q&A that I had made up (including a name and city for the supposed writer), and a "fast fact" pertaining to nutrition (for example, that 40% of consumers eat vanilla ice cream). No one ever asked where my "fast facts" came from. [*Editor's note:* Fact-checking can improve accuracy, but does not guarantee it. When checkers limit their contact to people mentioned in the article, errors originating from inaccurate or misleading sources may go undetected. The only way to ensure accuracy is expert prepublication review—a process few media outlets utilize.]

In addition to a catchy headline and good sources, the article must "lay out well" on the page. Typically this means using sidebars and boxes, with cute little quizzes ("What's Your Nutrition IQ?"; "Are You An Emotional Eater?"), fascinating facts ("Did You Know..."), or 2-day "starter menus" for special diet stories. It's a plus if the article itself can be done up in an easy-to-swallow format, such as "Your A-Z Guide To Fighting Fat," "Seven Secrets Every Thin Person Knows," or "Nutrition Myths That Keep You Fat." Editors seem to assume that straightforward stories won't be read, that readers must be entertained, and that "text-heavy" pages will intimidate them.

The women's magazine writer must also understand an editor's mandate to "work with the art director." In many cases, this means the writer must include points in the text to validate the accompanying photos. For example, if the art director thinks a story on summer fruit would "look great" accompanied by a photo of bananas, grapefruit, and kiwi fruit, then the writer must make sure these fruits are mentioned in the article. Sometimes the photography is planned or even executed before the article is written.

The power of the art director was carried *ad absurdum* in one article I wrote on eating "mini-meals." I had paid a registered dietitian to plan meals that would meet all the Recommended Dietary Allowances for adult women. Imagine my shock when my editor called to demand that a meal be changed to include the foods that the art director thought would "look good on the page." "Luscious strawberries" and "juicy orange slices" would have to replace raisins and bananas!

The final ingredient in a "good" nutrition story is the writing style. Three tones are permitted:

1. Bouncy two-year-old: "Don't wait! Start now on our power-packed, energy-boosting diet."

2. Concerned parent: "Eclairs are tempting, so have one—very occasionally . . . If you do have one, make it your only indulgence that day"; "If you must use white sauce, remember: the thinner the sauce, the thinner *you'll* stay."

3. Pseudosophisticated "friend": "Of course you can diet and lose weight. You've done it before . . . and before that . . . but each time the pounds you shed creep back, causing you to groan with disappointment when you step on the scale. Yet we all know women whose weight rarely fluctuates more than a pound or two and former fatties who managed to lose weight and *keep it off* for good . . . Now, we bring you the *real* secrets behind their success."

Once a writer has these chatty tones down pat, she simply asks which style the editor wants, and bingo! Another successful assignment!

No Journalistic Skills Required

What probably helped me most in becoming a successful women's magazine writer was the fact that I had no journalism training whatsoever. I have never taken a writing course in my life.

In 1980, I went into business for myself as a freelance public relations person for various agencies in New York City. The skills I acquired made it easy to shift from press kits into women's magazine writing. These included: (1) the ability to write headlines and opening paragraphs that were punchy and attention-grabbing; (2) an unquestioning attitude towards "experts"; and (3) the ability to produce unfailingly upbeat, inoffensive copy.

Writing press kits for new diet pills, migraine medicines, and blood pressure drugs, for example, required me to digest complex information and spew it back in easy-to-swallow, bite-size pieces, rarely using words of more than one syllable and remaining as one-dimensional as possible (sound familiar?). Snappy headlines and subheads were more important than hard information—after all, my primary responsibility was to help ensure that our material wasn't hurled immediately into the "circular file."

I made my first women's magazine contacts when pitching editors with story ideas that would include whatever clients I happened to be handling at the time. If the editors wanted more, I would send a press kit or bulleted list of article ideas that could be built around the client. Some of the "low-end" women's magazines willingly take articles provided by public relations firms, which I promptly produced for them. Several even gave me bylines—a joy to someone starting out in the field.

These assignments, paid for by the public relations agencies I worked for, provided me with "clips" which I then used to approach larger publications. Soon editors of women's magazines were asking me to write for them on assignment. Within a year, I had so much magazine work that I stopped doing public relations work altogether.

After a number of years playing at this kind of writing, I grew incredibly bored. Women's magazines like to pigeonhole writers (e.g., "health writer," "travel writer," "money writer"). Even though I managed somewhat to defy definition by writing in all three of these categories, editors who gave me "regular work" really wanted me to write the same stories issue after issue, year after year: How to shed five pounds in five days; Think yourself thin; De-stress yourself; Eat right over the holidays; Get in shape for summer; How to stick to your diet while eating out; Why your food diary is your best friend, etc, etc. These are women's magazine "staples"—the stories readers presumably want to read over and over.

Perhaps it's true. Maybe all those women out there really do want to read that stuff. But if that's the case, at least I have the satisfaction of knowing I no longer contribute to the propaganda that feeds such a mindset. And I can't help but believe that women's magazine readers are capable of taking in a healthy dose of hard information, meaningful speculation, and controversy—about food, nutrition, health, life—if their favorite magazines would only make the effort, and take the risk, of presenting them.

This article is based on my experiences in writing for more than a dozen women's magazines and talking with fellow journalists. There is no question that some women's magazines have more editorial "depth" than others. Those that cater to "educated" women generally offer less simplistic-sounding articles than those catering to "the secretary in Middle America." And magazines with bigger editorial budgets are apt to subject articles to more scrutiny than those with small budgets and little money for editorial content. Nevertheless, all operate under pressure from the market forces I have described.

Cars. Desk jobs. Escalators. It's hard to be active these days. Yet researchers now know that when it comes to health, the single most important thing you can do is live your life on the go.

REBEL AGAINST A SEDENTARY LIFE

By Katherine Griffin

A DECADE AGO MOST of my ideas about exercise came from my housemate John, a former cross-country runner. For exercise to do you any good, he told me, you have to get your heart pounding and keep it that way for at least 20 minutes, or even better, an hour. John's endless energy made him a persuasive advertisement for long runs and killer bike rides. I was sufficiently impressed that I allowed him to haul me out of bed at 6:30 several times a week to go running, a feat I haven't repeated since.

These days John lives nearby, and I still see him bounding off for two-hour runs. But I'm now paying more attention to a neighbor who embodies a strikingly different approach. Her name is Emma, and she's 92 years old. Every morning as I'm drowsily returning to consciousness, the *skritch-skritch* of a rake outside lets me know that Emma has started her workout. She spends a couple of hours each day raking everybody's leaves, up and down our block and around the corners. Her back is bent and her hair a white, wispy puff, but from a distance, watching her stab the rake at the leaves, stuff the leaves into bags, and haul the bags away, you'd swear she wasn't a day over 50.

Emma is modest about her labors. "Don't have anything else I have to do," she says, with a slightly embarrassed shrug. But in my eyes, she's doing more than defying expectations about how someone her age behaves. She's living proof, in my front yard, of the most important health finding of the decade: Just working movement into everyday life can be a veritable fountain of youth.

The irony is, we've discovered this just as we've created a society that compels us *not* to move. Today the average person going about her everyday life burns a whopping 800 fewer calories a day than she would have 20 years ago. That's the equivalent of three hours of daily walking that have simply vanished. Take even a cursory look at how most of us live and it's not hard to see why we move less. Most jobs require nothing more physically taxing than pecking at a computer. Growing numbers of us live in suburbs laid out so it's practically impossible to

HOW "Go for the Burn" BECAME "Easy Does It"

AFTER SOME FALSE STARTS, in 1978 the high priests of fitness declared the road to health was paved with three to five hard workouts a week. The then-20-something boomers dashed out to do right. But just as that dictum became a burden for a generation facing 50, the experts gave everyone a new goal to chase: exercise lite.

1951 Fifteen years after opening the nation's first health club, Jack LaLanne airs "The Jack LaLanne Show." "I'm going to build a new and lovelier you!" he tells his 6 million viewers before putting them through his workout. "We're going to reduce"—pause to touch his rump—"the old back porch!"

1963 Alarmed that baby boom children are weaker than European kids, the new President's Council on Physical Fitness instructs schools to get us exercising. Setting an example, the Kennedys turn family touch football games into a national pastime.

1968 In his best-selling *Aerobics*, Kenneth Cooper of the Cooper Institute argues that four workouts a week prevent heart disease. "I've been called a zealot, yes. But this is an idea that could reshape the lives of millions." Not until 1984 will a study finally tie exercise to longevity.

1977 Once-chubby ex-smoker Jim Fixx brings Cooper's message to the masses with his evangelical *Complete Book of Running*. Everyone perceives an irony when he later dies of a heart attack while running, but he had inherited heart disease.

1982 Jane Fonda's Workout video kicks off the aerobics craze. "Namby-pamby little routines that don't speed up your heartbeat and make you sweat aren't really worth your while."

1987 By touting beauty benefits, the *Buns of Steel* videos trigger another hard-core fitness wave and go on to sell 13 million copies. But when a study finds people who just walk or garden regularly earn exercise's health dividends, experts rethink their advice.

1991 Despite more than a decade of pleas from fitness experts, two in three women get no regular exercise—more than in 1985.

1993 A study at Tufts University finds that lifting weights reverses muscle and bone loss, and may be as important to good health as walking, jogging, swimming, or other aerobic exercise.

1993 Taking the just-get-moving cue, 14 million Americans now go walking at least twice a week, up almost 40 percent in six years. Leading the way is girl-next-door walking enthusiast Kathy Smith.

1996 The surgeon general's report on exercise makes it official: Doing any moderate exercise for 30 minutes a day can help unclog arteries, lower diabetes risk, delay osteoporosis, and lengthen life.

---

go anywhere without getting into a car. There are drive-through restaurants, banks, even liquor stores. In a thousand ways both big and small, our landscape shouts, "All right, nobody move!"

Some 15 percent of us, including my friend John, have compensated for this immobilization by making time for hard workouts. But for the great majority of us who have failed at that, the only answer is to become more active without formal exercise. And that calls for no less than an outright rebellion against the conveniences that cushion our lives.

Emma, for her part, refuses to pay for a gardener—or to let her neighbors hire one. How will the rest of us revolt? I don't know, but we'd better start plotting. Because either we move, or we die.

RESEARCHERS AREN'T JUST playing cheerleader when they say that movement is a genuine magic pill. They've piled up a mountain of proof that activity can stave off the killer diseases that steal vitality and life from millions every year. In 1996 the first surgeon general's report on physical activity exhaustively detailed that evidence. Think of an illness that someone you love has died from—cancer, heart disease—or an ailment that has hobbled someone you're close to—high blood pressure, osteoporosis, diabetes, depression—and chances are that moving around helps prevent it.

Meanwhile, the dangers of a sedentary life have become alarmingly clear. We're used to thinking of cigarettes as the number one health threat, but overused recliners are just as treacherous. Last July Steven Blair, an epidemiologist at the Cooper Institute for Aerobics Research in Dallas, published the first comprehensive study to compare the effects of a lack of exercise with other health dangers. Following 32,000 people for eight years, he found that those whose only risk was inactivity were more likely to die prematurely than those who had high cholesterol, high blood pressure, *and* a smoking habit but who got some exercise each day.

And forget "no pain, no gain" and all those eighties-style exercise mantras. In 1984 University of Pittsburgh epidemiologist Ronald LaPorte found that mail carriers who merely *walked* seven miles a day were as healthy as distance runners. "Workouts" like Emma's are where the vast majority of benefits lie. This means at least 30 minutes per day of activity that's as demanding as a brisk walk. Being about that active, Blair has found, cuts your odds of an untimely death by more than half. The risk for those who follow a hard-core regimen declines further but not by much more. In addition, the experts say, you can pile up activity in short bursts throughout the day.

It sounds simple: Get back to moving

ARE YOU ACTIVE ENOUGH?

DON'T WORRY IF you can't find the time to get to the gym, experts now say. Accumulating 30 minutes of vigorous movement—taking the stairs, mowing the lawn, pedaling your bike around the block—can offer the same benefits as a full-fledged workout. The trouble is, our lives have become so convenient that even getting bits and pieces of exercise takes a concerted effort. To find out how well you're doing, circle true or false for each of the statements below.

I always take the stairs instead of the escalator.
TRUE or FALSE

I usually walk or ride my bike to do errands.
TRUE or FALSE

I do my own housecleaning and laundry.
TRUE or FALSE

My job involves a lot of walking or lifting.
TRUE or FALSE

I do my own yard work.
TRUE or FALSE

I play active games with children a lot.
TRUE or FALSE

I resist the impulse to find the closest parking space.
TRUE or FALSE

I have stairs in my house.
TRUE or FALSE

I often do exercises while watching TV—at least during commercials.
TRUE or FALSE

My hobbies involve a lot of activity.
TRUE or FALSE

I take a 30-minute walk or go to the gym five times a week.
TRUE or FALSE

.... Total number of trues

SIX OR MORE TRUE
You're probably managing to work in at least 30 minutes of activity a day.

FIVE OR FEWER TRUE
You need to get moving. Make some small changes to rally yourself.

Walking Away From Convenience

Get out of the car. Whenever possible, go partway to your destination by car, park, then walk the rest. Or even if you simply trade time in the car for time on a bus or train, the walk to and from the station will add valuable active minutes to your day.

Go on three-minute walks. Piling up short periods of activity appears to be as good as exercising all at once, so take "moving" coffee breaks or lunchtime walks.

Swear off E-mail. Communicating by computer is sure to keep you in your chair all day. Walk over and talk to your coworkers face-to-face.

Make chores your workout. Scrub the floor. Weed the garden. Bike to the store. Everyday activities count as exercise as long as they're strenuous enough to leave you slightly winded.

Shun escalators. Elevators may be hard to forswear if your office is on the eighteenth floor. But escalators are usually only a flight or two long—and they're often right next to the stairs.

around, a little bit here, a little bit there. But don't fool yourself. The promise of the 20th century was that technology would transform our lives, freeing us from the drudgery of manual labor. For most Americans that promise has been fulfilled, and we aren't begging to chop wood and haul water again. "All through the course of evolution, people had to be active to survive," says Philip James, an obesity researcher at Rowett Research Institute in Aberdeen, Scotland. "Now, for the first time, we have constructed a world in which you have to go out and make a conscious decision to be active."

It was James who calculated that the average person now burns 800 fewer calories each day than she did in 1975. The main culprits? Cars, freeways, offices, and suburbs spreading willy-nilly across the land (the typical American spends 45 minutes each day sitting behind the wheel of a car); televisions glowing in every home (three hours per day); and computers humming in every workplace.

The evils of automobiles and desk jobs are frighteningly familiar to 46-year-old Susan Donahue of Davis, California. Until three years ago her job as a veterinary technician at the local university kept her hopping. "I was always chasing sheep around or carting stuff to the lab," she says. But since becoming the editor of the university's veterinary newsletter, she spends her days behind a terminal, chasing deadlines instead of sheep.

Once movement was gone from her job, she was appalled to realize that she'd turned into the stereotypical sedentary American. "I'd drive to work, drive home, and that was it," she says. Years earlier she had gardened during the week and hiked or skied on weekends. But as she got busier and added a computer to her home, those hobbies slipped out of Donahue's schedule. "When life speeded up," she says, "exercise was the first to go."

Having too much to do, of course, is the epidemic of our era. And Americans pinched for time can find mechanized ways to make any chore far less time-consuming. Can't spare an hour for the lawn? Invest in a sit-down mower and a leaf blower. No time to scrub the car? Drive it through the car wash. Even conveniences that seem innocuous contribute to the decline in activity: Just adding a second phone in your house means you may walk 70 fewer miles a year.

"Everything we do—cleaning, cooking, yard work—burns fewer calories than it used to," says Blair. "It's the accumulation of tiny little increments, but they add up to a lot."

Eventually Susan Donahue got fed up. After casting a critical, almost subversive eye on her surroundings, she seized one big opportunity for movement: She gave up the sticker that allowed her to park on campus and started cycling the flat, four-mile round-trip to work. "Instead of mindlessly driving along with all the other driver-drones, I just told myself that I was going to make this happen," she says. "Everything else would have to adapt to it." No more excuses about being too busy, no more oversleeping and flying out the door late.

Three years later she still bikes every day, rain or shine. Sometimes it's a hassle. She has to allow more time to get to work. Her skirt gets stuck in the spokes. Rainy days find her wearing plastic bags over her shoes and looking, she admits, like a fashion outcast. But she won't give up her daily ride. "It's a wonderful thing to work into my day," she says. "Now when I get home I feel energized." So much so that she also takes evening walks with her husband, keeps up with the yard work, and goes on weekend rides with a local bicycle club.

How did Donahue manage to buck the system? Researchers who study why people get moving would ascribe it to some combination of her self-confidence, enjoyment of the activity she chose, and support from others. As a student years before, Donahue had bicycled everywhere, so there was a part of her deep down that knew she could switch from car to bike. And once she was back to cycling, the joy of being outdoors, seeing things she'd otherwise miss, motivated her to stick with it even on cold, windy mornings when the car tempted her. Finally, Donahue's husband was a longtime cycling enthusiast who was thrilled when she started to ride and got her involved with the bike club.

Donahue's path was further smoothed by the fact that she lives in Davis, a town where visionary planners had created a network of bike lanes and greenbelts. Today one in four commuters in Davis cycles to work, compared with 3 percent nationwide.

When Donahue bicycles in other cities, though, she can see why everyone drives. Exhaust fumes and traffic too often make human-powered transport unpleasant and even dangerous. And when she has to hunt around the back of a building before she can find its dirty and poorly lit funneling highway money into bike and walking paths, requiring office buildings to have centrally located and attractive stairs, and restricting driving in downtown areas to get people out walking.

This kind of social engineering may sound preposterous, but think back 20 years. Who would have imagined no-smoking restaurants and bars, or forlorn smokers huddled outside office buildings? Now that we know sitting around is as perilous as smoking, shouldn't we, as a society, create opportunities to bustle about, so it's not just the determined few who make movement routine?

In the meantime, those of us who want to thrive at Emma's ripe age will have to change our lives on our own, each find-

> Now that we know sitting around is as perilous as smoking, why don't we create more opportunities to bustle about?

stairwell, she understands why everyone takes the elevator. Such barriers help explain why people don't make the effort to move and why many experts think that the only sure way out of our bind will be to change our environment.

"Ideas have been floated that range from feasible to ridiculous," says Blair, who mentions levying a tax on recliners, ing her own carpet of leaves to attack on sunny—as well as chilly—mornings.

"Don't like to sit around all day," Emma says.

Such a simple idea. Why does it have to be so complicated?

Katherine Griffin has been a staff writer at the magazine since 1989.

Diet Pills
Are Millions of Women Playing Russian Roulette with Their Health?

Suddenly, diet pills seem to be everywhere. Prescriptions for "fen-phen"—the nickname for the unapproved combination of fenfluramine (Pondimin) and phentermine (Ionamin and others)—reached 18 million last year alone, and doctors wrote more than 3 million prescriptions for dexfenfluramine (Redux) during its first year.

Used along with calorie restriction and moderate exercise, fen-phen and Redux do appear to offer a weight-loss advantage over lifestyle changes alone. But the drugs are far from perfect—and for some unlucky women, they've proven to be deadly.

Handle with Care
To begin with, most people find that once they go off the drugs, the weight returns. "Everything we know indicates that when you stop the drug, you stop the effects," says James O. Hill, Ph.D., codirector of the Center for Human Nutrition at the University of Colorado Health Sciences Center in Denver. "If we're going to use drugs [to treat obesity], treatment is going to have to be chronic."

The catch is that no one has thoroughly studied either the safety or effectiveness of giving diet drugs over

the long haul. Moreover, the risk of one very rare but deadly complication appears to rise with increased duration of use.

That complication is primary pulmonary hypertension (PPH), a disorder that permanently damages blood vessels in the lungs. Studies have linked both fenfluramine and dexfenfluramine to an increased risk of PPH.

PPH is exceedingly rare in the general population. It has few early symptoms, is difficult to diagnose, and has no consistently effective treatment. Half of those who develop the condition die of heart failure, usually within five years.

No one quarrels with the fact that PPH is deadly, and fenfluramine and dexfenfluramine now carry clear warnings about the disorder. The debate heats up over the degree of risk posed by the drugs and whether the benefits of the medications outweigh their risks.

A Looming Crisis?
Last year's approval of Redux seemed to signal a new era in the treatment of obesity. But shortly after the drug's approval, a study published in the *New England Journal of Medicine*

found that people who took fenfluramine-based drugs for longer than three months were 23 times more likely to develop PPH than someone who had never used them (*WHA*, October 1996).

If those figures are correct—and not everyone agrees that they are—then 23 to 46 cases of PPH could be expected for every 1 million people who take a fenfluramine-based drug.

Those numbers have some observers worried that cases of the deadly disorder will increase dramatically as more and more people—primarily women—take fen-phen and Redux.

In the March *American Journal of Respiratory and Critical Care Medicine*, three lung specialists wrote that "physicians such as ourselves dealing with pulmonary hypertension are simply scared. We have little doubt that we will see new cases of PPH."

But many obesity experts believe the PPH risk has been overblown and that media coverage of the issue has been irresponsible. They caution against using one study as the basis for condemning potentially useful medications. Moreover, they point out that obesity is itself a risky condition, especially when potentially fatal complications such as heart disease and cancer are taken into account.

Disagreements over risk estimates aside, physicians on both sides of the issue worry about overuse and misuse of fenfluramine-based drugs. "These medications aren't for cosmetic weight loss. They're for people at serious risk of health problems," says Dr. Hill.

Unfortunately, far too many people aren't giving these drugs the respect they deserve. "People treat them as if they're 'just' diet pills—as in, 'It's no big deal, you don't have to worry about side effects,'" he says. "But these are serious medications. They really should be used only when we know that the patient will get some benefits and is already at some risk to begin with."

Food for Thought

If you're tempted to take fen-phen or Redux, here are some questions to ask yourself:

• How much do you want to lose? See the chart to see if you can even be considered a legitimate candidate for the drugs.

• How committed are you to making healthy long-term changes? Fen-phen and Redux may help you lose weight initially. However, they don't work for everyone—and even when they do, weight loss tends to plateau around the six-month mark.

Moreover, the rebound statistics are dismal. That doesn't mean it's impossible to keep the weight off once you stop taking the drugs, but be prepared to make major changes in your eating habits and a solid commitment to daily exercise.

• Who will be monitoring you? This isn't the time to take your prescription and run. You should be *closely* monitored by your personal physician or a reputable obesity specialist.

If you pursue long-term treatment, be aware that studies generally have been limited to one year. No one knows whether taking diet medications indefinitely is effective or safe.

As far as PPH is concerned, women in their 30s and 40s appear to be at highest risk, but there's no reliable way to predict who might develop the condition. Symptoms include shortness of breath, decreased exercise tolerance, fainting, chest pains, and swollen ankles.

In addition, other side effects can occur: Phentermine's side effects include nervousness, insomnia, and hypertension; side effects of fenfluramine and dexfenfluramine include drowsiness, lethargy, dry mouth, and diarrhea. In addition, about 15% of those who take fenfluramine-based drugs complain of short-term mental fuzziness or forgetfulness. Most of

these effects dissipate within a few weeks.

The issue of long-term brain toxicity with fenfluramine and dexfenfluramine was raised by studies of monkeys given dexfenfluramine. But differences in brain physiology lead to far higher levels of the drug in animal brains, says Richard L. Atkinson, M.D., professor of medicine and nutritional sciences at the University of Wisconsin in Madison. To date, there have been no reports of such toxicity in people, but the issue is being studied.

So, based on what's currently known, here's the bottom line: If you're significantly overweight and are already facing serious obesity-related health problems, these drugs may be worth a shot. But if you're slightly overweight and your biggest health problem is tight jeans, the drugs are an expensive shot in the dark—one that isn't worth the risk.

Weighing the Risk

Body mass index (BMI) is a standard used to measure obesity. If your BMI is 30 or greater (see the darker area), the benefits of treatment with diet drugs may outweigh the risks. The same is true if your BMI is between 27 and 30 and you also have diabetes, high cholesterol, or hypertension (see the lightly shaded area). But if your BMI is less than 27, don't even consider diet drugs.

Body Mass Index*

Weight \ Height	5'0"	5'2"	5'4"	5'6"	5'8"	5'10"	6'0"
140	27	26	24	22	21	20	19
150	29	27	26	24	23	21	20
160	31	29	27	26	24	23	22
170	33	31	29	27	26	24	23
180	35	33	31	29	27	26	24
190	37	35	33	31	29	27	26
200	39	36	34	32	30	28	27
210	41	38	36	34	32	30	28
220	43	40	38	35	33	31	30

* If your height or weight isn't shown on this chart, here's how to figure your BMI: Multiply your weight by 700, then divide that by the square of your height in inches.

Update '97

News and our views

'Fen-phen' therapy may be associated with heart problem

If you're taking a combination of the weight-loss medications fenfluramine and phentermine—commonly known as "fen-phen"—Mayo Clinic physicians recommend that you talk to your doctor. Mayo physicians have observed an unusual form of heart valve disease in 24 women taking fen-phen. In light of this finding, Mayo physicians suggest you discuss with your doctor the benefits and risks of continuing fen-phen therapy.

The heart valve damage was discovered during routine medical visits. Subsequent testing showed that the valves were thickened and blood was "leaking" backwards (regurgitating), making the heart work harder to pump blood through the body. In some of the women, more than one heart valve was affected. Five of the women needed heart surgery to repair or replace damaged valves.

The women, who were free of cardiovascular disease prior to taking fen-phen, had been using the medications for an average of one year. Eight were also found to have pulmonary hypertension, a serious disease of the heart and lungs. So far, none has died.

Mayo investigators say they don't know how the medications may cause heart valve damage, but the findings raise significant concern. More comprehensive study is needed and planned.

Fenfluramine and phentermine are each approved by the Food and Drug Administration for treatment of obesity. The combination of the two drugs is not FDA-approved, even though the medications are commonly prescribed that way. Last year, doctors wrote 18 million monthly prescriptions for the drugs.

From *Mayo Clinic Health Letter,* August 1997, p. 7.

DYING TO WIN

*For many women athletes, the toughest foe is anorexia.
Gymnast Christy Henrich lost her battle*

Merrell Noden

Christy Henrich's fiancé, Bo Moreno, loved her for her sweet side, but he also knew her demons. That's why, when Henrich's parents were preparing to check her into the Menninger Clinic in Topeka, Kans., two years ago for treatment of her eating disorders, Moreno warned them to inspect her suitcase carefully. "It had a false bottom," he says. "She had lined the entire bottom of the suitcase with laxatives. That was part of her addiction." Henrich weighed 63 pounds at the time.

At another treatment center about a year later, the staff had to confine her to a wheelchair to prevent her from running everywhere in an attempt to lose weight. "Another part of the addiction," says Moreno. "Constant movement. Anything to burn calories."

At the peak of her career as a world-class gymnast, the 4' 10" Henrich weighed 95 pounds. But when she died on July 26, eight days past her 22nd birthday, of multiple organ failure at Research Medical Center in Kansas City, she was down to 61 pounds. And that actually represented improvement. On July 4, the day she was discharged from St. Joseph's (Mo.) Medical Center, she had weighed 47 pounds.

"She was getting intensive supportive care," says Dr. David McKinsey, who treated Henrich during the last week of her life, the final three days of which were spent in a coma. "But a person passes the point of no return, and then, no matter how aggressive the care is, it doesn't work. The major problem is a severe lack of fuel. The person becomes so malnourished that the liver doesn't work, the kidneys don't work, and neither do the muscles. The cells no longer function."

Henrich had been in and out off so many hospitals over the past two years that Moreno lost count of them. Her medical bills ran to more than $100,000. There were occasional periods of hope, when she would gain weight and seem to be making progress. But for the most part, as Henrich herself told Dale Brendel of *The Independence* [Mo.] *Examiner* last year, "my life is a horrifying nightmare. It feels like there's a beast inside me, like a monster. It feels evil."

Henrich's funeral was held last Friday morning at St. Mary's Catholic Church in Independence. Her pink casket sat at the front of the church as several hundred mourners filed in. Some were fellow gymnasts; some were friends and relatives; some were former classmates at Fort Osage High, where Henrich had been a straight-A student. In his eulogy Moreno asked those present to do what most people had always had trouble doing when Henrich was alive: to think of her as more than just a gymnast. "She was a talented artist and an unbelievable cook," he said. "But I must admit, her favorite hobby was shopping, for herself and others."

Moreno closed by reading the lyrics to *I Believe in You*, a song he wrote and recorded for Henrich last summer:

America's sweetheart brought to her knees
Willing to do anything to please
A product of our country
Pushed too far
You've got to be Extra-Tough, little lady
Now look this way and grin
Remember to hold your head up high
And hold the pain within

Eating disorders are easily the gravest health problem facing female athletes, and they affect not just gymnasts but also swimmers, distance runners, tennis and volleyball players, divers and figure skaters. According to the American College of Sports Medicine, as many as 62% of females competing in "appearance" sports (like figure skating and gymnastics) and endurance sports suffer from an eating disorder. Julie Anthony, a touring tennis pro in the

1970s who now runs a sports-fitness clinic in Aspen, Colo., has estimated that 30% of the women on the tennis tour suffer from some type of eating affliction. Peter Farrell, who has been coaching women's track and cross-country at Princeton for 17 years, puts the number of women runners with eating disorders even higher. "My experience is that 70% of my runners have dabbled in it in its many hideous forms."

Eating disorders, however, are by no means limited to athletes. The Association of Anorexia Nervosa and Associated Disorders reported before a U.S. Senate subcommittee hearing earlier this year that 18% of females in the U.S. suffer from eating disorders. The illnesses tend to strike women who, like Henrich, are perfectionists, and they often seize those who seem to be the most successful. In 1983 singer Karen Carpenter died following a long battle with eating disorders, and for years Princess Diana waged a well-publicized fight against bulimia.

Girls or women who suffer from depression or low self-esteem are particularly susceptible to eating disorders, as are victims of sexual abuse. The expectations of society, particularly those regarding beauty, also play a role. Not coincidentally, the ideal of the perfect female body has changed dramatically in the past several decades. Marilyn Monroe, as she sashayed away from Jack Lemmon and Tony Curtis in *Some Like It Hot,* looked like "Jell-O on springs." Lemmon's description was a compliment in 1959. A decade later it would make most women cringe.

Given the importance that sport attaches to weight—and, in the subjectively judged sports, to appearance—it isn't surprising that eating disorders are common among athletes. Nor is it surprising that they exact a far greater toll among women than men. In a 1992 NCAA survey of collegiate athletics, 93% of the programs reporting eating disorders were in women's sports. It is true that some male athletes—wrestlers, for example—use extreme methods of weight loss, but there is an important difference between these and the self-starvation practiced by anorexics. A wrestler's perception of his body is not distorted. When he is not competing, he can return to a healthy weight. That is not the case with anorexics, trapped as they are behind bars they can't see.

A study conducted a few years ago at Penn found that while both men and women tend to be unrealistic about how others perceive their bodies, men's perceptions tend to be distorted positively, while women's are more likely to be negative. "Someone feeling really good about herself isn't going to find her self-worth in her looks alone," says Farrell. "But how many girls between the ages of 16 and 22 [when eating disorders tend to strike] feel really good about themselves?"

"Men grow into what they're supposed to be," says Mary T. Meagher, the world-record holder in the 100- and 200-meter butterfly events. "They're supposed to be big and muscular. A woman's body naturally produces more fat. We grow away from what we're supposed to be as athletes."

Though laymen tend to lump anorexia and bulimia together—perhaps because experimentation with bulimia often leads to anorexia—the two are markedly different. "In a way bulimia is more dangerous," says Pan Fanaritis, who has coached women's track at Georgetown, Missouri and Villanova and is now the men's and women's coach at Denison. "Anorexia you can see."

What you see is frightening. Anorexia is self-starvation driven by a distorted perception of one's appearance. It is not unusual for an anorexic who is 5′ 8″ to weigh 100 pounds or less—and still think she's too fat. In the women's distance races at the Penn Relays this April, it was not hard to pick out the anorexics: Their arms were shrunken like the vestigial forelimbs of some dinosaurs. And on some a thin layer of downy fur had begun to form as their bodies struggled to compensate for the layers of fat they had lost.

The long-term consequences of anorexia are catastrophic. Deprived of calcium, the body steals it from the bones, leading to osteoporosis. "I've seen X-rays where the bones look like honeycomb," says Fanaritis. "X-rays of an anorexic of four or five years and those of a 70-year-old are very similar." Anorexics have suffered stress fractures just walking down the street.

Bulimia is a binge-purge syndrome in which huge quantities of food—sometimes totaling as much as 20,000 calories in a day—are consumed in a short period of time and then expelled through self-induced vomiting, excessive exercise, the use of diuretics or laxatives, or some combination of those methods. Stomach acids rot the teeth of bulimics and, if they are sticking their fingers down their throats to induce vomiting, their fingernails. Their throats get swollen and lacerated. Electrolyte imbalances disrupt their heart rates. But since bulimics are usually of normal weight, years may pass before a parent, roommate or spouse learns the terrible secret.

"You can always find an empty bathroom," says one recovering bulimic who was an All-America distance runner at Texas. During her worst period of self-abuse she was visiting bathrooms five or six times a day, vomiting simply by flexing her stomach muscles. "It's like a drug," she says of the syndrome. "It controls you. An overwhelming feeling comes over you, like a fog."

In the 1992 NCAA survey 51% of the women's gymnastics programs that responded reported eating disorders among team members, a far greater percentage than in any other sport. The true number is almost certainly higher. Moreno says he knows of five gymnasts on the national team who have eating disorders. Bob Ito, the former women's gymnastics coach at Washington, has estimated that on some of his teams 40% of the athletes had "outright eating disorders." One world-class gymnast has admitted that while she was at UCLA the entire team would binge and vomit together following meets. It was, she said, a "social thing."

Why might gymnasts be more vulnerable to eating disorders than other athletes? The subjectivity of the judging system can't help; nor can the fact that to reach the top, gymnasts must sacrifice having normal childhoods. Moreno also points to authoritarian coaches.

"A large percentage of coaches tell the girls how to count calories, how to act, what to wear, what to say in public," he says. "It becomes a control issue for the girl. They feel the only thing they control is the food they put in their bodies."

Anorexia offers a convenient antidote to what young gymnasts dread most—the onset of womanhood. Not only do anorexics keep their boyish figures, but many go months or even years without their menstrual periods, a side effect that contributes to osteoporosis. "This is a matter of locked-on adolescence," says Scott Pengelly, a psychologist from Eugene, Ore., who has treated athletes with eating disorders. "Chronologically, they may be adults. But they have a 13-year-old's way of looking at life."

In the Lilliputian world of gymnastics, arrested development seems to be an occupational necessity. Women gymnasts "are the most immature people on a college campus," says Rick Aberman, a psychologist and a consultant to the University of Minnesota's athletic department. "They're treated like little kids. When you have 18- or 19-year-old women trying to deny they've matured, you get problems. If [gymnasts] have hips or breasts, it creates inner turmoil that's so destructive. They're trying to deny something that's natural."

No one knows that better than Cathy Rigby, who 20 years ago was the darling of U.S. gymnastics and paid for it with 12 years of bulimia. "As much as [the news of Henrich's death] makes me sad, it makes me angry," Rigby says. "This sort of thing has been going on for so long in our sport, and there's so much denial."

When Rigby competed, every story celebrated her girlishness, which she worked so hard to maintain that she pinned her pigtails back from her face, fastening them so tightly that she got headaches. And the image of the world-class gymnast as waif has only become more exaggerated in the two decades since. The average size of the women on the U.S. Olympic gymnastics team has shrunk from 5' 3", 105 pounds in 1976 to 4' 9", 88 pounds in 1992. At last year's world championships the all-around gold medalist, 16-year-old Shannon Miller, was 4' 10", 79 pounds.

What chance would Vera Caslavska have had in such company? Caslavska, who won the all-around titles at the 1964 and '68 Olympics, was a geriatric giant by today's standards. In Mexico City the 26-year-old Czech was 5' 3", 121 pounds. What's more, she and Ludmila Turischeva of the Soviet Union, who succeeded Caslavska as all-around champion, looked like women. Gold medal

or not, Turischeva was upstaged in '68 by 13-year-old Olga Korbut, who was 4' 11" and 85 pounds. Gymnastics has not been the same since.

At its highest levels gymnastics has evolved in a direction that is incompatible with a woman's mature body. That was plain when Nadia Comaneci, the darling of the 1976 Olympics, showed up at the world championships two years later having grown four inches and put on 21 pounds. She had become a woman, and as John Goodbody wrote in *The Illustrated History of Gymnastics,* "We learnt that week how perfection in women's gymnastics can be blemished by maturity."

By the 1979 world championships, where she won the combined title, Comaneci was her old svelte self, having lost nearly 40 pounds in two months. Eating disorders originate in the mind, and like any disease of self-deception, they are difficult prisons to escape. That was suggested in 1990, in Barbara Grizzuti Harrison's story on Comaneci in LIFE magazine. "I am fat and ugly," Comaneci, then 28, told the writer, although she was a size 6. When they went to dinner, Grizzuti Harrison wrote, "Her appetite for food is voracious. She eats her own food and [her companion] Constantin's too. After each course, she goes to the bathroom. She is gone for a long time. She comes back, her eyes watery, picks her teeth and eats some more. She eats mountains of raspberries and my crème brûlée. She makes her way to the bathroom again. When she returns, she is wreathed in that rank sweet smell."

Henrich's career followed a pattern not unlike that of thousands of little girls who fall in love with gymnastics the first time they see it on television. Henrich started at the age of four. When she was eight she enrolled at the Great American Gymnastics Express in the neighboring suburb of Blue Springs. Al Fong, a 41-year-old former LSU gymnast, founded Great American in 1979, one year before Henrich joined. Even in a sport dominated by monomaniacal men, Fong's determination to produce champion gymnasts is extraordinary. "I work at this seven days a week," he told a reporter last year, "and I look forward to doing it for the next 25 years. It's an obsession with me."

Fong's elite gymnasts are renowned for the hours they train: one three-hour session at six in the morning and then four more hours at five in the afternoon. On meet days they are in the gym to work out two hours before the meet begins. "He pushed them really hard," says Sandy Henrich, Christy's mother. "He wanted them to train no matter what. He didn't want them to get casts [for fractures] because it took away their muscle tone."

For intensity Fong met his match in Henrich. Her nickname at the club was E.T.—hence the Extra-Tough allusion in Moreno's song—and she more than lived up to it, competing with stress fractures and placing second all around in the U.S. nationals just three months after she broke her neck in 1989. "No one can force someone to train 32 hours a week unless they really want to," Fong said last week. "The sacrifices are too great. Christy worked five times harder than anybody else. She became so good because she worked so hard and had this kind of focus."

Henrich made sensational progress. In 1986, at age 14, she finished fifth at the national junior championships and competed in her first international meet, in Italy. In early 1988, when she finished 10th in the all-around competition at the senior nationals, her dream of making the U.S. team at that year's Olympics seemed attainable.

"What's a [high school] dance compared to the Olympics?" she said when she was 15. "It's what I want to do. I want it so bad. I know I have a chance for the Olympics, and that gets me fired up." But Henrich didn't make the Olympic team in 1988. She missed a berth by 0.118 of a point in a vault in the compulsories.

About the same time, her best friend, Julissa Gomez, saw her Olympic dream vanish forever, in devastating circumstances. Gomez broke her neck while performing a practice vault at a meet in Tokyo in May 1988, then went into a coma when an oxygen hose hooked to her respirator became disconnected after she had been given a tracheotomy. She died three years later without ever regaining consciousness.

"Julissa's death devastated Christy," says Moreno. "Christy's condition went downhill after this. She went to the gym and got a photo of Julissa and hung it in her room. It's still there."

Despite the tragedy that had befallen Gomez, in 1989 Henrich had her best year as a gymnast. She finished second in the all-around at the U.S. championships and fourth in the world championships in the uneven parallel bars. By that time she also had a serious eating disorder.

Its inception can be traced in part to an incident in March 1988, at a meet in Budapest, when a U.S. judge remarked that Henrich would have to lose weight if she wanted to make the Olympic team. Sandy Henrich recalls meeting her daughter at the airport upon her return: "The minute she got off the plane, the first words out of her mouth were that she had to lose weight. A judge had told her she was fat. Christy was absolutely devastated. She had a look of panic on her face. And I had a look of panic on my face. She weighed 90 pounds and was beautiful."

Henrich began eating less and less, an apple a day at first, and then just a slice of apple—this while continuing to work out six, seven hours each day.

In one important respect Henrich was different from many anorexics, who tend to live solitary existences. During her junior year at Fort Osage High she began to date Moreno, a friend of her older brother, Paul, and a wrestler on the Fort Osage team. "She was always very tough on herself," says Moreno, "and I could relate

to that." Indeed, he recalls that Henrich got jealous when she learned that his body fat was 8%, while hers was 9%. "I had to tell her men just have lower body fat," he says. They got engaged in 1990 and were to be married later that year, but the wedding had to be postponed when Henrich fell ill. "She wanted to live in Florida and become a nurse," says Moreno. "We'd even named our children. Jesse Joseph and Maya Maria."

Soon after they began dating, Henrich asked Moreno how wrestlers lost weight. "I told her we'd wear plastic. Run in the shower with the steam on. Take Ex-Lax. And," he recalls with a wince, "every one of the things I told her, she tried. That laid real guilt on me, but I had no idea she'd do it. I had always told her how stupid it was."

Moreno says Fong might have spotted the danger signals of anorexia and bulimia earlier. "I find it hard to believe Al would not notice that every day Christy would work out, run five miles and come back. She truly loved Al and would have done anything for him. He'd say, 'Tuck your stomach in. You look like the Pillsbury Doughboy.'"

Kelly Macy, the 1991 NCAA champion on the uneven bars who trained regularly with Henrich at Fong's gym when both were in their early teens, recalls, "Everything was weight, weight, weight. He'd say, 'You could do this if you weighed less.'"

Fong denies ever harping on Henrich's weight or making the Doughboy comment. "It's just not true," he says. "I've heard those comments. Where in the world does that come from?"

Moreno and Sandy and Paul Henrich agree that the blame for Christy's obsession with weight should not fall only on her coach. "It's the whole system," says Sandy. "No matter what you do, it's never, never enough. The whole system has got to change—parents, coaches, the federation."

Christy lived at home, and a former USA Gymnastics official suggests that her parents might have pushed harder for intervention. As Christy's weight dropped precipitously, "they had to be aware of it," the official says, adding that the federation received no complaints from the family. Some of Henrich's friends question if they, too, should have seen the signs earlier.

"I think Christy had a problem a long time before [the obvious symptoms appeared]," says Macy, who herself suffered from anorexia while competing for Georgia and now travels the country speaking about the dangers of eating disorders. "I just didn't realize it. She was always working out, always doing extra stuff after practice. We'd finish, and she'd jump right on the exercise bike. Even my mother commented on it. She said, 'That Christy Henrich looks like she puts 150,000 percent into everything.'"

Moreno has come to understand Henrich's compulsion. "Christy's also to blame for her perfectionist attitude," he says. "The disease strikes people like that. I can remember Christy telling me, 'There's only one first place. Second place sucks.'"

Gail Vaughn, the director of Reforming Feelings, a counseling service in Liberty, Mo., worked with Henrich for six months last year. "Probably one of the things that worked against her most was that label, E.T.," says Vaughn. "She learned to deny pain. She competed in one of her biggest meets with a stress fracture. So when her body broke down and screamed in pain, she ignored it. Because she had learned to push past the pain."

For women, eating disorders are "like steroids are for men," says Liz Natale, a recovering anorexic who was a member of the Texas team that won the 1986 NCAA cross-country title. "You'll get results, but you'll pay for it."

For a time you do get results. That's part of the seduction. As an athlete's weight falls, his or her aerobic power increases. And psychologically there is no lash like anorexia. "To be a great competitor, you need that tunnel vision that anorexia feeds on," says Farrell. "Anybody who can starve herself can run a 10,000 really well."

But ultimately eating disorders exact a severe psychological toll. Distance runner Mary Wazeter was so tormented by constant thoughts of food that in February 1982, after withdrawing from Georgetown in her freshman year, she jumped from a bridge into the ice-covered Susquehanna River in her hometown of Wilkes-Barre, Pa. Her suicide attempt failed, but she broke her back and will spend the rest of her life in a wheelchair.

It does not take much to trigger an eating disorder. Natale recalls watching the mile run at the 1983 NCAA championships while sitting in the stands with her coach. "I remember her telling me to notice how thin all the women in the final were," says Natale. "I hadn't qualified, and I felt bad because I hadn't. I remember thinking if I wanted to run well, I needed to lose weight."

Many coaches aren't that subtle. Some divide their athletes into Lean Machines and Porkers. Tonya Chaplin, an assistant gymnastics coach at Washington, recalls that her club coach would punish female team members if they went much over their assigned weight by abusing them verbally, withholding meals and confining them to a "fat room." Before she quit the team, Chaplin was vomiting 12 times a day.

Regrettably, too many coaches see only what they want to see. Says Fanaritis: "How about the football coach who has the kid come back from summer vacation and he's gained 60 pounds and his neck has grown two inches, and the kid says, 'I lifted my ass off'? It's the same issue. You're not the one who said, 'Go home and use steroids.' You're not the one who said, 'Get skinny so you can run fast.' But you're in that middle ground."

Spurred by Henrich's case, USA Gymnastics has begun to take measures seeking to help prevent eating disorders. Last year the federation measured the bone density of all 32 national team members and found that three of them had deficiencies. It says it is trying to teach young gymnasts that they can say no if they feel too much is being asked by a coach. But how realistic is it to expect children to stop themselves from doing something they love? Especially when, as famed women's gymnastics coach Bela Karolyi once put it, "The young ones are the greatest little suckers in the world. They will follow you no matter what."

Christy Henrich was buried at St. Mary's Cemetery in Independence last Friday afternoon. A line of cars half a mile long moved slowly through the tombstones, which marked the graves of those who had lived 70, 80, even 90 years. For Henrich the time was tragically short. The inscription on her stone will read: 1972–1994.

Who *Isn't* on a Diet?

In search of sensible eating. BY MICHELLE STACEY

Show me a woman who spreads real butter heedlessly on a baguette and I'll show you a woman of uncommon independence (or uncommon genes). She is also a member of an ever-diminishing minority: women who don't diet. We have reached, in the last decade or so, a remarkable turning point in the annals of dieting, a point of redefinition that threatens to turn the universe of eating on its head. In short, restricting one's intake in some fashion has become so common that "normal eating" is no longer, well, normal eating.

"Normal" eating used to be a fairly simple affair. You got hungry, you ate; you got full, you stopped. American culture devised patterns that most people followed: breakfast started the day, lunch kept it going, dinner (once called supper) finished it off. Sometimes, of course, in the face of tradition (Thanksgiving) or great temptation (chocolate cake) one overindulged and kept eating past satiety. Normal, after all, essentially means "the norm," or what most people have decided is sensible, and once upon a time the norm was not to skip meals or to skim fats but to eat in a manner that might be called natural—that is, being attuned to one's internal signals of hunger and fullness, rather than attuned to external expectations of slenderness or self-denial.

Those impossible expectations, and the feast-or-famine behaviors they give rise to, have slowly been severing our ties with our previous, well-fed notions.

Consider this: a friend of mine confessed to a "big lunch" that necessitated skipping dinner entirely. The big lunch consisted of a roll with butter, three-quarters of a plate of gnocchi, two diet sodas and a *gelato* shared among four women. Our mothers would consider that normal (albeit not exactly nutritionally balanced), maybe even on the skimpy side—after all, she didn't clean her plate. Or consider this: an advertisement touts "Now you can have a sliver this big"—showing a piece of cheesecake that fills a magazine page—because the cake is made from nonfat cheese. Is that normal?

Eating-disorder researchers Janet Polivy and C. Peter Herman of the University of Toronto put it this way in an article in the *Journal of Consulting and Clinical Psychology:* "It is now 'normal' for individuals in our society to express concern about their weight and to engage in fitful attempts to change it. . . . Normal eating now requires periodic dieting." Polivy and Herman simply established what those of us sitting at the table have long known in our hearts about women and eating: it is becoming more and more difficult to eat without neurosis. Years, even decades, of power struggle with food—denying our hunger, trading off a dressingless salad for lunch with a chocolate mousse dessert at dinner, fretting and stewing over whether we had one smidgen of toast too much—have forced a sea change not only in the language of food but in its very reality.

2. NUTRITION AND FITNESS

Here are some of the voices of the new normality, or abnormality, about food. Not surprisingly, they are anonymous. Who would want to admit to these utterances?

- "I love the kind of vacation where you work out a lot, because then you don't have to worry about what you eat."
- "I weigh myself every day, because otherwise I'd be at the mercy of my subjective feelings about whether I'm heavier today: I would drive myself crazy."
- "I eat a Wasa cracker with lunch because if I eat bread it tastes so good I just can't stop."

Writer Barbara Grizzuti Harrison believes dieting has become one of the defining rituals of our lives. "We live in a time largely devoid of ritual: dieting is the ritual of the secular cult of fitness," writes Harrison, a self-described fat person. The ritual brings a sense of control; it sometimes feels oddly cleansing and comforting. Underlying that clarity, however, are confusion and some free-floating anxiety: what on earth are we supposed to eat? Any coherent answer to that question can be worth literally millions: *In the Kitchen With Rosie: Oprah's Favorite Recipes,* which describes the food that helped engineer Oprah Winfrey's seventy-two-pound weight loss, became the fastest-selling hardcover in history two years ago, selling 1.4 million copies even before its official publication date.

There are several ironies in all of this. Americans are, on average, fatter now than they were even ten years ago; one-third qualify as obese, up from one-quarter, according to the National Institutes of Health. Yet we have never before been as well informed (or as confused) about nutrition and weight loss. Yo-yo dieting is indicted, then cleared. Low-fat, high-carbohydrate diets are universally touted as the only key to weight loss, then we start hearing about something called insulin resistance and the dangers of eating too many carbohydrates. We are barraged with facts: fat contents, calories per ounce, sodium, transfatty acids. Perhaps the greatest irony of all in this orgy of obsessing and restricting is that the word "diet" has completely fallen out of favor. Diets don't work, proclaim an increasing number of obesity experts (and headlines). What you need is an "eating plan," a "lifestyle change," not a temporary restriction in calories. So why are most of us dieting, secretly or shamelessly?

To understand that conundrum, it may be comforting (or not) to know that although diet mania is hitting a new high, it is not something born of recent neuroses. Historians have traced a trail of "reducing" (America's first term for dieting) back to the 19th century. An early hint of body consciousness occurred at the end of the 18th century, when the fashion was simple Empire-style dresses that draped straight from the bustline to the ankle (though the bodies beneath these often revealing dresses were still rounded).

The first wholesale move toward an ideal of slenderness, in the 1830s, came at the prompting of a fashion magazine, *Godey's Lady's Book,* according to Roberta Pollack Seid in *Never Too Thin: Why Women Are at War With Their Bodies.* The newly fashionable slim body carried a moral message as well: all bodily appetites were coarse and impure, and good women were expected to be above the desires of the flesh. These ideas gained force during the Victorian era, when it was considered indelicate for women to consume hearty foods like meat. Salads, breads and cakes were appropriate feminine foods, and among young girls the pallor and languor caused by iron-deficiency anemia (then called chlorosis) were considered signs of beauty.

The first diet book, William Banting's *Letter on Corpulence,* appeared in 1864; anorexia nervosa was first diagnosed, as a mysterious, psychologically induced loss of appetite that usually appeared among upper-class adolescent girls, in 1873. Although the ideal female form swelled to larger proportions at the turn of the century, the Edwardian woman—wearing a bustle to exaggerate her hindquarters—proved to be the last stand for the rounded figure. Fashions became more revealing, and the infrastructure of undergarments—corsets, hoop skirts, crinolines, bustles—that had helped shape the out-of-shape disappeared (only to make a fanciful reappearance in the 1990s via such designers as Karl Lagerfeld, Vivienne Westwood, Valentino and Dolce & Gabbana, but not in any manner meant to be of help to the hefty). The culture of dieting had begun. By 1914, a writer for *Living Age* magazine was describing a "cult of slimness," and after World War I, flapper styles brought in the first truly androgynous look. The first best-selling weight-loss book, *Diet and Health,* with "Key to the Calories," was published in 1917; by 1959, ninety-two diet books were in print.

The '50s marked the beginning of the modern diet age, according to Seid. The decade also ushered in fad diets (the Revolutionary Rockefeller Diet, the dextrose diet), diet foods (low-cal sodas, Metrecal), a perfectly formed Barbie doll that came with her own scale (set at 110 pounds) and a televised Miss America contest (in 1954). In the '60s we got Dr. Taller's *Calories Don't Count* (1961), the Stillman diet (1968), Tab, Diet-Rite, Overeaters Anonymous (1960), Weight Watchers (1963) and Twiggy (5 feet 7½, 91 pounds). The '70s brought Dr. Atkins' *Diet Revolution* (1972, one million copies sold in seven months) and *Fasting as a Way of Life* (1977), the exercise imperative and cellulite.

You know the rest: a steady slide into Lycra dresses, nonfat cookies and Stairmaster addiction. We seem at least to have acquired some skepticism about the craziest of fad diets (Oprah's Optifast may have been the final loss of innocence), and membership in organized diet programs has dropped significantly in the last few years (Nutri/System has half the number of centers it had five years ago; the number of new participants in Jenny Craig dropped by one-third between 1993 and

1994; Weight Watchers saw a 15 percent decline in membership in 1992 and 1993).

Yet this seeming modification of the dieting impulse is up against a powerful force in shaping women's collective self-image; depictions of ideal female forms that are, for most women, unrealistic or even unattainable. A study of Brandeis University a few years ago found that female models are 9 percent taller and 16 percent thinner than the average woman. "Models fall at the extreme of the distribution of body types in the population," explains Joseph Cunningham, a professor of psychology at Brandeis, who helped conduct the study.

Can we blame media images for our permanently restrained, or at least self-conscious, eating patterns? Certainly there's a connection, but nothing is quite that simple. "I think it's pretty clear that the Twiggy and post-Twiggy models through the '70s and into the '80s did create a lot of pressure on the average woman to diet," says Richard Gordon, a professor of psychology at Bard College and author of *Anorexia & Bulimia: Anatomy of a Social Epidemic*. "This kind of look is a very dangerous thing, a very negative kind of image to be beaming, and I think it's been a contributing factor in what appears to be an increase in disorders over that period. But you can't totally blame the fashion industry, because while fashion leads and creates imagery, it also reflects."

What exactly is this ambient thinness reflecting? Perhaps, some social critics suggest, there is a strain of misogyny, a horror of female fleshiness, in our glorification of slim-hipped, boyish figures. Look at how models and actresses rebound from pregnancies. And, just as in Victorian days, the act of eating is saturated with moral meaning: chocolates are "sinfully delicious"; we are naughty when we eat meat or butter; we are pure and "doing the right thing" when we consume oatmeal or some other fibrous, low-fat food. The very act of self-restraint brings with it a sense of mastery and status. ("It makes me feel powerful to be hungry," a thin Ivana Trump announced bluntly in 1986.) Only the well-to-do, after all, can afford not to eat, and only an exceptionally self-controlled woman can turn down what every cell in her body is screaming for. Eating well—high-veggie, low-fat, slenderizing—has become a stylish must, a politically correct choice.

But the control that goes into making such choices has a way of backfiring. Perhaps this is why we are, in this age of food obsession, gaining weight. Diet experts say binging is not a naturally occurring phenomenon: it happens only after previous starvation and is the expression of a powerful physiological drive to refeed. "The bottom line is that the research shows very clearly that very restrictive diets don't work," says John Foreyt, director of the Behavioral Medicine Research Clinic at Baylor College of Medicine and coauthor of *Living Without Dieting*. "What happens is that physiology overwhelms psychology—hunger and

---

Fear of Fat

If every decade or so has its diet mantra, the '90s dictum is clear: "Fat makes you fat." Or, conversely, if you drain the fat out of your diet you will—effortlessly, almost automatically—lose weight. The bible of this movement is Dr. Dean Ornish's 1993 bestseller *Eat More, Weigh Less*, in which he advocates a 10-percent-fat diet that excludes all meat, fowl, fish and dairy (allowing only nonfat yogurt). Ornish's message is echoed by the less-credentialed but even more high-profile diet-and-exercise maven Susan Powter, author of *Stop the Insanity!*: "It's not food that makes you fat. It's fat that makes you fat."

Fat mania has driven SnackWell's fat-free cookies to the top of the grocery-store hierarchy, along with the hundreds of other reduced-fat, low-fat or nonfat products that are introduced each year. Fat paranoia has also led to such absurdities as reduced-fat peanut butter (which still has six grams of fat per tablespoon) and reduced-fat cake (if you're going to eat it, why not go for the real thing?). Now, predictably, we are entering a backlash period, in which experts are worrying that those on super-low-fat diets may not get enough of certain fatty acids, and others are suggesting that such dieters may actually put on weight by eating too many simple carbohydrates.

The bottom line as usual, moderation. Eating less fat can help you lose weight because fat is more calorie-dense and also may be stored more easily as fat in your body. But you must replace the fat you cut out with complex carbohydrates—fruits, vegetables, whole grains—not simple carbs like those in sugary nonfat goodies. Many experts also agree that a 10-percent fat diet is so low that it's hard to maintain, and suggest that 20 percent is just as effective and a lot more tasty. Two other caveats: you must still keep portion size within reason (just because pasta and breads are low- or nonfat doesn't mean their calories don't count) and, for any weight-loss regimen to produce lasting results, you must add physical activity.

— M.S.

feelings of deprivation will overwhelm will power." Indeed, the failure rate of old-fashioned low-calorie diets is about 95 percent. And worse, chronic dieting—the new "normal eating" that has self-restraint as its byword—makes it ever harder to get back in touch with the reality of food. "The dieter learns to ignore signals from her body about hunger," explains Janet Polivy, a professor of psychology at the University of Toronto and coauthor of the "normal eating" theory. "Hunger and eating no longer go together. When people lose track of their hunger through dieting, it makes them more prone to overeat and binge eat."

But if expert opinion seems to be coalescing nicely in opposition to restrictive dieting, the question of what to put in its place—of how, after all, we ought to be eating—seems foggier than ever. Is there an "obesity gene"? Will everyone lose weight on a low- or nonfat diet? Even the experts seem confused.

There is a central mystery here that defies solution, that seems to deepen the more we learn about eating and our bodies. It now looks as it our bodies may have an intrinsic wisdom of their own, a "normality" they force upon us despite the blatant abnormality of our eating.

Some of that wisdom may come from simple hunger, once seen as a threat but now often a secret friend to be courted, a sign that we are doing the right (abstemious) thing. A thin friend of mine, who says she only feels anxious when she is full and comfortable when she is hungry, once moaned to me, "If only I could eat when I'm hungry and not eat when I'm not hungry. I'd be fine." Dr. C. Peter Herman, coauthor with Janet Polivy of the "normal eating" theory, calls this system "the Garden of Eden version of eating": what eating was before our loss of innocence, before we began to distrust our bodies' innate wisdom.

Many eating experts speak now of rediscovering the rightness of hunger. Several new nondiet weight-management books speak of "intuitive eating" and of "mouth hunger" versus physical hunger. New programs tout customized eating plans and the reorganization of goals: recognizing that, despite what Susan Powter screams at us, not everyone will be a size 4. The next wave in eating may involve making peace with food, this beleaguered pleasure that we have transformed from a comfort to an adversary. Perhaps we can learn to create our own culinary Eden, where the greatest sin would be to *not* savor every bite, be it of carrots or creme brûlée.

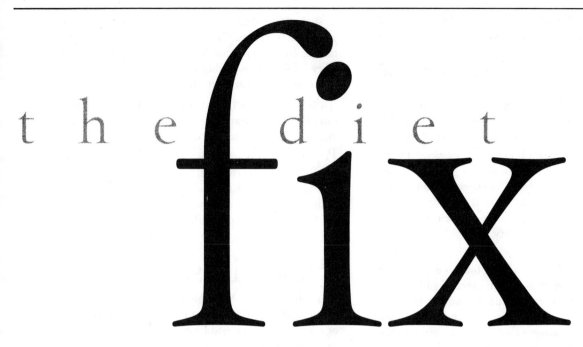

the diet fix

BY ELIZABETH SOMER, M.A., R.D.

EAT TO BEAT SEVEN OF THE BIGGEST HEALTH CONCERNS FOR WOMEN.

have you ever changed your diet to protect yourself against a certain health risk—and wondered if you were doing yourself any good? Just sifting dietary fact from fiction can be a full-time job. With each precious 24-hour day already packed with work, workouts, errands and *life,* even the most health-conscious person may find herself cutting corners when it comes to nutrition.

But that's a bad idea, since certain dietary strategies can help you reduce your risk for some of the biggest health problems affecting women today. And while current nutrition news remains complex, much of it can be distilled to a few surprisingly simple steps, such as emphasizing unrefined foods over processed foods.

"A main contributor to the diet/health issue is what we've done to our food supply," says Walter Willett, M.D., M.P.H., D.P.H., professor of epidemiology and nutrition at Harvard School of Public Health in Boston. "We've taken wholesome, nutritious foods such as corn and made corn oil and high-fructose corn syrup; then we throw away the good stuff. People would be much better off if they planned meals and snacks around minimally processed, wholesome foods."

And remember to include plenty of fresh produce. "Try to get at least five servings of fresh fruits and vegetables every day," recommends Susan Krebs-Smith, Ph.D., R.D., research nutritionist for the National Cancer Institute in Bethesda, Md. "If that's the only dietary change people

make, a number of other things will fall into line." For example, fruits and vegetables are rich in antioxidants and phytochemicals, substances that have been shown to protect against disease. Filling up with fruits and vegetables also leaves you less room for foods that are higher in fat and calories.

In addition to following those basic guidelines, you can get much more specific depending on which health issues concern you most. We've listed seven of the biggies—from breast cancer to stress—and provided the most important dietary strategies you can implement to help protect yourself.

Breast Cancer

Diet has been associated with up to 60 percent of cancers in women, according to estimates reported in the *Diet and Health Report* by the Food and Nutrition Board of the National Academy of Sciences. While women can cut their risks by exercising regularly and breastfeeding their babies, by far the greatest impact (aside from not smoking) comes from following some simple dietary guidelines. If you do nothing else, make sure you:

Include Soy Foods Consume weekly at least three servings of tofu and other soy foods, which are rich in phytoestrogens, substances that have been shown to reduce breast-cancer risk. Try adding tofu to enchiladas, salads and lasagna, or add isolated soy protein powder to muffin or cookie batter.

Use Olive and Canola Oils Cut down on fat intake, though the fat-breast cancer link is under fire and favor monounsaturated fat sources (such as olive and canola oils) over sources of both saturated fat (such as butter and red meat) and *trans* fatty acids (such as margarine).

Limit Alcohol Cut back on or eliminate alcohol from your diet. Even moderate consumption (three or more drinks per week) has been shown to increase breast-cancer risk. On the other hand, moderate intake of alcohol, especially red wine, also may reduce heart-disease risk, so consider your family's health history to decide which is a greater health issue for you.

Eat Like a Bunny At least three times a day, feast on a banquet of vegetables that contain cancer-fighting phytochemicals such as lycopene, lutein, indoles and sulforaphane. (Tomatoes, spinach, cabbage and broccoli are excellent examples.) Eating a diet rich in vegetables may cut your breast-cancer risk by as much as tenfold.

DURING THE COLD AND FLU SEASON, ADD THREE TO FIVE CLOVES OF GARLIC TO YOUR MEALS EACH DAY.

Colds and Flu

Gone are the days when people were considered simply *victims* of a cold or the flu. Today, the consensus among experts is that while we're constantly bombarded by bacteria, viruses and other "germs," whether or not we succumb to them has as much to do with the strength of the body's defense systems as it does with the force of the attack. During cold and flu season, you can reinforce your immunity by taking the following steps:

Treat Yourself to Fruit Replace high-fat treats with fresh fruits, which contain immunity-boosting vitamins and minerals, including vitamin C. Nibble on apple and orange slices instead of potato chips, grab a banana instead of a chocolate bar, or have a glass of orange juice instead of soda with your sandwich.

Vary Your Veggies Consume at least four servings of different vegetables each day to make sure you get the vitamins and minerals you need for good health, as well as the phytochemicals that may help ward off disease. "Women who often eat out should frequent restaurants that offer a selection of vegetables and soups," recommends Margo Woods, D.Sc., associate professor of medicine at Tufts University School of Medicine.

Use Garlic Add a total of three to five garlic cloves to your meals each day. Garlic contains numerous sulfur-containing compounds that have potent antibacterial effects. They inhibit germs' ability to grow and reproduce, similar to the way penicillin fights infection.

Take a Supplement Take a multiple vitamin and mineral supplement with extra antioxidants, including vitamins C and E and beta carotene.

Pop Extra Vitamin C At the first sign of a cold or the flu, supplement with 500 to 1,000 milligrams of vitamin C a day, ideally in small, multiple doses of about 200 milligrams each. Take vitamin C, along with plenty of fluids, for the duration of the illness.

Heart Disease

Heart disease is the No. 1 health concern for women, with 27 percent of all women and 50 percent of women over age 55 at risk. The good news is that lifestyle changes, including the following changes in eating habits, can help prevent this crippling disease, help stop its progress and help reverse damage that already may have been done:

Get into Legumes Choose legumes (such as beans and peas) and fish over red meat at least four times a week. Legumes are rich in saponins (phytochemicals that may lower cholesterol levels), and in soluble fiber, which also helps reduce cholesterol levels. The omega-3 fatty acids in fish help lower triglycerides and may lower LDL cholesterol levels, thus reducing heart-disease risk.

Choose Plant-Based Foods Make sure that three out of every four foods you eat are plant-based. "If people obtained most of their calories from fruits, vegetables, grains and legumes, they would be well on their way to good health," says William Connor, M.D., a professor at the School of Medicine at the Oregon Health Sciences University in Portland.

Watch Body Fat Avoid gaining excess body fat, especially around your waist and chest. The tendency to store body fat above rather than below the belt has been associated with an increased risk for cardiovascular disease.

Take a Supplement Use a supplement that provides extra antioxidants, including vitamins C and E and beta carotene.

Use Olive Oil Throw out the margarine (high in trans fatty acids) and butter (high in saturated fats), and instead use olive oil, which is a heart-healthier, monounsaturated fat.

Osteoporosis

Unless women of all ages start taking their diet and exercise habits more seriously, nearly one in three will develop spine or hip fractures as a result of osteoporosis. Many of the 20 million women already affected by osteoporosis

HOW WELL YOU EAT AFFECTS HOW WELL YOU HANDLE STRESS.

may have suffered needlessly, since a healthful diet and regular exercise may prevent or at least slow bone loss. Fortunately, it's never too late to improve your habits; make these yours:

Drink Milk or Take Supplements To ensure that you're getting enough calcium, drink three glasses of skim milk daily or take calcium and magnesium supplements in a 2:1 ratio (i.e., 800 milligrams of calcium with 400 milligrams of magnesium), plus 200 to 400 international units of vitamin D.

Eat Calcium-Rich Foods Include two daily servings of other calcium-rich foods, such as a snack of raw broccoli florets and nonfat dip or a cup of steamed spinach with dinner.

Limit Protein Eat meat (extra-lean), chicken (from the breast and drumstick, not the thigh and wing) and fish no more than two three-ounce servings a day. (Excessive protein intake increases urinary calcium loss and can contribute to osteoporosis.)

Avoid Sodium Throw out the salt shaker, since a high-sodium diet also increases urinary loss of calcium.

Stress

Stress and less than-optimal nutrition often go hand in hand. A vitamin or mineral deficiency is a physical stressor in itself, since suboptimal amounts of any nutrient place a strain on every body process that depends on it. On the other hand, how well your body is nourished affects how well you emotionally handle stress. But at those times when you're stressed out and your nutritional needs are at their greatest, your eating habits are likely to be at their worst. So when the going gets tense, make time for the following:

Don't Skip Meals Eat regularly, even if it's only a nutritious mini-meal or snack.

Avoid Caffeine Don't rely on coffee, tea, cola or other caffeinated beverages to keep you going, since they only aggravate stress. Instead, drink fruit or vegetable juices, sparkling water, herbal teas and all-roasted grain beverages (like Postum).

Eat Healthful Snacks Snack on baby carrots or low-fat popcorn for crunch and naturally sweetened starches (such as an English muffin topped with all-fruit spread) rather than sugary or fatty commercial snack foods.

Take a Supplement Take a moderate-dose, well-balanced multiple vitamin and mineral supplement with extra vitamins C and E. (Supplements taken in small, multiple doses are better absorbed than once-a-day supplements.)

Find Nonfood Comforts Listen to your body and pay attention to why you're eating. If you're overeating to

soothe stress and troublesome emotions, find a nonfood way to nurture yourself.

PMS

Yesteryear's "grin and bear it" approach to PMS management has been replaced with a take-charge approach that begins with diet. To lessen the incidence and strength of symptoms, take the following dietary steps during the two weeks leading up to your period:

Curb Cravings With Carbs But Not Sweets While it's common to address cravings with chocolate and other sweets, a high sugar intake actually may aggravate the mood swings and depression that can accompany PMS. "Instead, treat yourself to specialty breads such as onion or black olive bread topped with salsa," recommends Woods. By making bread tasty, interesting and flavorful, you won't need butter, and you'll satisfy your urge for something sweet.

Limit Sodium Eat salty foods in moderation to manage the swelling and breast tenderness associated with fluid retention.

Eat More Fiber Eat two fiber-rich fruits, vegetables, whole grains or legumes at each meal and at least one with each snack, for a total of 10 or more servings daily. Imbalances of the hormones estrogen and progesterone can contribute to PMS, but a high-fiber diet enhances estrogen excretion and can improve hormonal balance and ease PMS symptoms.

Avoid Alcohol and Caffeine Don't drink caffeine and alcohol during the 10 to 14 days before your period starts. While fluid intake is crucial, some fluids can do you in. Caffeine consumption has been linked to the prevalence of PMS. And although alcohol may slightly reduce the discomfort associated with PMS, it also aggravates mood swings and other emotional problems.

Take a Supplement Consider taking a moderate-dose vitamin and mineral supplement that contains 100 percent of the daily requirement for calcium, magnesium, iron, zinc and the B-complex vitamins, and no more than 400 international units of vitamin E. Some women report that supplementing with 50 to 150 milligrams a day of vitamin B_6 during the premenstrual phase eases their symptoms.

Fatigue

Maintaining steady levels of blood sugar and nutrients is vital to everyday performance, both physical and mental. Without a regular supply of nutritious foods, blood sugar drops and the body runs out of fuel the same way a car runs out of gas. But most people turn to so-called pick-me-ups like coffee and candy, which inadvertently fuel their fatigue. Instead, try the following:

In a Nutshell

If you're looking for the absolute bottom line on eating for better health, here are the eight most important dietary steps you can take. These comprehensive guidelines take into account that the advice for preventing one health problem, such as heart disease, could contradict the recommendations for fighting another, such as cancer.

1. Cut fat to no less than 20 percent and no more than 30 percent of total calories. Cur saturated fat intake to no more than 10 percent of total calories.

2. Maintain a healthy weight *and* body fat percentage (between 20 and 25 percent for women, 12 and 20 percent for men).

3. Consume five to nine servings of fresh vegetables and fruits each day. At least two of them should be dark green or orange in color, and at least two should be rich in vitamin C. Include three or more vegetables from the cabbage family (broccoli, brussels sprouts, asparagus, cauliflower or cabbage) each week.

4. Get at least six servings of grain foods, preferably whole-grain, daily.

5. Include at least three servings of low-fat, calcium-rich foods each day, including low- or nonfat milk, yogurt and cheese; dark green, leafy vegetables; and calcium-fortified soy milk.

6. Limit refined and added sugars to less than 10 percent of total calories or fewer than eight teaspoons a day based on a 2,000 calorie-a-day diet. (Keep in mind that a single can of cola contains up to 9 teaspoons of sugar.

7. If you consume fewer than 2,000 calories a day, take a moderate-dose vitamin and mineral supplement that contains extra vitamin C, vitamin E and beta carotene.

8. Drink at least eight glasses of water a day.

Don't Skip Meals Eat four to six small meals and snacks throughout the day to keep energy levels in balance. Don't skip breakfast, and don't dip below a daily intake of 1,500 calories, even if you're trying to lose weight. "Make eating well easy by keeping a stockpile of quick and simple-fix foods in the kitchen, like frozen vegetable mixes, packaged fresh vegetables, canned beans and pasta," advises Woods.

Eat Iron-Rich Foods Consume several iron-rich foods daily, including extra-lean meat, dark-green leafy vegetables, legumes and dried apricots. Low iron levels can starve your tissues of oxygen, resulting in fatigue, poor concentration and reduced productivity. For exercisers, iron deficiency can reduce muscle strength and cause you to tire more easily and recover from exercise more slowly. To maximize iron absorption, include vitamin C-rich foods like orange juice or strawberries with your meals, and cook in cast-iron pots.

Limit Sugar and Caffeine Consume energy drainers such as sugary foods and caffeinated beverages in moderation.

Take a Supplement Because fatigue also can signify deficiencies of nutrients other than iron, consider taking a moderate-dose vitamin and mineral supplement if you consume fewer than 2,000 calories a day, or just on days when you can't eat as well as you'd like.

Drink Plenty of Liquids Since fatigue may indicate dehydration, have a glass of water every two hours; have one every hour if you exercise, if you live or work in a hot climate or if you drink diuretics like coffee and tea.

Elizabeth Somer, M.A., R.D., *is author of* Food and Mood (*Henry Holt & Co., 1995*).

Weighty Matters in Women's Health

By Eric Houston

OBESITY, THE EXCESS accumulation of body fat, strikes half of all African–American women, putting them at increased risk for diabetes, heart disease, hypertension, respiratory problems and some forms of cancer. According to the third National Health and Nutrition Study conducted by the Centers for Disease Control, Black women's obesity rate, at 50 percent, is well above that of the rest of the nation. Compare it with 33.5 percent for White women, 31.5 percent for African–American men and 32 percent for White men.

"Obesity is really at the root of a lot of these health problems, but people don't usually connect their health problems with their weight status," says Shiriki K. Kumanyika, a University of Illinois–Chicago professor who heads the school's human nutrition and dietetics department. Kumanyika cites a recent study by the Association of Black Cardiologists in which 36 percent of African–Americans questioned could identify salt as a contributor to high blood pressure but only 8 percent knew the condition also was linked to obesity. "There are so many overweight people that the connection isn't being made," Kumanyika says.

Explanations for the prevalence of obesity among African–American women include heredity, lack of physical activity, and eating habits that favor foods high in fat content, such as fried foods, eggs and macaroni with cheese. Socioeconomic factors play a part as well, forcing many families to consume whatever is available at low cost, sacrificing more expensive fresh fruits, vegetables, lean meats and fish.

Whites and are less likely to see themselves as obese. Black girls tend to view heavier bodies as more attractive — and healthier. "There is evidence that at 9 or 10 years old, African–American girls picture their ideal selves as a heavier version than what we see occurring with the non–African-American population," explains Lillie Williams, a Howard University nutrition professor.

Stress and societal pressures also play key roles in weight issues, according to Kathy Sanders-Phillips, a Los Angeles psychologist who has studied eating habits among African–American and Latino women under a grant from the National Cancer Institute.

Of course, when it comes to health, the problem is not physical appearance—looking heavy—but excess fat on the body. That is what leads to medical problems, such as hypertension, a condition in which the heart is forced to work harder to pump blood through the body.

Doctors and scientists commonly agree that women with more than 30 percent body fat and men with more than 25 percent body fat are obese. One measurement used to determine fatness is the body mass index (BMI), which is arrived at by dividing a person's weight in kilograms by height in meters squared. When a woman's BMI exceeds 27.3 or a man's is more than 27.8, that person is considered overweight. For example, a woman who is 5–feet–5–inches tall (1.65 meters) and weighs 185 pounds (83.9 kilograms) would have a BMI of approximately 30.8. That would make her moderately obese based on the

may lead to overestimates of fatness using the BMI.)

Nutrition experts and doctors who have examined obesity among African–American women say the remedy is not an obsession with thinness or chronic dieting. Indeed, such obsessions among White women have generated bulimia and anorexia nervosa — eating disorders that Black women generally have avoided.

Cultural differences about food account for much of the obesity.

Cultural differences in attitudes about weight and food also account for much of the obesity among African–American women. Some studies suggest that many Blacks have higher preferred weights than

BMI method. (The BMI has been criticized as racially biased because it does not take into account the larger frames and heavier bones attributed to Blacks in anthropologic classifications. Heavier bones and frames

Try Dieting for Health

Clearly, the focus for African-American women has to be healthier lifestyles, rather than the latest fad diet.
Some suggestions:

Cut down on foods high in fat, sodium and sugar—cakes, fried foods and greasy snacks such as potato chips—and replace them with fresh fruits, vegetables, lean meats and seafood. Substitute fattening foods such as cheese with a reduced-fat version.

Cook healthy. Salmon is low-fat, but deep-fried salmon cakes are not. Deviled eggs can be made less wicked by using fat-free ingredients and replacing the yolk with a vegetable puree.

Substitute herbs and spices such as garlic and cumin for salt, which can contribute to weight and health problems.

Incorporate physical activity into daily routines. Take the stairs instead of the elevator and walk instead of drive.

Form support networks with friends to adopt and stick to healthier lifestyles.

For more information about healthy eating habits or to find a registered dietitian, contact the American Dietetics Assocation at (800) 342-2383.

Gynecological
and Sexual Health

For a long time gynecological and reproductive health issues were what most people thought of when asked about women's health. While the definition of what is covered by women's health has expanded, gynecological issues are still a cornerstone of the discussion. In this section we have tried to provide a range of gynecological concerns from everyday pain to the burning national question of abortion.

Part of the key to awareness associated with being familiar with one's body is a knowledge of the tests needed for preventive screening. Most women take the Pap test for granted. However, the test can have false positives and false negatives. Either of these can have serious consequences. Cathy Perlmutter reviews what women can do to ensure a valid result in "The Smart Pap." This information is particularly important for women who may be using a managed care system with a health care provider they may not know well. How can women in this changing system ensure for themselves the best possible care?

Women's health has seen any number of shifts in view of what constitutes appropriate care for "women's problems." Nowhere is this more clear than in the thinking on hysterectomy (surgical removal of the uterus). Once done as a routine cure-all for many types of "female complaints," hysterectomy has fallen into disfavor. Rita Rubin argues the controversial position that the pendulum has swung too far and that for some women hysterectomy may be the best solution to a long-term and painful problem.

For those women who are sexually active, the dual problems of contraception and prevention of sexually transmitted diseases (STDs) are an ever-present concern. Some STDs, such as AIDS, are life threatening. Others,

such as human papiloma virus, can cause long-term problems and may be linked to cervical cancer. Awareness of symptoms and prevention is critical for all women.

Even those women who are in long-term heterosexual, monogamous relationships need to think about contraception. The rate of unplanned pregnancies among women in their forties is the same for women in their twenties. Julia Califano's article, "Rethinking Birth Control," provides updated information on both old and new methods of contraception and discusses how each acts against STDs.

Condoms are one method that provides both STD protection and protection against an unplanned pregnancy. More women are taking the initiative and buying condoms for themselves and their partners. Yet Katherine Cottrell argues that not all condoms are created equally. Strength, sensitivity, lubrication, size, and style are all factors about which the condom-savvy woman and her partner should be aware.

Over 9 percent of the reproductive-age population in the United States is affected by infertility. In "Overcoming Infertility," Tamar Nordenberg looks at how infertility is diagnosed and at some of the technologies available to treat it. In addition to the clinical side of infertility, there is the emotional side. Infertility can threaten a woman's image of herself as well as have an impact on the emotional state of her partner and of their relationship.

Endometriosis, the abnormal growth of uterine tissue, affects 10 percent of reproductive-age women. It is often a factor in infertility. Previously thought of as something women just had to accept, new treatments are now available and are described by Joseph Anthony in the article, "Endometriosis: The Hidden Epidemic."

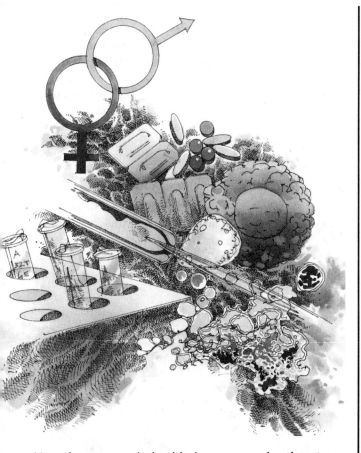

Very few women's health issues provoke the strong response that abortion does. Two articles discuss this controversial topic. The first article tries to find a middle ground on the abortion issue, one that supports women's reproductive choices and also works to make abortion less frequent through pregnancy prevention. Among the suggestions: improved sexuality education, better contraception, and insurance coverage for contraception. Indeed, these three items are at the heart of improving womens' reproductive health.

The last article, "Psychological Aftereffects of Abortion" revisits the research on abortion-related trauma. The quality of research is examined, and it is determined that while many women handle the emotional side of the abortion decision without psychological consequences, a few may need additional support.

Looking Ahead: Challenge Questions

What are some of the pros and cons of hysterectomy? When should it be done?

Abortion is a volatile issue. What do you believe should be done to resolve this question?

Contraception is often seen as a "woman's problem." Do you agree or disagree? What role should men play in contraception?

Sexually active women are at risk for STDs. What are some of the ways a woman can minimize her risk of contracting one?

If you could design a new contraceptive, what would it be? What factors would you take into consideration in designing it?

How does our cultural view of women have an impact on a woman's view of herself when faced with infertility? What about our view of children?

THE SMART PAP

How to wage a successful 'smear' campaign to improve the accuracy of your results

You know the routine. The doctor scrapes cells from your cervix (the opening to your uterus). Then the cells are "fixed" on a slide. Finally, that slide is sent to a lab where a specially trained technician—a *cytotechnologist*—analyzes it under a microscope for signs of trouble.

And the results? Lifesaving! In the 40 years since Pap smears were introduced, cervical cancer has dropped from being a leading cancer killer among women to tenth place. No other cancer-screening test can boast that lifesaving record.

But what every woman fears most is the small minority of Pap tests called "false negatives." That means she is told that her results are "negative"—meaning no abnormal cells or disease present—when in fact, there *is* cancer or precancer present. In other words, a potential or even a full-blown cancer gets missed.

Fortunately, in many cases abnormal cells never develop into cancer. Or sometimes a precancerous or cancerous condition is missed one year but caught on the following year's Pap test. But when this doesn't happen, a false negative can be devastating. Experts agree that every year some cervical-cancer deaths—although the number may be small—result from false-negative Pap smears that could have been prevented.

Clearly, reducing the rate of false-negative Pap tests can spare women's lives and tears. And now there's something you can do to spare yourself.

Just follow our four steps to the smartest Pap ever and increase the odds of an accurate Pap test in your healthy favor.

THE SMART PAP ...

1. ... REQUIRES A PAP PROFESSIONAL WHO'S A WHIZ

Most faulty Paps happen when your feet are in the stirrups. "More than 60% of erroneous Pap smears go wrong when the doctor takes cells from the woman's cervix and puts them on the slide," says Ellen Sheets, MD, gynecologic cancer specialist and director of the Pap Smear Evaluation Center at Brigham and Women's Hospital in Boston. If the doctor is rushed or inexperienced, for example, he or she may miss collecting cells from the whole cervical area. Or the sampling tools can miss an abnormal area that is unusually high in the cervix. These are called "sampling" errors—and even

the most careful lab screening is pointless once they're made.

Our experts' recommendation Go to someone skilled in taking Paps ... and that usually means a gynecologist or nurse clinician working with a gynecologist. "The medical literature clearly shows that gynecologists take better smears than family medicine doctors, general practitioners or internists," says David Wilbur, MD, director of cytology at the University of Rochester Medical Center. Data show that nurse clinicians in busy gynecology practices may actually take the best samples. "In both cases, that's probably because they do more of them and are better trained," explains Dr. Wilbur.

This doesn't mean that no other doctors or nurse-practitioners take careful Paps. Some undoubtedly do. But to make sure you're in good hands, watch the tools.

"If you see a doctor coming at you with a cotton swab, just say 'No, thank

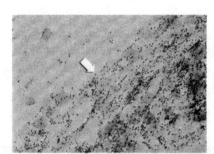 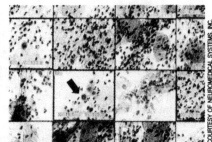

Once is not enough: Occasionally, difficult-to-spot abnormal cervical cells (*left, arrow*) may be missed on the initial microscope screening. That's why some labs rely on computer-assisted screening, like Papnet (*right*), to rescreen slides.

COURTESY OF NEUROMEDICAL SYSTEMS, INC.

you,'" says Dorothy Rosenthal, MD, professor of pathology and oncology at Johns Hopkins Medical Institutions in Baltimore. "It's worthless."

Your doctor should be using two tools to remove cells for testing: a small wooden or plastic spatula for the outside of the cervix and a small brush (looks like a pipe cleaner or mascara brush) for the inside. If you can't see what tools your doctor is wielding, ask.

An extra good sign: After taking your sample, the doctor immediately dunks her sampling tools in a little fluid-filled vial instead of smearing them on glass slides. That means she's using ThinPrep, approved last May by the Food and Drug Administration. That results in a larger collection of cells and helps make cells more readable at the lab. ThinPrep—expected to be widely available early next year—requires a special processor at your doctor's lab. Your doctor can call 1-888-844-6773 for more information. Probable fee: an additional $15 to $20.

To make a change If you want to see a gynecologist for Pap smears but you're in an HMO with rules that call for generalists to do Paps, you may have to pay for the visit yourself ... or perhaps you won't. Complain; when people make a fuss, they *can* win. Refer your HMO to the article "Variation in the Duration of Protection Given by

Screening Using the Pap Test for Cervical Cancer" (*Journal of Clinical Epidemiology*, vol 42, no. 10, 1989), which says: "[We found that] ... women who received their most recent Pap test from an obstetrician-gynecologist are protected significantly longer [from cervical cancer] than women receiving tests from other sources." Or show them this article.

2. ... IS CHECKED BY A GOOD LAB

Assuming your doctor has taken a good sample, the next vital link in getting an accurate Pap is the laboratory where the doctor sends your sample.

The lab cytotechnologists who analyze your smears spend their days peering through microscopes at Pap slides covered with thousands of cells that look like tiny dots. A given slide can hold 50,000 to half a million cells each, and the cytotechnologist is looking for perhaps one or two abnormal cells among all of them!

"Having done this job myself," says Leopold G. Koss, MD, professor and chairman emeritus of pathology at Montefiore Medical Center, New York, "I can tell you it is one of the most tedious, demanding occupations ever invented." Even the best cytotechnologist, being human, sometimes makes mistakes.

Unfortunately, some labs make more mistakes than others. "And in this day of managed care, some medical practitioners go to the cheapest lab they can, and those labs may be forced to cut corners," says Martha Hutchinson, PhD, MD, director of cytopathology, New England Medical Center Hospital, Boston.

Since 1992, the federal government has enforced minimum lab standards under the Clinical Laboratory Improvement Amendments of 1988 (CLIA)—but minimum standards don't mean all labs are great.

Our experts' recommendation To determine whether your Pap is being sent to a top-notch lab, ask your doctor the following questions:

■ "What's the name of the lab you use? Where is it?" (At the minimum, your doctor should be aware of this.)
■ "Do you talk to the lab a lot? Do they tell you if a smear is inadequate

for evaluation and that you need to do it over again?"
■ "How much confidence do you have in your lab?" Ideally, your doctor will be so enthusiastic about the lab he'll be delighted you asked. For example, Jonathan Berek, MD, chief of gynecologic oncology at UCLA Medical Center, tells patients, "We have a very good lab. I know the people there, and if anything is equivocal at all, they call me."
■ "In one day, how many slides does a cytotechnologist at your lab screen?" Good answer: 60 or fewer. Disaster (and illegal under CLIA): more than 100. And in between? In most cases, more than 70 or 80 slides on a daily basis is a strain on most cytotechnologists, says Patricia E. Saigo, chief, cytology service at Memorial Sloan-Kettering Cancer Center, New York City. Screener fatigue is considered the number-one cause of lab error. If your doctor doesn't know the answer to this question, it's worth your time to call the lab directly.

To make a change If you don't like the answers you get to these questions, maybe you should consider changing doctors. Or ask your doctor or insurer to send your slide to another lab. Request a lab at a teaching hospital or a major medical center, suggests Beth Y. Karlan, MD, director of gynecologic oncology, Cedars Sinai Medical Center, Los Angeles. "Often all the slides are looked at by more than one knowledgeable person, including residents, pathologists and technicians." Be aware you may have to pay out of pocket to use another lab—around $10 to $30, but this may vary.

3. ... IS A RESCREENED PAP

Experts know that if every "negative" slide—the slides that don't show a

---

PREPARE FOR YOUR PAP
To increase your chances of accuracy:
■ Avoid sexual intercourse in the 24 hours before your test. Semen can interfere with test results.
■ Time your Pap about two weeks after the start of your last period so you can avoid the days of your menstrual period. The background blood can obscure cells on the slide.
■ Don't wear a tampon for at least 24 hours before your Pap. You may reduce the cells available for sampling.
■ Postpone your Pap test if you have an active yeast infection. Inflammation can mask abnormal cells on your cervix.
■ Don't douche or use intravaginal lubricants or medications for 48 hours before you have the Pap smear taken. You may be washing away or hiding the cells of greatest interest.

---

problem—were examined twice, the rate of false negatives would go down. In a good lab, rescreening might drop the false-negative rate from 5–10% to 3–7%. In a less than good lab, the decrease might be even greater.

But under CLIA law, all labs must recheck only 10% of negatives. So chances are your negative slide won't get that second look.

Our experts' recommendation If you want extra insurance against a false negative, ask your doctor to have your negative slide rescreened. You will probably have to pay for this out of your own pocket, but it might be worth it.

Three options for rescreening:

■ If you're confident in your doctor's lab, you can ask your doctor to have the lab staff look at your slide twice. Probable fee: about $20.

■ If your doctor has agreed to send your slide to a university or medical-center lab, ask for your slide to be screened twice there. Probable fee: about $25 to $30, but may vary.

■ If you still have questions about the quality of the lab your doctor uses, you may want to ask your doctor to send your Pap smear for a computer-assisted rescreening, new technology recently approved by the FDA.

One procedure, called Papnet, works like this. Your Pap smear is taken at your doctor's office and then

at your request is sent to a local lab that offers Papnet testing. After this lab does a first screening and your slide is negative, it is sent to the Papnet scanning center (at Neuromedical Systems, Inc., in Suffern, NY). Papnet's automated microscopes scan your cells and a supercomputer identifies cells most likely to be abnormal. Magnified images of these cells are sent back to the originating lab for another look.

For more information about a Papnet rescreen, you or your doctor can call the company at 1-800-727-6384. A Papnet recheck costs about $35 to $40 and your insurer probably will not pay for it.

Another computer rescreening system approved recently by the FDA is AutoPap QC (made by Neopath, Inc., Redmond, WA). Unlike labs with Papnet, labs equipped with AutoPap can offer computer rescreening on site. Although AutoPap uses slightly different technology, as with Papnet, accuracy trials are encouraging.

After the initial screening by a cytotechnologist, your negative slide goes through the AutoPap system and is "scored." If the score indicates the possibility of abnormal cells, the cells on your slide get another look by a cytopathologist or pathologist.

A lab that uses AutoPap automatically rescreens all negative slides. You don't need to request it. But if your doctor's lab doesn't have AutoPap, he or she can arrange to have your slide sent to a lab that does. To find out more about AutoPap, you or your doctor can call 1-800-636-7284. The cost may vary from lab to lab but averages around $20.

Right now there's a raging debate among experts about whether humans, or humans aided by computers, recheck Pap smears best—with evidence for superior results on both sides. "This technology is in its infancy and there is tremendous potential for future applications," predicts Diane Solomon, MD, cytopathologist for the National Cancer Institute. Dr. Solomon thinks that as the technology evolves, computer-assisted screening will reach a point where it is clearly better than human screening alone.

4. ... HAPPENS EVERY YEAR
Fabulous fact: The more Paps you get, the safer you are. The chance of finding abnormal cervical cells on a single Pap smear is over 80%. But if you get Pap smears three years in a row—and they all turn up negative (no abnormal cells)—there's a 99% chance that you really have no cervical cancer or precancer, says Dr. Hutchinson. That's tremendous peace of mind! (But go right on getting Paps every year.)

The vast majority of cervical cancers—90%—grow very slowly and are curable in the early stages. A cancer missed by one year's Pap (a false negative) will likely be caught next year or two years later in time for successful treatment. But three or more years later, it may be too late.

Our experts' recommendation Instead of skipping a few years (as some organizations, including the American Cancer Society, allow under certain circumstances), get a Pap every year. This was *Prevention's* own recommendation back in July 1993. Of the 4,900 women who will die of cervical cancer in 1996, about half will not have had the benefit of Pap screening. Some insurers don't pay for annual Paps, so you may have to pick up the tab. It's worth it! Fee range: $15 to $30 plus the charge for the office visit.

LAST ADVICE FOR BLUE-RIBBON PAPS
■ Call your doctor for Pap results. Better still, ask him to send them to you.
■ Know the symptoms of cervical cancer: bleeding between periods, bleeding after intercourse, abnormal vaginal discharge. Even if your Pap comes back negative—no evidence of abnormal or atypical cells present—such symptoms are cause for concern; get another look.
■ Suppose you have to choose between paying for a Pap test every year or paying for a Pap test and a rescreening every other year? Go for the yearly Pap tests. Until computerized systems are perfected and proven, our experts agree that annual Pap tests, taken by competent doctors who use excellent labs, are your best safeguard for the smartest Pap possible. —by Cathy Perlmutter with Toby Hanlon

Politically Incorrect Surgery

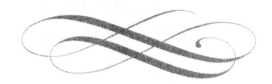

For years we've been told that hysterectomies are unnecessary, foisted on women by paternalistic doctors. But for some, the most drastic choice is the right one.

By Rita Rubin

KAREN TURSI HAD A hysterectomy on Day 57 of her last menstrual period. "I was ready to go out and buy stock in tampons," the marketing manager from Chicago says wryly.

She had experienced pain and bleeding from uterine fibroids and endometriosis since college. The two years before her hysterectomy were particularly bad. "From the day before my period to two days after it began, the pain was sometimes so intense that I could not stand up," she says. Yet some relatives and friends—not to mention a series of doctors—couldn't understand why a woman in her thirties would even consider having her uterus removed. "My sister-in-law, who does not understand female biology very well, was kind of freaked out by the whole thing," she says. Her regular gynecologist advised against the operation. So did three other doctors to whom she

turned for help. All argued that she was too young to become infertile, even though she had no desire to become a mother. "Some people cannot fathom a woman not wanting to have children," Tursi says.

Finally she convinced a fifth doctor that she was of sound mind and wanted a sound body. So, in April 1995, six weeks after her 36th birthday, Tursi had her uterus removed. "I was actually feeling better a week after surgery than I'd felt during the previous two years," she says.

Tursi isn't the only woman to maintain that a hysterectomy has improved the quality of her life. A small but growing body of research is challenging the notion that most hysterectomies are needlessly foisted upon women by paternalistic doctors. For many women, the new studies suggest, what may seem to be a politically incorrect operation is the physiologically correct choice.

Hysterectomies began developing a bad name in the 1970s, when feminists and consumer advocates sounded the alarm about unnecessary operations. Nearly 600,000 hysterectomies—a third of the world's total—are done in the United States each year. Although the U.S. rate has fallen since its mid-1970s high, it remains several times greater than the rate of hysterectomies in Europe.

A third of American women have had their uterus removed by the time they're 60. Only 8 to 12 percent of them had the operation because of cancer or a life-threatening infection. The rest have the surgery to treat a variety of lesser ills. These include unexplained heavy vaginal bleeding, which can cause anemia; a prolapsed (drooping) uterus, which can press on the bladder and lead to incontinence; and endometriosis, in which the uterine lining grows outside the uterus, causing pain and heavy bleeding.

But the most common reason for having a hysterectomy—accounting for more than a quarter of such operations—is fibroid tumors, whorled masses of muscle and fibrous tissue that grow out of the uterine wall, fed by the female hormone estrogen. It's estimated that at least 40 percent of all women will develop fibroids at some point in their lives, usually between the ages of 30 and 50. Often women don't know they have them. But when a fibroid grows as large as a plum or an orange, it can cause heavy menstrual bleeding, pelvic pain, and uncomfortable pressure on the bladder or bowels. The symptoms rarely threaten a woman's life, but they can make it miserable.

Despite the huge number of elective hysterectomies in the United States each year, until recently few researchers had carefully asked women what they thought about the operation. When two finally did, they were surprised. Harvard researcher Karen Carlson, for one, had read plenty about doctors' overreliance on the operation and about its effects on quality of life. Some studies—usually based on surveys of doctors—had found that hysterectomy reduces sexual responsiveness in a quarter of women. Other problems reported by doctors and dissatisfied patients included fatigue and depression. Worse, unless they take hormone replacement therapy, the 40 percent of hysterectomy patients who have their ovaries removed along with the uterus are plunged into premature menopause. Their bodies suddenly stop producing estrogen, which leads to hot flashes, mood swings, night sweats,

and other menopausal symptoms. A lack of estrogen also puts them at higher risk for osteoporosis, heart disease, perhaps even Alzheimer's disease.

Yet gynecologists kept telling Carlson, " 'Look, my patients thanked me for doing this procedure.' So we went into our research trying to be unbiased."

Even so, Carlson, a primary care doctor at Massachusetts General Hospital in Boston, did not expect the level of satisfaction she discovered when she interviewed 418 women before their hysterectomy, then three, six, and 12 months later. "Symptom relief following hysterectomy is associated with a marked improvement in quality of life," Carlson and her colleagues concluded in their 1994 paper published in *Obstetrics and Gynecology.*

In Carlson's interviews, few women reported problems as a result of the hysterectomy. Only 7 percent felt any loss of sexual responsiveness, and just 8 percent experienced depression—rates far lower than previous estimates. What's more, the operation alleviated *preexisting* sexual problems as well as fatigue, urinary incontinence, and pelvic pain in most women.

In related research, Carlson's team found that women who opted for drug treatment (either hormones or anti-inflammatory medicine) instead of hysterectomy frequently reported that their pelvic pain, bleeding, or incontinence persisted after a year. Of those with severe pelvic pain, half still suffered. Of those with heavy menstrual bleeding, a quarter got no relief from drugs. Hence nearly a fourth of the 380 women in this study went on to have hysterectomies.

A more recent study of 1,300 hysterectomy patients in Maryland backs up Carlson's findings. Kristen Kjerulff, an associate professor of epidemiology and preventive medicine at the University of Maryland Medical Center in Baltimore, found that these women, all of whom

had severe symptoms for at least two years, *chose* hysterectomy as their best option. And more than 95 percent were generally happy with the results, even two years later, when memories of the pain and bleeding had dimmed. "I was surprised, because hysterectomy has had such bad press, and I sort of was expecting to discover that many women were being taken advantage of by the medical community and being pushed into this surgery," says Kjerulff.

These startling findings do not mean women shouldn't be concerned about the overuse of hysterectomy. Women today have a growing number of less drastic surgical alternatives in which a surgeon removes either the fibroids alone or the lining of the uterus. And no one has yet compared women's satisfaction with those treatments to their feelings after a hysterectomy. "There are other good options available 80 percent of the time," says Joseph Gambone, head of reproductive endocrinology at the University of California at Los Angeles Medical School. "If nothing else has been tried, and you're told you need a hysterectomy, you should be suspicious, unless, of course, it's an emergency or cancer."

Carlson hopes to study how the newer procedures stack up, but results are years away. Meanwhile women who experience heavy, painful menstrual bleeding want to end their discomfort now. Carlson's research doesn't mean that hysterectomy is the right answer for every woman but that the operation should remain an option. And that women needn't feel like they've betrayed their sex if they choose it. What follows are the stories of three women with fibroids. None wanted to bear more children, so a hysterectomy was one possibility. Each made a choice that she believes was right for her.

KAREN TURSI
CHOSE A HYSTERECTOMY OVER
LESS INVASIVE OPTIONS
Between sick days and doctor's appointments, Karen Tursi missed three weeks

More than 95 percent of women were happy even two years later, when memories of the bleeding that led to the hysterectomy had dimmed.

of work the year before her hysterectomy. On the worst days she was in such agony that she had to crawl to the bathroom. Her menstrual cycle was dictating every part of her life. "I travel a lot on business," she says. "It seemed like the minute I walked on a plane I got my period. It was quite embarrassing." The problem took its toll on romance as well. "Sex was sometimes very painful, not to mention messy."

Tursi had about half a dozen fibroids; the biggest was nearly three inches thick. They crowded her cervix. They grew into the lining of her uterus.

Drug therapy helps some women but did little for Tursi. Birth control pills can reduce pain and bleeding by replacing a woman's natural surges of estrogen and progestin with lower, synthetic doses; the lower doses prevent the accumulation of prostaglandin, a hormone linked to menstrual pain and cramps. Other drugs such as Lupron, which block estrogen production altogether, can temporarily shrink fibroids. Birth control pills did lighten the flow of Tursi's periods for a while, but during the four years before her hysterectomy she switched formulas every six months searching for one that would relieve her increasing torment. She didn't want to try Lupron because it shuts down estrogen production abruptly, which can cause severe mood swings. Finally, on her doctor's advice, she injected Depo-Provera, the long-acting contraceptive that suppresses natural estrogen. For two months she had no period, then the one that lasted 57 days.

Throughout these years Tursi relied on powerful painkillers—Darvocet and Tylenol with codeine—to get through difficult days. As each analgesic gradually lost its effectiveness, she thought more seriously about a hysterectomy.

Tursi first asked about the surgery when she was 32, a stunningly young age to have one's uterus removed. Four doctors in as many years advised against it. The fifth doctor, who reluctantly agreed to perform the operation, suggested Tursi first try less invasive surgical procedures. A dilatation and curettage (D & C)—in which the cervix is widened and tissue is scraped from inside the uterus—might have temporarily stopped her bleeding but wouldn't necessarily have ended the pain. Her doctor also suggested a myomectomy, in which fibroids are cut away from the uterus. This operation, which preserves fertility,

IS A HYSTERECTOMY THE RIGHT CHOICE FOR YOU?

IF HEAVY MENSTRUAL BLEEDING caused by fibroids is taking over your life, you may have many options. (See "New Ways to Be Free of Fibroids.") The best one for you depends on your age, your symptoms, the size of your growth, and most of all, how you feel about the consequences. Consider the following.

HOW IMPORTANT IS IT TO YOU TO KEEP YOUR UTERUS?
Even a woman who doesn't intend to have children may feel that keeping her uterus is a priority—either for emotional or sexual reasons. Some women report that the removal of the uterus makes it more difficult to achieve orgasm. Others say they simply feel less feminine. For others, however, heavy bleeding so disrupts their sex life that having a hysterectomy is actually liberating.

ARE YOU CLOSE TO MENOPAUSE?
If so, consider a procedure that removes or shrinks your fibroids; they rarely return after the body stops producing estrogen. But there's a caveat: If you plan on taking hormone replacement therapy to protect your heart and bones, only a hysterectomy will ensure that your fibroids won't grow back.

HOW DO YOU FEEL ABOUT SURGERY?
You may not think that having heavy periods warrants major surgery that will require weeks of recovery and leave a big scar on your abdomen. The alternative procedures are less traumatic, though sometimes temporary, solutions. If your symptoms are severe, however, you may decide you need the immediate and permanent relief that only a hysterectomy can provide. —*Kate Lee*

is popular in Europe. But when a woman has many fibroids, the surgery can take hours and carries a greater risk of dangerous blood loss than a hysterectomy.

Tursi would have none of it. "I know my body better than anyone does," she says. "I wanted a life. I was tired of being in pain."

For Tursi, a drastic measure was perhaps the wisest choice. Less invasive techniques are not as successful in stemming symptoms as some doctors boast, according to a review of insurance claims data conducted by UCLA's Gambone. Some studies show that fibroids grow back in one out of four women who have a myomectomy, frequently making a second operation necessary. Women who undergo endometrial ablation—in which the doctor cuts away only the tissue lining the uterus—also sometimes need more surgery. "The studies that get into the scientific literature are done by people who are best at the procedures," Gambone says. "Not everybody can go to these doctors. Quite frankly, sometimes the studies exaggerate the procedures' success rates. In reality, these procedures work well about 50 to 60 percent of the time."

Tursi wanted a permanent solution. And only a hysterectomy could ensure that she would remain free of fibroids,

uterine pain, and excessive bleeding. So her doctor removed the organ most identified with womanhood but didn't take her ovaries, which continue to produce estrogen. "I feel fantastic," Tursi says. "It is the smartest thing I've ever done."

BARBARA PICCOLI
DECIDED A HYSTERECTOMY WASN'T FOR HER

Doctors often advise women like Barbara Piccoli to ride out the inconvenience of fibroids until menopause, when ovaries stop producing the estrogen that feeds them. Piccoli, a mother of two who lives in New Jersey, was untroubled by pain or heavy bleeding. She didn't even realize she *had* fibroids until her doctor felt them during a routine exam. But as her fibroids grew, so did her concern.

A dance teacher and choreographer, Piccoli wears form-fitting leotards almost every day. Her fibroids bothered her mainly because they were expanding her usually flat abdomen. And since her body was giving her no indication that menopause was near, waiting it out meant having a bloated tummy protruding from her trim figure for years.

She wanted a solution, but she didn't want a hysterectomy. Yet five doctors over a span of 18 months offered just two options: Wait it out or yank it out.

"They're extremely condescending when you're 49 years old," says Piccoli, now 52. "The physicians asked me, 'What would you need your uterus for?'" Their attitude incensed her: "If they had warts on their penis, would they want their penis removed? I don't think so. But if we have a fibroid on our uterus, they say to take everything else."

In Piccoli's case, doctors wanted to remove her ovaries as well as her uterus, a common combination for women over 40. The medical reasoning goes like this: Ovaries almost completely stop producing estrogen at menopause anyway, but they remain a risk for ovarian cancer, which kills nearly 15,000 American women each year. That didn't persuade Piccoli, who feared the mood swings, bone loss, and aging associated with menopause. Moreover, some scientists speculate that the ovaries perform a beneficial but as yet unknown function after menopause. Finally, she was concerned about the operation itself. "I'm extremely vain, so I didn't want a scar," she says. "I didn't want to be cut from stem to stern."

The Hysterectomy Education and Referral Service (HERS), which tends to steer women away from hysterectomies, directed Piccoli to a doctor in Philadelphia who performs myolysis, a new alternative to both hysterectomy and myomectomy. In myolysis, a surgeon makes a small cut in the navel and one to three more in the abdomen. A narrow viewing tube slips through the cut in the navel; through the other incisions, a laser or electrified needle enters and burns the tissue connecting a fibroid to the uterus. Cut off from its blood supply, the fibroid gradually withers away. Because burns on the uterine wall might affect fertility, doctors don't recommend myolysis for women who want to bear children. Nor is it suggested for women with more than four fibroids or with a fibroid larger than an orange. But for women like Piccoli who can temporarily shrink their fibroids with estrogen-blocking drugs, myolysis is the difference between major, scarring surgery and a day trip to the hospital. Women go home a few hours after the operation; recovery averages a week.

"There was some discomfort," Piccoli says. "After all, your body's being invaded. No matter what procedure you have, there's going to be a recuperation period." Still, she was back at work two weeks later (recovery from hysterectomy takes five weeks), and she has just two tiny scars, one on each side of her pelvis.

NEW WAYS TO BE FREE OF FIBROIDS

For Women Who Want to Preserve Their Fertility

ELECTROSURGICAL VAPORIZATION

This new option is the least risky, least complicated way to remove fibroids without losing the uterus. A long, thin electrode is inserted into the uterus through the vagina, and its high heat melts the fibroid cells and seals blood vessels at the same time. Vaporization works even for women with large fibroids growing on the surface of the uterus, though not for fibroids embedded in the uterine wall.

LAPAROSCOPIC MYOMECTOMY

This procedure allows doctors to remove the most embedded fibroids without major abdominal scarring. A surgeon makes a slit in the navel and inserts a hollow tube and viewing instrument (laparoscope) into the uterus. The doctor then slides a tiny laser or scalpel through the laparoscope, chops up the fibroid, and removes the bits through the tube. But sewing up the incisions in the uterine wall through the laparoscope's small opening can be difficult; sometimes doctors must make a second, two-inch incision to finish the operation. Some surgeons are using a new laparoscopic "sewing machine" to solve the problem.

For Women Who Don't Plan to Bear Children

MYOLYSIS

By cauterizing the tissue between the uterus and the fibroids—thereby cutting off blood supply—myolysis can shrink all but the largest fibroids enough to relieve symptoms. When performed by a skilled physician using two electric needles and a laparoscope, this new surgery can be the safest option. But uterine scarring from myolysis can cause pain and other complications, including infertility. Doctors at Yale University are experimenting with myolysis equipment that freezes—rather than burns—fibroids, which could someday make the procedure also an option for women who plan to have children.

DRUG THERAPY

Drugs called GnRH agonists are sometimes prescribed to shrink fibroids until a woman reaches menopause, when the growths often get smaller on their own. The drugs can be taken only for six months, however, because they block estrogen production, making women vulnerable to osteoporosis. Unfortunately, the fibroids usually begin to grow back about six months after the drugs are discontinued. To avoid this problem, doctors are now offering GnRH agonists along with low-dose hormone replacement therapy to keep bones from thinning. But this treatment is expensive—$400 a month—and rarely covered by health insurers. Thus it may be a realistic option for older women who won't need the drugs for long because they don't intend to take hormones after menopause.

VAGINAL HYSTERECTOMY

It's less invasive than abdominal hysterectomy, requires less than half the hospital stay and recuperation time, and causes little scarring. Yet only 25 percent of hysterectomy patients have the simpler procedure, even though studies suggest up to 80 percent could. The problem is that many doctors are still inexperienced with the technique, in which the surgeon slides a scalpel through the vagina, cuts the uterus free, and removes it through the vagina. To make the process easier, doctors have begun performing part of the surgery through a laparoscope inserted into the uterus through the navel. Vaginal hysterectomy is the best option for any woman who needs her uterus removed, unless she has severe endometriosis, dense uterine scar tissue, or very large fibroids. —K.L.

Piccoli's fibroids could eventually return, especially if she decides to take hormone replacement therapy when she reaches menopause. In addition, myolysis, like myomectomy, can miss tiny fibroids and sometimes must be done again. But for now her dancer's body is svelte, her ovaries still produce the hormones that help keep her bones strong, and Barbara Piccoli feels whole.

THERSA O'ROURKE
TRIED ALTERNATIVES BEFORE DECIDING A HYSTERECTOMY WAS THE RIGHT CHOICE

For about three or four hours every month, Thersa O'Rourke bled so heavily because of fibroids that she couldn't leave the bathroom. At 46, though, she would not consider a hysterectomy. She felt no pain, and as a nurse-midwife in solo practice, she didn't have time for major surgery. Who would look after her patients while she recuperated for five weeks? In the back of her mind, she also worried that her sex life would suffer. The uterus often contracts during orgasm, heightening the experience. "I think this is one area that isn't adequately discussed with patients," she says. "I had one woman friend tell me having a hysterectomy was a terrible mistake. I had other women tell me it made no difference." Of course, O'Rourke couldn't know in advance whether her sexual pleasure would diminish, but she didn't want to take the chance.

O'Rourke happened to work with Milton Goldrath, the director of gynecology at Detroit's Sinai Hospital and a pioneer of endometrial ablation, a technique of burning or cutting away the uterine lining, which is the primary source of menstrual bleeding. Unlike myolysis, ablation is done without an incision. A doctor inserts a thin scope through the vagina into the uterus, then uses a laser or an electrified needle to destroy the lining (called the endometrium). Women with small fibroids are good candidates for ablation; so are those with endometriosis and excessive bleeding. But because this technique permanently destroys part of the uterine lining, it is not a choice for women who want to become pregnant. With a daughter approaching college age, however, O'Rourke was far more concerned with preserving her romantic life with her husband.

Her fibroids, Goldrath told her, were small enough to qualify for an endometrial ablation, though he cautioned her that the procedure ends bleeding in just 30 to 40 percent of women, and merely reduces it in the rest. As with myolysis, the fibroids could grow back. Still, for many women, the procedure turns torturous symptoms into manageable ones.

ies showing that hormone replacement therapy seems to protect women against heart attacks. Trying to avoid her family's fatal path, she began taking estrogen. Consequently, her remaining fibroids grew, until her uterus swelled to the size of an 18-week pregnancy. "It began to ache and hurt. It was sticking up halfway to my belly button," she says. Her uterus, once essential to her sex life, became too painful to keep.

In 1994, grateful for the eight years the endometrial ablation had bought her, O'Rourke had a hysterectomy. Ideally, she would have had the operation vaginally, which halves recovery time, but she couldn't because a ruptured ectopic pregnancy years earlier had scarred her uterus. So, to make the most of an unpleasant necessity, she had a tummy tuck while still under anesthesia.

She does find it harder to achieve an

> "I was surprised. Hysterectomy has had such bad press that I was expecting to discover that women had been pushed into this surgery," says Kjerulff.

O'Rourke figured, "Why go in and have a major operation when this is far less traumatic to the body?"

On a Thursday afternoon she checked into the hospital. She went home the next morning and, after resting over the weekend, returned to work on Monday. "I had one year with no periods at all," recalls O'Rourke, now 56. "Then a year later I started having a very light menses that was more than acceptable."

A few years after the ablation, however, O'Rourke felt the hot flashes of menopause. Heart disease runs in her family, and she had read about the stud-

orgasm these days, although she wonders whether that change might have followed menopause anyway. Regardless, she says the trade-off is now worthwhile: She believes she'll live longer and better by taking the hormones that help keep her bones strong and her arteries clear. Like the women in Kristen Kjerulff's study, O'Rourke *chose* to have a hysterectomy—and did so only when it became the best option for her. That has made all the difference in her satisfaction.

Rita Rubin is a writer in Washington, D.C.

Prevent

SEXUALLY

TRANSMITTED

DISEASES

Lauren Picker

Shortly after graduating from college in 1988, Sara Lewis* noticed a constellation of small red bumps on her vagina. She assumed they'd go away by themselves, but instead they became larger and more plentiful. She finally went to her gynecologist, who diagnosed a sexually transmitted disease (STD)—in her case, genital warts.

"I just lay there crying in the stirrups," recalls Lewis. At 21, she'd had few sexual partners and she had never seriously considered the risks of sex beyond an unwanted pregnancy. "This shouldn't happen to me—I'm a 'good girl,'" she remembers thinking. It's an attitude that's all too common.

"Most people think of STD's as something that happens to the other guy, but they're really everybody's problem," says Dr. H. Hunter Handsfield, director of the STD control program at the Seattle–King County (Wash.) Department of Public Health. "It's a fair bet that half of us acquire an STD at least once by age 30."

AIDS is the STD that receives the most attention. This lethal and incurable disease is caused by a virus, HIV, that currently has infected more than 1.2 million Americans, killing more than 220,000 of them. But the AIDS plague has overshadowed other important STD's that are spreading at a rate of 12 million new infections per year in the U.S., with two-thirds of new cases affecting people under 25.

Name has been changed.

The most worrisome of these are, like AIDS, caused by viruses and are incurable. These viral STD's can have devastating health impacts and can even prove fatal. Genital warts, for example, are caused by the human papilloma virus, the most common STD. HPV is now believed responsible as well for most cases of cervical cancer, a disease that kills more than 4,000 American women each year. Add in cases of herpes and hepatitis B, and the proportion of Americans infected with an incurable viral STD other than HIV may approach 50%. For just one STD, genital herpes, "we know that about a quarter of all Americans become infected by age 35," says Handsfield.

Unfortunately, someone with almost any STD runs a much greater risk of contracting AIDS through sex with an HIV-infected partner. Herpes and syphilis cause sores or ulcers that facilitate HIV's entry into the body, but even nonulcerative STD's such as chlamydia and gonorrhea promote HIV infection, presumably because they allow the virus to enter the body through the microscopic lesions they cause. In fact, these much more common diseases, says Handsfield, "may contribute more to HIV transmission than do the ulcerative STD's." Preventing and controlling them, he adds, "is emerging as one of the most important but least appreciated ways of preventing the transmission and spread of AIDS."

STD's are blatantly discriminatory. Not only are women likelier than men to become infected (through sex with an

HALF OF ALL AMERICANS WILL ACQUIRE AN STD AT LEAST ONCE BY AGE 30

infected partner), but the consequences of those infections for women are also much more severe.

A woman has a greater susceptibility than a man to almost all STD's, including AIDS, for two reasons: She has a larger genital surface area that can be breached by microbes; and during sex, the man's secretions are deposited directly into the woman's body. In a single act of unprotected heterosexual intercourse with an infected partner, for example, a woman has a 50% or greater chance of contracting chlamydia, while a man runs only a 20% to 40% chance of being infected by a woman with the disease.

Once infection occurs, effective treatment for women is often delayed, partly because early symptoms of STD's are usually more subtle in women, so they don't seek treatment as promptly as men do. And when a woman does seek medical attention, the diagnostic tests don't work as well as they do for men, so an infection can persist for months or even years and cause extensive damage, particularly to reproductive organs, before being detected and treated.

"Women *far* more than men have serious long-term consequences from STD's," says Handsfield, who lists as examples infertility, life-threatening tubal pregnancies, sick infants and cervical cancer. "Unfortunately, women can't assume that their sexual partners will assume responsibility for the woman's sexual health."

Not all the news about STD's is bleak. Some bright spots:
● STD's are preventable by using latex or polyurethane condoms. The first male polyurethane condom, Avanti, is now available west of the Rockies and will be nationally distributed this fall. The FDA approved these "plastic" condoms so that people allergic to latex could have a way to prevent STD's, as well as pregnancy. Because testing has been limited, however, product labels state that "the risks of pregnancy and STD's ... are not known for this condom." Polyurethane condoms are thinner than latex and therefore provide greater sensitivity and heat transfer between partners. The new male condoms cost $1 to $1.50 each, or about twice the cost of a latex condom. Reality, the female condom, also made of polyurethane, has been available since 1994.
● While rates of viral STD's (genital herpes, hepatitis B, genital warts) are rising or showing no signs of decline, rates of some key *bacterial* STD's (syphilis, gonorrhea and possibly chlamydia) have fallen significantly in recent years, due to behavioral changes as well as public health efforts to educate people about prevention and screen them for infection. Another reason for the falling rates is that bacterial STD's can be cured with antibiotics once they're detected.

● A new detection test is available for chlamydia, and another one should be widely available soon. The new tests require just a urine specimen and will encourage many more people to be screened.
● Several vaccines for preventing genital herpes are being tested in clinical trials. Experts predict that a herpes vaccine will receive federal approval within a few years.
● A very effective vaccine for hepatitis B has been available since 1982, though it is vastly underused.

Here's a guide to some of the most important STD's.

CHLAMYDIA
During her senior year of college in 1984, Nancy Hartman* was stricken with such severe abdominal pain she could barely walk. She didn't connect her agony to a brief fling several weeks earlier. Then the campus doctor told Hartman that her pain was due to pelvic inflammatory disease caused by a chlamydial infection.

Chlamydia, a bacterial infection, strikes more often each year—about 4 million cases in the U.S.—than any other bacterial STD. The infections respond readily to antibiotics, but if they persist, they can cause devastating complications, especially for women.

"I was lucky the pain got severe," says Hartman, who was promptly treated and cured with antibiotics. Actually, she was lucky to have felt any discomfort at all. As many as 75% of women and 25% of men with chlamydia have no idea they're infected, a situation that can lead to unwitting spread of the microbe as well as to serious complications.

For many women, the first sign of a chlamydial infection is an inability to get pregnant. An examination may then reveal chronic tubal inflammation, a sign the infection has festered in the genital tract and scarred the fallopian tubes. Chlamydial infections account for up to 40% of all cases of female

5 tips for foiling STD's

1 Be selective in choosing sex partners. "Meeting people in bars as opposed to being introduced by a friend increases your risk for sexually transmitted diseases," says Dr. H. Hunter Handsfield, director of the STD control program at the Seattle–King County (Wash.) Department of Public Health.

2 Use condoms. "Condoms work, and the noise out there that they don't is flat-out false," says Handsfield. "Consistent use of latex condoms markedly reduces the risk of transmission of a variety of STD's." Recent studies show that no more than 2% of condoms break during intercourse.

3 Be aware of subtle symptoms. "Things that many of us might tend to disregard can be terribly important in indicating an infection that requires medical attention, to protect both your health and that of your partner," says Handsfield. For women, such symptoms may include increased vaginal discharge or an abnormal odor in the genital area; for men, a small amount of cloudy discharge from the penis; for both sexes, tiny painless sores in the genital area.

4 Be in a mutually monogamous relationship. Some data suggest that the person at highest risk for contracting STD's is someone who is monogamous (one partner at a time) in a relationship with someone who has many partners. The monogamous person, usually a woman, assumes her partner is also monogamous and takes no precautions.

5 Get screened periodically. Go to your doctor, a family-planning clinic or a public STD clinic and ask to be tested for the common STD's. Remember, it's not the infection itself that's so bad but rather the complications that can occur if an STD persists undetected and untreated.

69

infertility and also increase the risk for ectopic pregnancy (when the embryo develops in one of the fallopian tubes rather than in the uterus).

For the one in four infected women who experience them, symptoms generally appear one to three weeks after exposure and may include an abnormal vaginal discharge, a burning sensation while urinating, abdominal pain or pain during intercourse. Men may notice a discharge from the penis or burning when urinating.

Since symptoms so often are absent, all sexually active women should have a chlamydia test as part of a yearly pelvic exam and whenever suspicious symptoms appear. Experts also recommend frequent testing for men and women under 25 who have more than one partner.

Until recently, doctors tested for chlamydia by culturing genital secretions, an accurate but time-consuming (up to one week) procedure that is uncomfortable for men. The two tests recently developed for chlamydia can detect the microbes in a couple of days. Treatment of chlamydia has also improved, with just a single dose of the antibiotic azithromycin able to cure most infections.

GENITAL WARTS/HPV

HPV, the infection that caused Lewis's genital warts, is the most prevalent viral STD. As many as 40 million Americans have it, and up to a million more contract it each year. A 1991 study found that 46% of the women who used a health clinic at the University of California at Berkeley were infected with this highly contagious virus: If someone is infected with HPV, there is at least a 70% chance that his or her partner is also infected.

Genital warts generally appear as fleshy, cauliflower-like growths on the genitals or around the anus. Warts tend to surface within three months of exposure, but they sometimes don't appear until several years later. Although the warts HPV causes sometimes clear up on their own, more typically, people have them removed, because they often itch and are unattractive.

Treatments to remove warts include liquid nitrogen (freezing), electrocautery (burning), podophyllin (a caustic liquid) and, when warts are widespread, surgical or laser excision. The immune compound alpha interferon, which is injected into warts, has also received FDA approval, but it can cause flu-like symptoms. Unfortunately, getting rid of visible warts may not get rid of the virus particles, which are much more extensive, and so many patients who have warts removed need repeat treatments for new ones.

The main danger from HPV infection is not warts but cervical cancer. In a recent international study, more than 85% of women with cervical cancer were found to be infected with HPV. Ironically, an HPV infection expressed as warts is relatively good news. "As a rule, warts don't turn into cancer," notes Dr. Mark Schiffman, a medical epidemiologist at the National Cancer Institute and an expert on HPV.

Of some 70 types of HPV that have been identified, the two mainly responsible for genital warts, types six and 11, are only rarely implicated in cervical cancer. At least 10 other types of HPV cause cervical lesions that may ultimately develop into cancer.

These precancerous lesions usually don't cause symptoms, and the first sign of infection is often an abnormal Pap test. "I thought if I contracted something there would be some form of warning," says Alisa Spitler, a 32-year-old woman from Oakman, Ga., who was stunned to learn she had HPV after a Pap test detected abnormal cells.

Fortunately, regular Pap tests can detect cervical cell abnormalities, or dysplasia, well before the condition progresses to cancer. Mild dysplasias often go away on their own, without treatment. But if lesions persist or worsen, physicians can remove them, greatly reducing the risk of cancer without impairing a woman's ability to bear children.

HEPATITIS B

In 1982 Joe Brown* went to his university health center complaining of dizziness and fatigue and assuming he had mononucleosis. But a blood test revealed that his problem was hepatitis B, a viral infection that damages the liver.

Few people think of hepatitis B as an STD, but more than half of the 200,000 new infections each year are contracted through sex. This highly contagious virus, which is much hardier than HIV, can also spread through casual contacts such as sharing a toothbrush or razor blade. Like Brown, half of people newly infected with hepatitis B become acutely ill (about 5,000 of them die from it each year). The rest of those infected show no symptoms (or trivial ones perhaps mistaken for a cold) and don't realize they're infected.

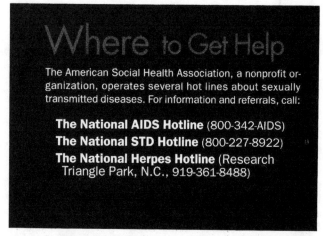

Where to Get Help

The American Social Health Association, a nonprofit organization, operates several hot lines about sexually transmitted diseases. For information and referrals, call:

The National AIDS Hotline (800-342-AIDS)
The National STD Hotline (800-227-8922)
The National Herpes Hotline (Research Triangle Park, N.C., 919-361-8488)

Whether they get sick or not, the great majority of infected people manage to lick the disease completely. But 5% to 10% of infected adults can't shake the virus and become hepatitis B carriers; they not only can transmit the infection to others but also may develop chronic hepatitis, a progressive disease that kills an additional 5,000 people each year, mostly from cirrhosis (scarring of the liver), but also from liver cancer.

Brown, who went on to become a carrier, was upset to learn there is a vaccine that could have prevented his infection. In fact, the safe and highly effective hepatitis B vaccine has been available from family doctors and many public health clinics since 1981, but it hasn't been widely used.

Those who could benefit most from the vaccine are sexually active young adults, both straight and gay, since three-fourths of all cases affect people between 18 and 39. Yet only 1% of Americans in this age group have been vaccinated against hepatitis B. In an effort to protect young adults, the American Academy of Pediatrics recommends that all adolescents be routinely immunized against hepatitis B. The Centers for Disease Control and Prevention takes things a step further by recommending that all infants be vaccinated.

The Major STD's

CHLAMYDIA
Estimated New Cases Yearly: 4 million.
Who's at Risk: People with multiple sexual partners; most prevalent among young people; cuts across all socioeconomic groups.
Symptoms: None in most infected women and up to half of infected men, but abnormal genital discharge or burning during urination (in both sexes); abdominal pain or pain during intercourse (women); testicular pain or swelling (men).
Consequences: For untreated women, pelvic inflammatory disease, which can lead to chronic pelvic pain, ectopic pregnancy or infertility; for untreated men, may lead in rare cases to sterility. Increased risk of HIV infection if a person with chlamydia is exposed to the virus.
Treatment: Antibiotics (azithromycin, doxycycline, ofloxacin).
Prevention: Condoms; probably some protection from spermicides.

GENITAL WARTS/HUMAN PAPILLOMA VIRUS
Estimated New Cases Yearly: 500,000 to 1 million.
Who's at Risk: People with multiple sexual partners; most prevalent among young people.
Symptoms: Fleshy, cauliflower-like growths or warts on and inside the genitals and anus; may appear on the throat when acquired through oral sex; abnormal Pap test.
Consequences: Some strains of HPV believed to cause cervical cancer; HPV also linked to vulvar, vaginal, penile and anal cancers.
Treatment: Warts removed by freezing with liquid nitrogen, burning with electrocautery, applying caustic liquids or by surgical or laser excision for cases where warts are widespread. The precancerous lesions caused by HPV can also be removed.
Prevention: Condoms, though they offer no protection against uncovered lesions.

GONORRHEA
Estimated New Cases Yearly: 500,000.
Who's at Risk: People with multiple sexual partners; most common among teens and young adults in poor inner city areas and in rural southeastern U.S.
Symptoms: None in many cases, but discharge from the vagina, penis or rectum; burning or itching during urination; low abdominal pain (women).
Consequences: Same as with chlamydia.

Treatment: Antibiotics; some strains are resistant to penicillin, but alternatives (such as cefixime and ceftriaxone) are available.
Prevention: Condoms; probably some protection from spermicides. Vaccine in development.

HEPATITIS B
Estimated New Cases Yearly: 200,000, with slightly more than half of them sexually transmitted.
Who's at Risk: (sexually transmitted cases only): gay men; people with multiple sexual partners.
Symptoms: None in about one-third of those infected, but fever, muscle aches and fatigue and, as the disease progresses, dark urine and jaundice in the skin and eyes.
Consequences: For the chronically infected, possibly cirrhosis of the liver or liver cancer.
Treatment: No effective one.
Prevention: Condoms; hepatitis vaccine.

GENITAL HERPES
Estimated New Cases Yearly: 200,000 to 500,000.
Who's at Risk: People with multiple sexual partners.
Symptoms: Recurring blisters or sores usually in the genital area; fever, nausea and genital pain often occur during the first episode; in two-thirds of those infected, herpes symptoms are so mild they don't realize they have the virus.
Consequences: Increased risk of HIV infection if a person with herpes is exposed to the virus.
Treatment: Acyclovir to reduce symptoms and outbreaks.
Prevention: Condoms, though they offer no protection against uncovered sores. A vaccine could be available by 1998.

SYPHILIS
Estimated New Cases Yearly: 120,000.
Who's at Risk: People with multiple sexual partners; most commonly occurs in poor urban communities.
Symptoms: Syphilis sores, or chancres, in the primary stage of the disease; can appear anywhere on the body but are often hidden from view.
Consequences: If untreated, can lead to mental illness, blindness, heart disease and death. Increased risk of HIV infection if exposed to the virus.
Treatment: Penicillin.
Prevention: Condoms, though they offer no protection against uncovered sores.

Sources: Centers for Disease Control and Prevention and the Alan Guttmacher Institute

GENITAL HERPES

In a 1982 cover story, *Time* magazine proclaimed herpes "today's scarlet letter." Though AIDS soon pushed herpes out of the headlines, the ranks of herpes sufferers continue to swell. Today about 60 million Americans, or one in four, are believed to be infected with herpes simplex type 2, the virus that causes genital herpes. In 1992 Megan Smith* contracted the disease from her boyfriend.

"We always used a condom, but somehow I got it," says Smith, 29. Her symptoms: swollen glands and a lesion so tiny that "I practically had to use a magnifying glass to see it," she says.

Herpes symptoms usually show up two to 21 days after exposure and can vary enormously in severity from one person to the next. Many people associate genital herpes with recurring bouts of blisters or sores in the genital area, accompanied by pain, fever and nausea. But it's now clear that most people with herpes are not seriously affected.

Some two-thirds of herpes cases are so mild that people don't even know they're infected. Although herpes is most contagious during an outbreak, when sores are visible, it can also be passed by asymptomatic shedding of viruses from someone who feels perfectly fine, a fact that helps explain why up to half a million new infections occur each year.

The oral drug acyclovir, available since 1985, can reduce the frequency, duration and severity of outbreaks. A vaccine against genital herpes is now in clinical trials and could be available by 1998.

GONORRHEA

Although gonorrhea is waning, it still causes more than half a million new infections each year, primarily in impoverished urban areas and in rural southeastern communities, where nearly one in ten 15- to 19-year-olds may have it. Women have a 50% chance of contracting gonorrhea in a single act of unprotected intercourse with an infected partner.

Symptoms of gonorrhea, which is caused by gonococcus bacteria, mirror those caused by chlamydia and usually surface two to five days after infection. In fact, the two infections are virtually indistinguishable without a microscopic exam of genital discharge (for men) or a culture of cervical secretions (for women).

Untreated, gonorrhea can lead to fever, pain and, in women, pelvic inflammatory disease, which can cause infertility. Infectious disease experts are concerned about the growing number of gonorrhea cases that are resistant to one or more antibiotics.

The antibiotics penicillin and tetracycline have historically been used to cure the infection, but cases resistant to these drugs have risen rapidly, from fewer than 1% of infections in the U.S. in 1980 to 10% at present. Work on a gonorrhea vaccine is under way.

SYPHILIS

The introduction of penicillin in the 1940s sharply curtailed syphilis as a public health problem. But from 1970 to 1985, syphilis surged among gay men, and in the late 1980s cases soared once again, to their highest level in 40 years, due to the practice among crack addicts of trading sex for drugs. Syphilis cases are now declining rapidly again in most of the country. But they remain prevalent among blacks in lower socioeconomic groups, who have an infection rate more than 60 times higher than whites. The good news about syphilis: A course of penicillin can still cure the disease.

The condom report

What's new in sheath chic

Katherine Cottrell

If you're in a new relationship or still searching for Mr. Right, condoms should be a fact of life. In fact, they may even save your life. Latex condoms help prevent transmission of the human immunodeficiency virus (HIV) which causes AIDS. They also help to protect against other sexually transmitted diseases, including gonorrhea, syphilis, hepatitis B, genital warts, herpes and chlamydia. Condoms can be up to 95 percent effective in protecting against these diseases (most failures result from user error) and enjoy a similar success rate as a contraceptive, when used as directed with a spermicidal foam or jelly.

But with all this going for it, the lowly condom still has an uphill struggle for acceptance by women, particularly those who have weathered the storm of STDs from the shelter of a monogamous relationship. "Our ability to experience pleasure increases when we are comfortable with our sexuality," says Marsha Olinski, sexual-health counselor at the Hastings and Prince Edward Counties Health Unit in eastern Ontario. And being informed about the whys and hows of condom use will go a long way toward increasing your comfort level.

If you feel shy about buying condoms, you're not alone.

Safe purchases If you feel funny milling around that certain aisle in the drugstore, you're not alone. While 60 percent of women whose partners wear condoms are involved in the purchase decision, only one in four women buys her own condoms, according to Hélène Carty of Johnson & Johnson, marketer of Ortho Shields and Legend condoms. When you do pull that box off the shelf, a quick glance should give you the minimum requirements: material (it should always say latex);

a valid expiry date; a lot number and the manufacturer's name, address and telephone number.

All reputable brands list this information on the box, but that doesn't necessarily mean you're getting a safe condom. Health Canada's Health Protection Branch sets minimum standards and does random testing for strength and leakage. But the onus is on manufacturers to comply with the set standards, so they regularly do their own testing. Results are available by calling the number on the package. But there's no

CONDOM DOS & DON'TS

• DON'T use a condom that's been opened or exposed to heat or friction—stored in a wallet or back pocket, for example.

• DO try a few "dry runs" to get used to putting a condom on. (You could make a banana your silent partner for this.) Familiarity will help make using a condom part of your foreplay; just make sure your hands aren't cold when you move on from your banana to the real thing.

• DON'T use a condom with oil-based lubricants such as baby oil or petroleum jelly; they weaken the latex. Many cream or suppository medications for conditions such as yeast infections are oil-based. Check the label, or rub the preparation between your thumb and forefinger and then rinse with water. If it doesn't wash clean away, it isn't a safe water-based product.

• DO use extra water-based lubrication if you like. Your partner may find that a drop of lubricant inside the condom heightens his enjoyment too.

• DON'T rely on lambskin condoms to protect against STDs. If you or your partner are among the less than 1 percent of the population affected by latex allergies, sexual-health counselor Marsha Olinski suggests wearing a latex condom over the lambskin one which lies against the skin. "Some people wear two condoms to reduce risk anyway."

guarantee that a defective batch of condoms won't make it to drugstore shelves. The safest course: stick to the major brands.

Don't be fooled by marketing claims. "Strong" condoms aren't always more durable, and "sensitive" condoms may not be thinner.

Strength and leakage The key test for breakage is air inflation. A condom must hold a minimum 25 litres of air, which inflates it to watermelon size, without bursting. If the Health Protection Branch finds five or more condoms burst out of 20, the batch must be recalled. To test for leakage, the condom is filled with 300 millilitres of water and examined for visible leaks. Then, it's sealed off, like a giant water balloon, and rolled around on colored blotting paper to doublecheck for pinprick-size leaks. If more than two condoms out of 50 fail the test, the batch is recalled.

But don't be fooled by marketing claims. "Strong" on the box doesn't necessarily mean it holds up any better under pressure. A survey in a recent issue of Consumer Reports magazine showed that most condoms marked "strong" did not have higher burst volumes than their regular counterparts.

Sensitivity Likewise, so-called "sensitive" condoms may not be any thinner than the rest. And if they are, the Consumer Reports survey suggests they may not meet test requirements for strength. It found that 25 to 30 percent of thinner condoms failed the 25-litre burst test, and those that passed had some of the worst burst scores. (U.S. standards only require a 16-litre air-burst test, but the Consumer Reports survey stuck to Canadian standards.)

Lubrication For your comfort and his, Olinski recommends lubricated condoms. Do your own testing to discover which works best for you, or add your own water-based lubricant such as K-Y jelly. Avoid oil-based products such as petroleum jelly or baby oil, which can degrade latex and make condoms unsafe. Some lubricants contain spermicide which may offer extra protection against pregnancy, as well as kill a number of the viruses and bacteria responsible for sexually transmitted diseases. But all condoms—even the pretreated kind—should be supplemented with spermicidal foam or jelly for maximum protection. On the downside, says Olinski, spermicide-laced condoms can cause vaginal irritation.

Getting it on

BEFORE Open the package carefully so you don't tear the condom.
• Pinch the reservoir tip to remove air. This leaves room for the semen and keeps the condom from bursting. • Place the unrolled condom over the tip of the penis, reservoir out, and unroll it down to the base of the penis.
AFTER Grasp the base of the condom to avoid slippage, and withdraw the penis while it is still hard. • Remove the condom carefully to avoid leakage and dispose of it. Never reuse. • Pat yourself and your partner on the back for having enjoyed safer sex.

SAFE BETS

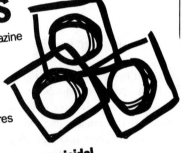

In May 1995, the U.S. magazine Consumer Reports tested 37 different brands of condoms for strength and durability. The top three performers, listed below, inflated well beyond 25 litres without bursting*:

1. **Sheik Excita Ribbed, spermicidal**
2. **Ramses Ribbed, spermicidal**
3. **Sheik Elite**

Health Canada standards require condoms to hold at least 25 litres of air.

Size One size usually fits all. But if a man complains that a condom is uncomfortable or too tight, says Olinski, odds are he's not just trying to impress you. Buy him a large; width and length vary from brand to brand, but a few extra millimetres may make all the difference to his comfort level—and a good fit is a safer fit. There's no maximum size. But if a condom is falling off, it's too big.

Styles Condoms come in every color, flavor and scent imaginable. There are condoms that glow in the dark, and condoms with various textures, such as ribbing, which promise to boost sexual pleasure. Have fun with your choices, but avoid novelty condoms which do not protect against STDs or pregnancy. Look for a warning on the box.

Rethinking Birth Control

If you still believe the IUD is dangerous and the Pill is for women under 35, you may be stuck in a contraception rut. Here's a roundup of the most effective methods for midlife women.

JULIA CALIFANO

Through two years of dating, 10 years of marriage and two kids, Chris, a college professor in Syracuse, NY, relied almost exclusively on a diaphragm for birth control. Indeed, this 40-year-old would still be putting up with the hassle and mess if, at her last checkup, her doctor hadn't suggested she try an intrauterine device (IUD). Persuaded by his argument that it was highly effective, long-lasting and, for most women, nearly free of side effects, she switched. She hasn't regretted her decision. "It's such a pleasure not to have to plan ahead or get out of bed in the heat of passion," she says. "We don't even think about birth control anymore."

By the time a woman turns 35, she's moved an average of eight times, switched jobs seven times and had two children, yet there's only a 50–50 chance that she has ever thought about changing her method of birth control, according to a survey by Ortho Pharmaceutical. But the truth is she should. "A woman's contraceptive needs change as her life changes," says Anita Nelson, M.D., medical director of the Woman's Health Care Clinic at Harbor UCLA Medical Center in Los Angeles. "A barrier method may be great when you're 21 and concerned about AIDS and other sexually transmitted diseases [STD's], but it's probably not ideal when you're 35 and married with kids."

Perhaps more surprising is the staggering rate of unplanned pregnancies among women in their 40s: According to the Alan Guttmacher Institute in New York City, eight out of 10 pregnancies in this age group are unintended—the same rate as for women under age 20.

How can you tell if your current choice is still your best choice? Reassess your birth control periodically, taking your lifestyle, health, sex life and desire for children into consideration. Here's a guide to the options, plus expert advice on what to use when.

The IUD: Unfounded fear

What it is: The current IUD of choice is ParaGard, a piece of plastic with copper inside it that's put into the uterus to stop sperm from reaching eggs for up to 10 years. Another IUD called Progestasert contains hormones; it works for one year.

Benefits: Long-term, reversible, worry-free protection, and an insertion process that's only slightly more involved than a Pap smear. Progestasert also reduces menstrual cramps and the flow of monthly bleeding.

Drawbacks: The copper IUD can cause heavier than usual periods, won't protect you from STD's and shouldn't be used if you're not in a mutually monogamous relationship. Users with multiple partners are at increased risk for pelvic inflammatory disease (PID), an infection that can cause infertility.

What you may not know: Though most people still associate this device with the dreaded Dalkon Shield (an IUD that caused infection and infertility in thousands of women, along with a few deaths, in the '70s), ParaGard is considered one of the best and safest birth control options. In fact, it's the most popular form of reversible contraception outside the U.S., with 85 million users worldwide.

When to consider it: If you're in a mutually monogamous, long-term relationship and have had at least one child (for childless women there's a small risk that the device will be expelled). "An ideal time to switch to the IUD is when you've completed your family but don't want to take the irreversible step of sterilization," says nurse practitioner Kara Anderson, a medical consultant to the Planned Parenthood Federation of America in New York City.

The Pill: Now for Older Women

What it is: This oral contraceptive is a combination of two hormones, progestin and estrogen, that suppresses ovulation.

Benefits: Easy, reliable and offers a wealth of health benefits. After five

A Field Guide to Cost and Effectiveness

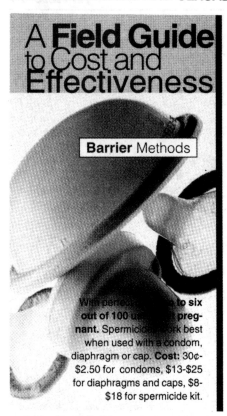

Barrier Methods

With perfect use, up to **six out of 100 [users] get pregnant.** Spermicides work best when used with a condom, diaphragm or cap. **Cost:** 30¢-$2.50 for condoms, $13-$25 for diaphragms and caps, $8-$18 for spermicide kit.

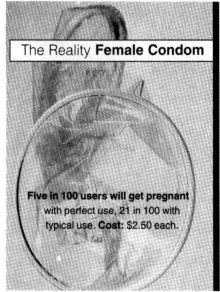

The Reality **Female Condom**

Five in 100 users will get pregnant with perfect use, 21 in 100 with typical use. **Cost:** $2.50 each.

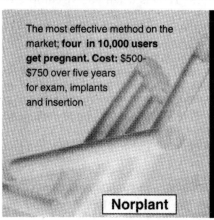

The most effective method on the market; **four in 10,000 users get pregnant. Cost:** $500-$750 over five years for exam, implants and insertion

Norplant

years the Pill halves your risk of endometrial and ovarian cancers, an effect that, for endometrial cancer, may last as long as 15 years after you stop using it. [Experts aren't sure how long the protective effects last for ovarian cancer.] It also reduces the risk of benign breast lumps, ovarian cysts, iron-deficiency anemia and PID.

Drawbacks: Side effects include breast tenderness, nausea, weight gain and headaches (though these usually clear up after two to three months). The Pill must be taken every day, and it doesn't protect against STD's. In addition, studies show it increases the risk of heart attack and blood clots in women over 35 who smoke. Some studies have also shown that the Pill increases breast cancer risk, though a recent analysis of 150,000 users found this risk to be negligible. In most cases, say experts, the health benefits far outweigh the risks.

What you may not know: A study at San Francisco State University found that women who use triphasic pills such as Orthonovum 7/7/7 (in which hormone levels vary throughout the course of the month) experience heightened sex drive compared with women on other types of pills.

When to consider it: If you're in a committed relationship and want a highly effective form of contraception. Contrary to what many believe, the Pill can be ideal for fortysomething non-smoking women. It eases the transition to menopause, says David Grimes, M.D., vice chairman of the department of obstetrics and gynecology at the University of California at San Francisco. "The Pill helps regulate periods, prevent hot flashes and protect against bone loss," he explains.

Norplant: A Five-Year Plan

What it is: Six flexible, matchstick-sized capsules inserted by a doctor just beneath the skin of the upper arm. They release progestin to suppress ovulation for five years.

Benefits: It's effective and convenient—you can't mess up. Norplant is also easily reversible; after removal, any remaining drugs leave the body in about three days. In addition, experts believe Norplant may be as good as the Pill at reducing the risk of endometrial and ovarian cancer.

Drawbacks: Norplant won't protect you from STD's, and it can cause ir-

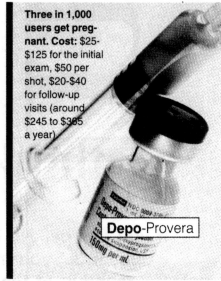

Three in 1,000 users get pregnant. Cost: $25-$125 for the initial exam, $50 per shot, $20-$40 for follow-up visits (around $245 to $365 a year)

Depo-Provera

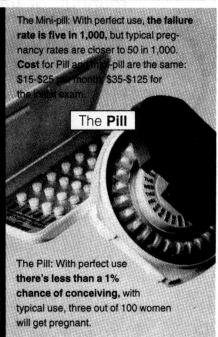

The Mini-pill: With perfect use, **the failure rate is five in 1,000,** but typical pregnancy rates are closer to 50 in 1,000. **Cost** for Pill and mini-pill are the same: $15-$25 per month; $35-$125 for the initial exam.

The **Pill**

The Pill: With perfect use **there's less than a 1% chance of conceiving,** with typical use, three out of 100 women will get pregnant.

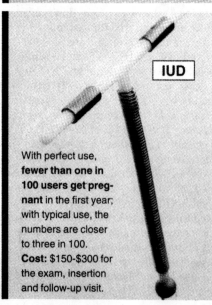

IUD

With perfect use, **fewer than one in 100 users get pregnant** in the first year; with typical use, the numbers are closer to three in 100. **Cost:** $150-$300 for the exam, insertion and follow-up visit.

Among women who are in their 40s, a staggering eight out of 10 pregnancies are unintended—the same rate as for women under age 20.

regular bleeding during the first year. There have also been a number of lawsuits filed by Norplant users, primarily because of problems such as pain or scarring upon removal. Despite the bad press, experts say such problems shouldn't arise if you use an experienced doctor. (For referrals, call your local Planned Parenthood clinic.)

What you may not know: Norplant is very expensive if used for fewer than three years.

When to consider it: If you're breastfeeding (unlike estrogen in the Pill, progestin doesn't reduce milk flow) and plan to wait several years before having another child or if you've completed your family. You also may want to try it if you absolutely don't want to worry about an accidental pregnancy.

Depo-Provera: Convenience Without Long-Term Commitment
What it is: This injection of synthetic progestin suppresses ovulation for 11 to 13 weeks.
Benefits: Depo-Provera provides many of the health perks of the Pill, and you don't have to take it every

day. After about a year, periods may stop completely, which many women consider a welcome side effect.
Drawbacks: Doctor's visits are required four times a year to get the shots, and the effects are not immediately reversible (fertility may not return for an average of 10 months after the last dose). Side effects may include headaches, weight gain, depression and heavier, more frequent periods. Depo-Provera also provides no protection against STD's.
What you may not know: Though many American women think of this method, approved here in 1992, as new, Depo-Provera has been used by more than 30 million women in 100 other countries over the past 30 years.
When to consider it: If you're nursing or trying to space out the arrival of new children, or you can't remember to take the Pill every day.

The Reality Female Condom: Women in the Driver's Seat
What it is: The Reality Condom is a floppy polyurethane tube with an in-

ner ring at the closed end that fits over the cervix, like a diaphragm, and an outer ring at the open end that hangs outside the vagina.
Benefits: Protection against AIDS and other STD's; more spontaneity than with male condoms, since it can be inserted in advance.
Drawbacks: It has about as much sex appeal as a sandwich bag.
What you may not know: The device is reputed to squeak during use (adding a little extra lubricant can alleviate this distraction).
When to consider it: If you're not in a stable relationship or you have a partner who refuses to wear a condom.

Tubal ligation: No More Hassles
What it is: This surgical procedure blocks the fallopian tubes so that sperm and egg never meet.
Benefits: No-worry, contraceptive-free sex for the rest of your life. And, after the cost of the surgery ($1,000-$2,500), you'll never spend another dime on birth control.
Drawbacks: This procedure isn't foolproof: Though only five in 1,000 users become pregnant in the first year, surprisingly, over 10 years the failure rate is one in 50 (2%). And, as with any surgery, the procedure carries risks. Finally, depending on how it's done it can't easily be undone.
What you may not know: Sterilization is the most popular method of birth control in the U.S., chosen by a whopping 42% of contraceptive users.
When to consider it: If you're *sure* you don't want any more children.

The Mini-Pill: Fewer Annoying Side Effects
What it is: This pill contains no estrogen and a very small dose of progestin—hence the name.
Benefits: Since it contains no estrogen, the mini-pill has fewer side effects than the Pill and is not associated with any increased risk of blood clots or breast cancer. It also causes lighter than normal periods, making it a good choice for women who are anemic or who tend to bleed heavily.

Contraception 911

Condoms break, diaphragms slip and even the most responsible woman sometimes misses a Pill. The good news is that post-coital contraceptive options are expanding. An FDA advisory panel recently agreed unanimously that the Pill can safely be used as a morning-after contraceptive. The procedure—taking two doses of two or four pills each, depending on the brand, within 72 hours of unprotected sex—reduces the risk of pregnancy by 75%, though nausea and vomiting are common side effects. Several different Pill brands can be used; check with your doctor for specifics. Note: Don't try this on your own.

An emergency IUD insertion can also be done within five to seven days of unprotected sex and is more than 99% effective. Contact your doctor or Planned Parenthood, or call the new 24-hour Emergency Contraception Hotline (800-584-9911) for a list of doctors who provide emergency contraception in your area. You'll also find a list of local providers on the Internet at http://opr.princeton.edu/ec/.
Alternatives to surgical abortion are on the way. The long-awaited French abortion drug mifepristone, better known as RU 486, is expected to be available in this country later this year. The drug blocks progesterone and causes the uterus to discard its lining

along with the implanted egg. It can be used up to nine weeks into pregnancy and may also be used as emergency birth control up to three days after unprotected sex, with fewer side effects than oral contraceptives.
On the horizon: Two FDA-approved drugs already on the market, methotrexate (a chemotherapy drug) and misoprostol (used to prevent stomach bleeding), induce abortion when combined. Since research is still limited on this method, few doctors use it, but that may soon change. Planned Parenthood has received FDA clearance for a large-scale clinical trial to test the technique's safety and effectiveness.

Women who use triphasic birth control pills report experiencing a heightened sex drive.

And it doesn't require a waiting period to get pregnant after you stop taking it.

Drawbacks: It can cause irregular bleeding, offers no protection against STD's and has a significantly higher failure rate than combined oral contraceptives, particularly if you have trouble remembering to take a pill every day.

What you may not know: This method has almost no margin for error. Missing even one day can result in a pregnancy.

When to consider it: If you're nursing (which naturally reduces—but doesn't rule out—fertility); it also seems to slightly increase the quantity and quality of breast milk.

Barrier Methods: STD Protection

What they are: This group includes condoms; diaphragms and cervical caps used with spermicidal jellies or foam; inserts and film. All prevent sperm from reaching eggs.

Benefits: They're safe, cheap and available without a prescription; barrier methods also guard against STD's. Latex condoms provide the best protection against the AIDS virus.

Drawbacks: They interfere with spontaneity and can be messy, and your partner may complain of lessened sensation during sex with condoms. Also, caps can be tricky to insert and diaphragms may increase the risk of urinary tract infections in women.

What you may not know: Lubricated condoms and spermicides help counteract vaginal dryness, a common perimenopausal and postpartum problem.

When to consider them: If you're breast-feeding, planning to get pregnant relatively soon or having sex infrequently. Condoms are the best choice if you want iron-clad protection against AIDS and other STD's. Barrier methods are also handy backups when you forget to take a Pill.

Julia Califano is a writer in Hoboken, NJ

Six Reasons to Switch

If you've been using the same contraceptive since college, it's probably time to take a fresh look at your birth control options. Here are some compelling reasons to reconsider your method:

1. You've settled down with one partner. Provided neither one of you has a sexually transmissible disease, you can switch from condoms to a method you both like better and will use consistently.

2. Your health has changed. If you develop heart disease, high blood pressure or diabetes, you should re-evaluate your current method with your doctor.

3. You're breast-feeding. Consider a nonhormonal contraceptive, such as condoms, a diaphragm or a copper intrauterine device (IUD), or a progestin-only method, such as the minipill, Norplant or Depo-Provera.

4. You've completed your family. Sterilization is only one long-term option. Also consider Norplant, Depo-Provera, the IUD and the Pill.

5. You're contemplating pregnancy. If you're on the Pill, doctors recommend stopping two to three months before conceiving to re-establish your natural cycle. If you use Depo-Provera, it can take up to a year after your last shot to conceive.

6. You dislike your current method. If you hate inserting your diaphragm or can't remember to take the Pill every day, don't grin and bear it—switch.

ENDOMETRIOSIS

THE HIDDEN EPIDEMIC

Joseph Anthony

Joseph Anthony writes on social trends from Portland, Oreg.

Janice Nase of New York City would not admit to herself that anything was wrong. But with each menstrual period the pain became more intense. "Eventually I was spending a week at a time in bed with painkillers and heating pads," says the 38-year-old waitress. "I had joint pain, muscle pain, pain in my abdominal area and also in my legs and back. I wouldn't leave the house without a bottle of Advil."

Her fiancé (now husband) finally convinced her that something was seriously amiss. "He said, 'My God, you seem terribly ill all the time. A woman shouldn't accept the kind of pain you're going through.' " When Nase finally sought medical attention, she learned she had endometriosis.

Endometriosis is one of the most common yet least understood gynecologic problems. Women with the disease may experience debilitating pain, infertility or both. But it's still not clear what causes it, how it can best be treated, or even how many women have it, with estimates ranging from 1% to half of all women. Experts attending last year's "Endometriosis 2000," a federally sponsored exploration of causes and treatments, concluded that "as many as 10% of women of reproductive age" are affected by the disease, including millions of women who have endometriosis and may not know they do.

Each month the endometrium, the tissue that lines the uterus, builds up and is sloughed off during the menstrual cycle. But sometimes endometrial tissue turns up elsewhere in the body, most commonly on the ovaries, but also on the outer surface of the uterus, on fallopian tubes and elsewhere in the abdomen, including the intestines. In rare cases, endometrial tissue is found as far afield as the lungs and the nose.

This wayward endometrial tissue acts as if it were still part of the uterine lining, thickening, bleeding and then breaking down in sync with the menstrual cycle. Cysts, nodules and ultimately scar tissue form wherever these endometrial "implants" have invaded. Nase had cysts on both her ovaries, and endometrial tissue had wrapped itself around her colon and begun to invade it.

Diagnosing endometriosis requires direct examination of the pelvic cavity. That means general anesthesia and surgery, usually using a procedure called laparoscopy, in which miniature cameras and surgical instruments are inserted through small incisions in the abdomen. Typically women undergo laparoscopies because they're experiencing one or both of the disease's two main consequences: infertility and intense pelvic pain.

Endometriosis is a major cause of infertility, detectable in up to 60% of infertile women. Sometimes the damage caused by endometriosis is obvious, as when scar tissue clogs the fallopian tubes or when bands of scar tissue known as adhesions distort the shape of reproductive organs. In these cases, surgery to remove adhesions and scar tissue often restores fertility. But women with very mild cases of endometriosis may also have trouble conceiving. On the bright side: About three-quarters of women with mild cases who try to become pregnant eventually succeed; in-vitro fertilization has proved effective in helping women with endometriosis conceive; and pregnancy often helps relieve the disease's symptoms, at least temporarily.

Pain, the other hallmark of endometriosis, is usually most severe just before and during menstruation. (Oddly, severe endometriosis may cause little or no discomfort, while the pain from mild cases can be excruciating.) Other symptoms may include pain during intercourse, heavy menstrual bleeding, painful urination, lower-back pain, diarrhea or constipation.

Because endometriosis can cause so many different symptoms, doctors refer to it as "the chameleon disease of the pelvis." Lucy Hanna, a 36-year-old biostatistician at Brown University, spent more than a year going to doctors—two gastroenterologists, two urologists and three gynecologists—before her severe abdominal pains were correctly diagnosed. "I even had one doctor insist that I couldn't have endometriosis, because the pain wasn't coming at the right time of the month," she says.

A major problem, says Dr. Kevin Bachus, an obstetrician/gynecologist and a reproductive endocrinologist in Fort Collins, Colo., is "differentiating between someone who has painful periods that are not related to endometriosis and someone whose problem is related to endometriosis and is going to get worse, since endometriosis seems to be a progressive disease." But short of a laparoscopy, doctors clearly have trouble making that distinction.

A 1980 study in Boston involved 235 young women, mainly adolescents, who had long complained of painful periods and had been sent to psychiatrists because they were thought to be faking their complaints. After undergoing laparoscopies, nearly half of the women turned out to have endometriosis.

The cause of endometriosis remains a mystery. Most experts believe the disease stems from "retrograde menstruation," in which a woman's menses exits through the fallopian tubes into the pelvic cavity instead of through the vagina. Up to 90% of women experience some degree of retrograde menstruation, however, some other factors are clearly at work. Studies over the past 10 years suggest that an impaired immune response may be involved, perhaps disabling the body's ability to remove out-of-place endometrial tissue. Susceptibility may be inherited, since a woman whose sister or mother has endometriosis has a higher risk of developing it herself.

Exposure to toxic chemicals, particularly dioxins, is another possible cause. Dioxins are formed during incineration and as byproducts in the production of herbicides and pesticides; as a result, they're present in tiny amounts in the air and in many foods. In a 1993 study, rhesus monkeys developed endometriosis after being fed food containing a dioxin for four years. "The severity of endometriosis was directly correlated with the dose of dioxin administered," says Dr. Sherry Rier, an immunologist at Dartmouth Medical School and a lead author of the study.

Some experts contend that our exposure to dioxins and other toxic chemicals may be causing the apparent increase in the incidence of endometriosis since the 1920s, when the disease was first described. But a more likely explanation is that modern women are ovulating more than their predecessors.

"In earlier times, women were either pregnant or breast-feeding more often, and during that time they are not ovulating," says Dr. Stephen Corson, an ob/gyn at Jefferson Medical College in Philadelphia. "It has only been recently, with the introduction of mechanical barriers for contraception, that women have gone for five to 20 years with incessant, uninterrupted ovulation, which many people think is a factor in the development of endometriosis."

Ovulation fuels endometriosis by causing the menstrual periods that trigger new lesions. And estrogen released during ovulation stimulates lesions to grow, bleed, break down, inflame and ultimately damage whatever organs they've invaded. The drugs used to treat endometriosis all work by limiting ovulation in some way. (Symptoms usually disappear after menopause, when the ovaries stop functioning.)

Drugs and surgery, the basic treatments for endometriosis, can relieve pain, clear up endometrial deposits and restore fertility. But there is as yet no cure.

Drugs. Because they suppress ovulation and cause lighter periods, birth control pills can be helpful. While not effective against established cases of endometriosis, they can help prevent endometriosis from occurring and ward off recurrences in women who have been treated by other means. "It is very rare to see somebody on birth control pills experience a recurrence of endometriosis once she has been successfully treated," Corson says.

Other drugs relive pain by shrinking lesions. They include danazol, progestins, gestrinone and the GnRH analogs, the latest advances in drug treatment, which turn off estrogen production by preventing the pituitary's release of hormones that trigger it. The "Endometriosis 2000" meeting concluded that the GnRH analogs (including the drugs Lupron, Suprefact, Synarel and Zoladex) were "more effective" than other drugs at relieving the pain of endometriosis.

But drugs that treat the disease also cause a range of unpleasant side effects (hot flashes, mood swings, weight gain, increases in facial hair and decreases in bone density, among others), so they're usually prescribed for no more than six even years, but the lesions and pain often recur. And drug treatment appears to offer no help in improving a woman's fertility.

Surgery. The most common treatment for the disease is to remove endometrial growths. Surgery can help relieve pain and improve a woman's changes of becoming pregnant, especially in cases of moderate or severe endometriosis. But as with drug treatment, it's common for lesions to recur after surgery. A total hysterectomy (removal of the uterus and the ovaries) can successfully relieve the pain in 90% of women with severe endometrial pain that hasn't responded to other treatments.

Help Is Available

Mary Lou Ballweg of Milwaukee, Wis., underwent five operations, including a total hysterectomy, in the course of battling endometriosis. In 1980 she cofounded the Endometriosis Association, an international self-help organization for those with the disease. She offers this advice:

● Don't ignore severe pain, and don't assume it's "just normal." "Urination should not be painful," Ballweg says. "Sex should not be painful. Menstruation should not be painful."

● "Don't put up with patronizing and arrogant medical professionals who say your pain is psychosomatic and you should be on tranquilizers," Ballweg says.

Members of the Endometriosis Association have access to a crisis help line and receive a bimonthly newsletter, booklets and a listing of local chapters. To find out about joining the group or to order the kit "How Can I Tell If I Have Endometriosis?" call 800-992-3636. The association has also published *The Endometriosis Sourcebook* (Contemporary Books, 1995), available in bookstores or from the group.

If this were a disease affecting middle-aged white males, you'd see government money for research you wouldn't believe.

Women with endometriosis often go through several treatments before finding something that works for them. Nase, for example, underwent three years of drug treatment and three operations before getting relief. "People tell me it can come back, but all I know is that right now I can work every day, I take no painkillers and I feel great."

Despite the fact that endometriosis affects an estimated 5 to 10 million American women, research interest in the disease—and federal funds to support it—has been scarce until recently. Critics say sexism is the reason. "I believe that if this were a disease affecting middle-aged white males—like senators, for example—you'd see so much government money for research you wouldn't believe it," says Dr. David Olive, director of reproductive endocrinology and infertility at Yale University Medical School.

months at a stretch. With luck, a course of treatment will suppress endometriosis for months or

Overcoming Infertility

by Tamar Nordenberg

Myth or fact: If a couple is having trouble conceiving a child, the man should try wearing loose underwear? That's a fact, according to a study on "Tight-fitting Underwear and Sperm Quality" published June 29, 1996, in the scientific journal *The Lancet*. Tight-fitting underwear—as well as hot tubs and saunas—is not recommended for men trying to father a child because it may raise testes temperature to a point where it interferes with sperm production.

But couples having difficulty getting pregnant can tell you the solution is almost never as simple as wearing boxers instead of briefs. Lisa (who asked that her last name not be used) tried for more than two years to get pregnant without success. "Everyone gave me advice," she says. "My mother said I should just go to church and pray more. My friends said, 'Try to relax and not think about it' or 'You're just over-stressed. You work too much.' "

Actually, psychological stress is more likely a *result* of infertility than the cause, according to Resolve, a nonprofit consumer organization specializing in infertility.

"Fertility problems are a huge psychological stressor, a huge relationship stressor," says Lisa Rarick, M.D., director of the Food and Drug Administration's division of reproductive and urologic drug products.

So, while going on a relaxing vacation may temporarily relieve the stress that comes with fertility problems, a solution may require treatment by a health-care professional. Treatment with drugs such as Clomid or Serophene (both clomiphene citrate) or Pergonal,

Humegon or Metrodin (all meno-tropins) are used in some cases to correct a woman's hormone imbalance. Surgery is sometimes used to repair damaged reproductive organs. And in about 20 percent of cases, less conventional, high-tech options like *in vitro* fertilization are used.

Will the therapies work? "Talking about the success rate for fertility treatments is like saying, 'What's the chance of curing a headache?' " according to Benjamin Yonger, M.D., executive director of the American Society for Reproductive Medicine. "It depends on many things, including the cause of the problem and the severity." Overall, Younger says, about half of couples that seek fertility treatment will be able to have babies.

A Year Without Pregnancy

Infertility is defined as the inability to conceive a child despite trying for one year. The condition affects about 5.3 million Americans, or 9 percent of the reproductive age population, according to the American Society for Reproductive Medicine.

Ironically, the best protection against infertility is to use a condom while you are not trying to get pregnant. Condoms prevent sexually transmitted diseases, a primary cause of infertility.

Even a completely healthy couple can't expect to get pregnant at the drop of a hat. Only 20 percent of women who want to conceive become pregnant in the first ovulation cycle they try, according to Younger.

To become pregnant, a couple must have intercourse during the woman's fertile time of the month, which is right

before and during ovulation. Because it's tough to pinpoint the exact day of ovulation, having intercourse often during the approximate time maximizes the chances of conception.

After a year of frequent intercourse without contraception that doesn't result in pregnancy, a couple should go to a health-care professional for an evaluation. In some cases, it makes sense to seek help for fertility problems even before a year is up.

A woman over 30 may wish to get an earlier evaluation. "At age 30, a woman begins a slow decline in her ability to get pregnant," says Younger. "The older she gets, the greater her chance of miscarriage, too." But a woman's fertility doesn't take a big drop until around age 40.

"A man's age affects fertility to a much smaller degree and 20 or 30 years later than in a woman," Younger says. Despite a decrease in sperm production that begins after age 25, some men remain fertile into their 60s and 70s.

· A couple may also seek earlier evaluation if:
• The woman isn't menstruating regularly, which may indicate an absence of ovulation that would make it impossible for her to conceive without medical help.
• The woman has had three or more miscarriages (or the man had a previous partner who had had three or more miscarriages).
• The woman or man has had certain infections that sometimes affect fertility (for example, pelvic infection in a woman, or mumps or prostate infection in a man).
• The woman or man suspects there

may be a fertility problem (if, for example, attempts at pregnancy failed in a previous relationship).

The Man or the Woman?

Impairment in any step of the intricate process of conception can cause infertility. For a woman to become pregnant, her partner's sperm must be healthy so that at least one can swim into her fallopian tubes. An egg, released by the woman's ovaries, must be in the fallopian tube ready to be fertilized. (See diagram below.) Next, the fertilized egg, called an embryo, must make its way through an open-ended fallopian tube into the uterus, implant in the uterine lining, and be sustained there while it grows.

It is a myth that infertility is always a "woman's problem." Of the 80 percent of cases with a diagnosed cause, about half are based at least partially on male problems (referred to as male factors)—usually that the man produces no sperm,

a condition called azoospermia, or that he produces too few sperm, called oligospermia.

Lifestyle can influence the number and quality of a man's sperm. Alcohol and drugs—including marijuana, nicotine, and certain medications—can temporarily reduce sperm quality. Also, environmental toxins, including pesticides and lead, may be to blame for some cases of infertility.

The causes of sperm production problems can exist from birth or develop later as a result of severe medical illnesses, including mumps and some sexually transmitted diseases, or from a severe testicle injury, tumor, or other problem. Inability to ejaculate normally can prevent conception, too, and can be caused by many factors, including diabetes, surgery of the prostate gland or urethra, blood pressure medication, or impotence.

The other half of explained infertility cases are linked to female problems

(called female factors), most commonly ovulation disorders. Without ovulation, eggs are not available for fertilization. Problems with ovulation are signaled by irregular menstrual periods or a lack of periods altogether (called amenorrhea). Simple lifestyle factors—including stress, diet, or athletic training—can affect a woman's hormonal balance. Much less often, a hormonal imbalance can result from a serious medical problem such as a pituitary gland tumor.

Other problems can also lead to female infertility. If the fallopian tubes are blocked at one or both ends, the egg can't travel through the tubes into the uterus. Such blockage may result from pelvic inflammatory disease, surgery for an ectopic pregnancy (when the embryo implants in the fallopian tube rather than in the uterus), or other problems, including endometriosis (the abnormal presence of uterine lining cells in other pelvic organs).

A medical evaluation may determine

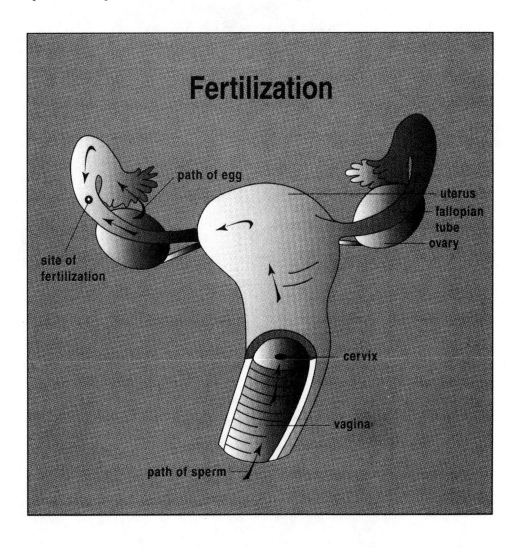

Fertilization

path of egg

site of fertilization

uterus
fallopian tube
ovary

cervix

vagina

path of sperm

Science and ART

Sometimes it may be necessary or preferable to get pregnant without intercourse. A woman may choose to get pregnant with the sperm of someone who is not her partner.

In some cases, a woman may not be able to become pregnant with her partner because his sexual problems make it impossible for him to ejaculate normally during sex, or because the sperm have to bypass the vagina if the vaginal mucus cannot support them, or for other reasons. In these cases, through artificial insemination, the semen is placed into the woman's uterus or vaginal canal using a hollow, flexible tube called a catheter.

New, more complex assisted reproductive technologies, or ART, procedures, including *in vitro* fertilization (IVF), have been available since the birth 18 years ago of Louise Brown, the world's first "test tube baby." IVF makes it possible to combine sperm and eggs in a laboratory for a baby that is genetically related to one or both partners.

IVF is often used when a woman's fallopian tubes are blocked. First, medication is given to stimulate the ovaries to produce multiple eggs. Once mature, the eggs are suctioned from the ovaries and placed in a laboratory culture dish with the man's sperm for fertilization. About two days later, three to five embryos are transferred to the woman's uterus. If the woman does not become pregnant, she may try again in the next cycle.

Other ART procedures, based on many of the same principles, include:
• *Gamete intrafallopian transfer, or GIFT:* Similar to IVF, but used when the woman has at least one normal fallopian tube. Three to five eggs are placed in the fallopian tube, along with the man's sperm, for fertilization inside the woman's body.
• *Zygote intrafallopian transfer, or ZIFT* (also called tubal embryo transfer): A hybrid of IVF and GIFT. The eggs retrieved from the woman's ova-ries are fertilized in the lab and replaced in the fallopian tubes rather than the uterus.
• *Donor egg IVF:* For women who, for example, have impaired ovaries or carry a genetic disease that can be transferred to the offspring. Eggs are donated by another healthy woman and fertilized in the lab with the male partner's sperm before being transferred to the female partner's uterus.
• *Frozen embryos:* Excess embryos are frozen, to be thawed in the future if the woman doesn't get pregnant on the first cycle or wants another baby in the future.

New treatments for male factors are fast-evolving. Intracytoplasmic sperm injection is one of the most exciting new procedures, according to Benjamin Younger, M.D., executive director of the American Society for Reproductive Medicine. A single egg is injected with a single sperm to produce an embryo that can implant and grow in the uterus.

About two-thirds of births from ART procedures are single births. Of the rest, almost all are twins, with about 6 percent resulting in the birth of triplets or more.

—T.N.

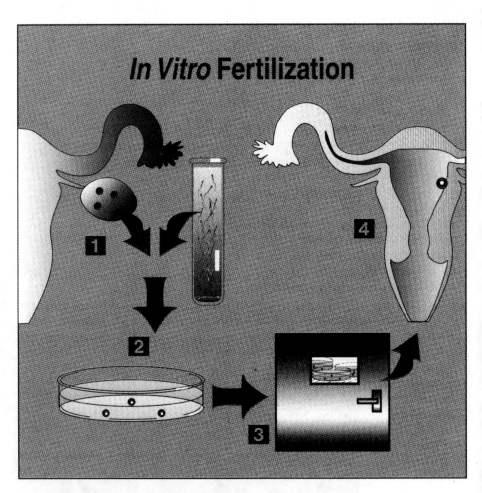

In Vitro Fertilization

1 The eggs are removed from the ovary.

2 The eggs and sperm from a donor are combined in a Petri dish.

3 The Petri dish is placed in an incubator.

4 If fertilization occurs, the embryo is transferred to the uterus.

It is a myth that infertility is always a "woman's problem."

whether a couple's infertility is due to these or other causes. If a medical and sexual history doesn't reveal an obvious problem, like improperly timed intercourse or absence of ovulation, specific tests may be needed.

Tests for Both

The man's evaluation focuses on the number and health of his sperm. The laboratory first examines a sperm sample under a microscope to check sperm number, shape and movement. Further tests may be needed to look for infection, hormonal imbalance, or other problems.

Male tests include:
• *X-ray:* If damage to one or both of the vas deferens (the ducts in the male that transport the sperm to the penis) is known or suspected, an x-ray is taken to examine the organs.
• *Mucus penetrance test:* Test of whether the man's sperm are able to swim through a drop of the woman's fertile vaginal mucus on a slide (also used to test the quality of the woman's mucus).
• *Hamster-egg penetrance assay:* Test of whether the man's sperm will penetrate hamster egg cells with their outer cells removed, indicating somewhat their ability to fertilize human eggs.

For the woman, the first step in testing is to determine if she is ovulating each month. This can be done by charting changes in morning body temperature, by using an FDA-approved home ovulation test kit (which is available over the counter), or by examining cervical mucus, which undergoes a series of hormone-induced changes throughout the menstrual cycle.

Checks of ovulation can also be done in the physician's office with simple blood tests for hormone levels or ultrasound tests of the ovaries. If the woman is ovulating, further testing will need to be done.

Common female tests include:
• *Hysterosalpingogram:* An x-ray of the fallopian tubes and uterus after they are injected with dye, to show if the tubes are open and to show the shape of the uterus.
• *Laparoscopy:* An examination of the tubes and other female organs for disease, using a miniature light-transmitting tube called a laparoscope. The tube is inserted into the abdomen through a one-inch incision below the navel, usually while the woman is under general anesthesia.
• *Endometrial biopsy:* An examination of a small shred of uterine lining to see if the monthly changes in the lining are normal.

Some tests require participation of both partners. Samples of cervical mucus taken after intercourse can show whether sperm and mucus have properly interacted. Also, a variety of tests can show if the man or woman is forming antibodies that are attacking the sperm.

Drugs and Surgery

Depending on what the tests turn up, different treatments are recommended. Eighty to 90 percent of infertility cases are treated with drugs or surgery.

Therapy with the fertility drug Clomid or with a more potent hormone stimulator—Pergonal, Metrodin or Humegon—is often recommended for women with ovulation problems. The benefits of each drug and the side effects, which can be minor or serious but rare, should be discussed with the doctor. Multiple births occur in 10 to 20 percent of births resulting from fertility drug use.

Other drugs, used under very limited circumstances, include Parlodel (bromocriptine mesylate), for women with elevated levels of a hormone called prolactin, and a hormone pump that releases gonadotropins necessary for ovulation.

If drugs aren't the answer, surgery

may be. Because major surgery is involved, operations to repair damage to the woman's ovaries, fallopian tubes, or uterus are recommended only if there is a good chance of restoring fertility.

In the man, one infertility problem often treated surgically is damage to the vas deferens, commonly caused by a sexually transmitted disease, other infection, or vasectomy (male sterilization).

Other important tools in the battle against infertility include artificial insemination and the so-called assisted reproductive technologies. (See accompanying [Science and ART] article.

Fulfillment Regardless

Lisa became pregnant without assisted reproductive technologies, after taking ovulation-promoting medication and undergoing surgery to repair her damaged fallopian tubes. Her daughter is now 4 years old.

"It was definitely worth it. I really appreciate having my daughter because of what I went through," she says. But Lisa and her husband won't try to have a second child just yet. "At some point you have to stop trying to have a baby, stop obsessing over what might be an unreachable goal," she says.

When having a genetically related baby seems unachievable, a couple may decide to stop treatment and proceed with the rest of their lives. Some may choose to lead an enriched life without children. Others may choose to adopt.

And no, according to Resolve, you're not more likely to get pregnant if you adopt a baby.

To get more information about infertility, send a self-addressed, stamped envelope to: Resolve, 1310 Broadway, Somerville, MA 02144-1731; call their National Helpline at (617) 623-0744; or visit their World Wide Web site at *http://www.resolve.org/.*

Tamar Nordenberg is a staff writer for FDA Consumer.

The national abortion debate:
Are both sides asking the wrong questions?

THE WAR OVER ABORTION WILL NOT end this year. The battles have turned internecine, with Republicans fighting over a "human life" amendment and Democrats disagreeing about whether *any* restrictions on the right to choose are acceptable. Meanwhile, clinics are still being picketed, doctors stalked, insults hurled.

If any of this is to change, partisans on both sides must recognize something important: We cannot keep discussing abortion as if the black-and-white question—legal or illegal?—is *all* that matters. While we argue our beliefs, 1.5 million abortions are performed every year, and, as Dan Ebener, a pro-life leader in Davenport, Iowa, observes, "All the name-calling is doing nothing to reduce the abortion rate." Even those who believe, as *Glamour* does, that women must have the right to choose should be working to create a world in which fewer women need avail themselves of that right.

When President Clinton campaigned in 1992, he envisioned a country in which abortion would be "safe, legal and rare." The *rare* part never really took off as a political goal—for either side. Pro-life advocates too often assume that outlawing abortion is the same as eradicating it—as if the crowded back alleys of pre–*Roe* v. *Wade* America had taught no lessons. For those in the pro-choice camp, preserving the right to abortion can easily seem the only pressing goal. When pro-choicers *do* express hopes of lowering the rate, they are sometimes accused of hypocrisy: If abortion is morally *right*, critics ask, why need it be *rare?* Such pro-choice reasoning, one conservative professor wrote earlier this year, "fails the moral giggle test."

Not in real life it doesn't. We often accept something as legal and still prefer to avoid it—divorce, for example. Not everyone who is pro-choice sees abortion in the same ethical light, but what they tend to agree on is this: Abortion is a right they will fight for but hope not to exercise.

Now it is time to put the same energy with which we support *or* oppose legal abortion into reducing the rate. Our first national priority should be to *treat the unplanned pregnancy rate as the scandal it is.* One in every ten women at risk of pregnancy (sexually active, fertile women who are not trying to have a baby) uses no birth control—and the resulting conceptions account for half of our country's abortions. "Sixty percent of pregnancies in this country are unintended," says Jane Johnson, interim co-president of the Planned Parenthood Federation of America. "If you left the house and 60 percent of the time you didn't end up where you were headed, wouldn't your family and friends say, 'Something's *wrong* with her'? Well, something is haywire in our country."

The problem may lie in our psyches, our self-esteem, our ability to think long-term. But as a society, there *are* steps we can take—and it is a mark of how off-target the debate has become that the same politicians who despair at the abortion rate often oppose the very measures that would help reduce it. Federal family-planning funds, which support the clinics millions of young women use, prevent about 516,000 abortions annually. Such funds were once considered a cornerstone of American public policy—not just by firebrand feminists but by President Richard Nixon, who in 1969 announced that "No American woman should be denied access to family-planning assistance because of her economic condition."

Yet funding for Title X, the family-planning program Nixon signed into law, has been declining year after year; in 1995 the House Appropriations Committee voted to eliminate Title X altogether. Thanks to pro-choice *and* pro-life members, that ban was later reversed by the

Of all women who obtain abortions each year:

9% are women ages 35 and over
14% are women ages 30–34
21% are teens
22% are women ages 25–29
34% are women ages 20–24

Chart source: National Center for Health Statistics. Numbers are for 1991, the most recent year available.

House. As Representative Susan Molinari (R–N.Y.) told *Glamour:* "Let's be honest. If we are against abortion ... we must stand up for family planning. We must give women a place to go."

Other measures to help curb the abortion rate: ● **Better insurance coverage of contraceptives** Just 15 percent of large fee-for-service plans and 39 percent of HMOs cover the five most effective reversible methods—even though most insurers *do* cover abortion. ● **Realistic sex education** The World Health Organization has found that countries that teach teens about birth control and reproductive health boast the lowest teen pregnancy rates. ● **Vigorous public support for contraceptive research,** which is now being conducted by just four major private companies *worldwide.* ● **Positive awareness of adoption**—an option too often dismissed as a tool of antiabortion forces.

Making these issues as urgent as abortion itself will require some adjustments on the part of the media, which sometimes see abortion as a juicier topic than earnest ideas about how to prevent it. Women in trouble—ooh! Violent confrontation—news! On the other hand: Better access to birth control—yawn. Sex ed for all—ho hum. Learning to say no—just wake us when it's over. As president of the National Abortion and Reproductive Rights Action League, which in 1994 expanded its mission to include *reducing* the abortion rate, Kate Michelman has seen this phenomenon up close. "When I talk about sex ed, there's a deafening silence," she says. "All journalists want to talk about is abortion. I can't get any traction on these other issues!"

It's up to all of us—on both sides—to help change that. If we do not, we will remain frozen in the same old shouting match over legal abortion, forever debating the solution, never addressing the problem.

Psychological Aftereffects of Abortion

The Rest of the Story

Joyce Arthur

British Columbia Coalition for Abortion Clinics (writer@direct.ca)

Over the last decade, a consensus has been reached in the medical and scientific communities that most women who have abortions experience little or no psychological harm. Yet, a woman's ability to cope psychologically after an abortion continues to be the subject of heated debates. Vocal anti-choice advocates claim that most women who have abortions will suffer to some degree from a variant of post-traumatic-stress disorder called "post-abortion syndrome," characterized by severe and long-lasting guilt, depression, rage, and social and sexual dysfunction. Why is there such a major discrepancy between the scientific consensus and anti-choice beliefs?

Conflicting studies done over the last 30 years have contributed to this atmosphere of confusion and misinformation. A 1989 review article that evaluated the methodology of 76 studies on the psychological aftereffects of abortion noted that both opponents and advocates of abortion could easily prove their case by picking and choosing from a wide range of contradictory evidence. For example, many studies, especially those done between 1950 and 1975, purport to have found significant negative psychological responses to abortion. Such studies, though, often suffer from serious methodological flaws. Some were done when abortion was still illegal or highly restricted, thereby biasing the conclusions in favor of considerable (and understandable) psychological distress. In some cases, research was based on women who were forced to prove a psychiatric disorder in order to obtain the abortion. Further, a large number of studies, both early and recent, consist simply of anecdotal reports of a few women who sought psychiatric help after their abortion. In short, many studies that favor anti-choice beliefs are flawed because of very small samples, unrepresentative samples, poor data analysis, lack of control groups, and unreliable or invalid research questions.

Researcher bias on the part of scientists and physicians has also been a serious problem. In earlier times, society's views on how women "should" feel after an abortion were heavily skewed toward the traditional model of women as nurturing mothers. In one study done in 1973, post-doctoral psychology students taking psychoanalytic training predicted psychological effects far more severe than those predicted by women themselves before undergoing an abortion. This might be because traditional Freudian theory teaches that a desire to avoid childbearing represents a woman's denial of her basic feminine nature.

Some psychiatric studies, along with much of today's anti-choice literature, tend to cast women who have abortions into one of two roles: victim or deviant (although these terms are not necessarily used). Victims are coerced into abortion by others around them, in spite of their confusion and ambivalence, and against their basic maternal instincts. Deviants have little difficulty with the abortion decision, which is made casually for convenience sake. Such women have no maternal instinct and are often characterized in a derogatory or pitying fashion as selfish, callous, unfeminine, emotionally stunted, and/or neurotic.

Books written by anti-choice advocates that deal with post-abortion effects are, by and large, heavily infected with bias. Not only is contrary evidence unrefuted, it is rarely even mentioned. Incorrect and out-of-date "facts" abound. The authors' pop psychology often seems to be based on little more than their own wishful projections about the nature of women and how they should feel. Here are two typical examples from essays in the anti-choice book *The Psychological Aspects of Abortion* (1979):

"It is interesting that women who need self-punishment do not abort themselves more often. . . . Abortion is done 'to' the woman, with her as only a passive participant. This is further indication of masochism." (Howard W. Fisher, *Abortion—Pain or Pleasure?*)

" . . . sooner or later [after the abortion], the truth will make itself known and felt, and the bitter realization that she was not even unselfish enough to share her life with another human being will take its toll. If she had ever entertained a doubt as to whether her parents and others really considered her unlovable and worthless, she will now be certain that she was indeed never any good in their eyes or her own. A deep depression will be inevitable and her preoccupation with thoughts of suicide that much greater." (Conrad W. Baars, *Psychic Causes and Consequences of the Abortion Mentality*)

With the advent of safe, legal, routinely performed abortion, a wealth of good evidence has come to light that is quite contrary to common anti-choice assertions. The typical abortion patient is a normal, mentally stable woman who makes a strongly resolved decision for abortion within a few days after discovery of the pregnancy, and comes through the procedure virtually unscathed. Several scientific review articles—published from 1990 to 1992 in highly respected journals such as *Science* and *American Journal of Psychiatry*—support this conclusion. The reviews evaluated hundreds of studies done over the last thirty years, noting the unusually high number of seriously flawed studies, and pointing out common methodological problems. Based on the more reliable studies, all the reviews concluded that although psychological disturbances do occur after abortion, they are uncommon and generally mild and short-lived. In many cases, these disturbances are simply a continuation of negative feelings caused by the unwanted pregnancy itself. Serious or persistent problems are rare and are frequently related to the circumstances surrounding the abortion rather than the abortion itself.

Further, many women who were denied abortion showed ongoing, long-term resentment, and their resulting unwanted children were more likely to have increased emotional, psychological, and social problems in comparison with control groups of wanted children. These differences between children widened throughout adolescence and early adulthood. Finally, many studies show that giving birth is much more likely than abortion to be associated with severe emotional aftereffects, such as post-partum depression.

The review articles largely concluded that the most frequently reported emotions felt by women immediately following an abortion (experienced by about 75% of women) are relief or happiness. Feelings of regret, anxiety, guilt, depression, and other negative emotions are reported by about 5% to 30% of women. These feelings are usually mild and fade rapidly, within a few weeks. Months or years after an abortion, the majority of women do not regret their decision. In fact, for many women, abortion appears to be a positive experience that improves their self-esteem, provides inner strength, and motivates them to refocus their lives in a meaningful way.

Studies on abortion are done primarily through self-report measures, however, and it is possible that some women may be reluctant to admit negative feelings after their abortion. To help quantify this, consider these figures: every year since 1977, 1.3 million to 1.6 million abortions are performed in the United States; about 21% of all American women between the ages of 15 and 44 have had an abortion. These are very large numbers indeed. The American Psychological Association has pointed out that, even if only 10% of the millions of women who have had abortions experienced problems, there would be a significant mental health epidemic, clearly evident by large numbers of dysfunctional women requesting help. There is no evidence of any such epidemic, thereby supporting the general reliability of self-report measures.

Some women who are disturbed by or unhappy with their abortion decision belong to support groups like Women Exploited by Abortion, and Victims of Choice. Several anti-choice studies and books purporting to demonstrate the overall harmfulness of abortion limit their sample to the membership of such groups. Not only does this introduce an immediate and fatal flaw to their argument, it shows deliberate obfuscation on the part of the authors. This does not mean that post-abortion support groups are valueless to women. The very existence of such groups points to the strong need for health professionals to identify and provide extra help to women who are most at risk for developing psychological problems related to abortion. Many studies have shown that women at greater risk tend to include:

- emotionally immature teenagers
- women with previous psychiatric problems
- women aborting a wanted pregnancy for medical or genetic reasons
- women who encounter opposition from their partner or parents for their abortion decision
- women who have strong philosophical or religious objections to abortion
- women who are highly ambivalent or confused about their abortion decision, and had great difficulty making the decision

- women who are coerced by others into having an abortion
- women undergoing second-trimester abortions

In spite of psychological problems suffered by a few women after abortion, the existence of "post-abortion syndrome" is doubted by most experts. There is little need to posit a unique disorder in this case, since abortion is not significantly different from any other stressful life experience that might cause trauma in certain people. Former Surgeon General C. Everett Koop, himself anti-choice, noted this in 1988. Unfortunately, facts, evidence, and common sense rarely get in the way of anti-choice advocates who are determined to prove that women suffer terribly from "post-abortion syndrome." Certainly, if this were true, it would be a lethal weapon in the fight to reverse Roe vs. Wade. This was, in fact, the motivation behind a 1989 Surgeon General's report on the health effects of abortion on women, which was called for by former President Ronald Reagan on behalf of anti-choice leaders. Although the report was duly prepared, the Surgeon General chose not to release it, apparently because it did not support the anti-choice position. Meanwhile, anti-choice literature continues to churn out the myth that women are severely harmed by abortion.

Because abortion is such a volatile issue, it is probably unrealistic to expect this aspect of the controversy to die down soon, if at all. However, by recognizing that a small subset of women may require increased counseling and support during their abortion decision and afterwards, the women's community and health professionals can do much to minimize the damage wrought by the anti-choice movement's dangerous and irresponsible campaign of misinformation.

Psychological Health

Although this unit offers a rather eclectic collection of topics—everything from empowerment via physical activity through the diagnosis and treatment of eating disorders—a closer examination reveals common themes. The first commonality is stress, resulting from multiple and often conflicting roles. Trying to divide time and attention among family, home, and work leaves precious little time for self-care. Another common thread is the all-too-common misdiagnosis of women's health problems. Since women are often dismissed as being hormonal, emotional, and irrational, their legitimate health concerns may be overlooked, placing their health in serious jeopardy. Next, the theme of personal responsibility emerges. It is not only advisable but necessary for women to become aware of their own physical and psychological states, to know what is normal and what is unusual for each individual.

Another common psychiatric disorder addressed in this section is depression. "Depression: Way beyond the Blues" begins by helping the reader to distinguish between a case of the blues and a real clinical depression. Author Sandra Arbetter offers a list of symptoms, information on antidepressants, and suggestions for how to help a friend who is depressed.

Certainly related to both stress and depression are eating disorders. Many women in the United States either suffer from an eating disorder or at least exhibit a dysfunctional attitude about food. "Treating Eating Disorders" provides a detailed description of anorexia (self-starvation) and bulimia (binge-purge syndrome). Treatment options are also discussed.

The two remaining articles in this chapter present a very different perspective on mental health issues. In "Childless by Choice," Katherine Griffin describes her personal odyssey in coming to terms with her decision not to have children. She summarizes studies of both personal and marital satisfaction in women who are childless. She argues persuasively against the notion that "women without kids are assumed to be either sad, barren spinster types, or career-crazed imitations of men."

The more upbeat side of psychological health is examined in "The New Rite of Passage." Here Susan Seligson examines the empowerment of women through rigorous physical activity, describing the hardy individual as one who feels committed to a goal, has a sense of control over her environment, and finds new situations to be challenging rather than threatening. Elements of all of these characteristics are evident in the women profiled here.

Looking Ahead: Challenge Questions

What is the relationship between multiple role demands and stress in the lives of women?

Why are emotional issues so frequently ignored or misdiagnosed in women?

Why do far more women than men fall victim to eating disorders?

Why was the article "Childless by Choice" included in this section?

Why would women find physical activity empowering?

UNIT 4

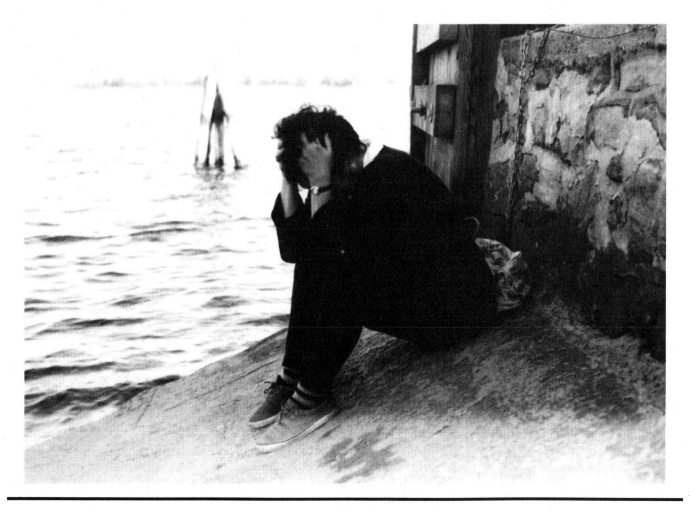

How Real Women Keep Stress at Bay

CATHERINE WALD

Some women just don't seem to be bothered by stress. They work, raise kids, run households, volunteer, stay in shape—and they seem to enjoy every minute of it. When you call them on the phone, they sound enthusiastic, rested and full of energy rather than harassed, exhausted and miserable. How do they do it?

"Of course, there is no such thing as a completely stress-free woman," says Valerie Raskin, M.D., assistant professor of clinical psychiatry at the University of Illinois at Chicago. "Life is an endless opportunity to have stress. Things can and do go wrong. But there are women who are able to handle it better than others, women for whom life doesn't *feel* stressful."

Who are these women, and what are their secrets? To find out, I spoke with five who are considered by their friends to be stress-free.

An Easy Grader

Judith Irvin, a professor and mother of two in Tallahassee, Florida, has decided that she can't be perfect at everything. So she focuses her efforts on the two most important areas of her life: teaching and mothering. "On many other things that aren't as important, I allow myself to do a B+ job," she says. "When I have to choose between having a clean house or spending time with my kids, I choose my kids. I love having a clean house, but I figure that's something I'll do later."

One thing she won't defer is taking a little time to herself every day. In the morning, as soon as her two teenagers leave for school, Judith gets a cup of coffee and sits in a special chair for 30 minutes of quiet meditation and thought. "It's the only time of day when my mind isn't on a zillion things. I've found it to be extremely valuable, both psychologically and emotionally."

Judith is also a firm believer in exercise, which takes the form of either long walks in her neighborhood or an occasional game of racquetball. In the privacy of a soundproof court, Judith plays her heart out—and curses like a stevedore.

A Flexible Flyer

For Jan Melnik, stress is something to manage, not something to avoid. "I personally think stress can be very positive if it's channeled in the right way," says the Durham, Connecticut, marketing consultant. "If you're running in ten different directions for things that are not important to you, then you'll feel the negative effects of stress. But if you are really doing what you *want* to be doing, you can have many balls up in the air."

To keep all her balls up in the air, Jan uses a planner and several computerized programs—as well as good old-fashioned pencil and paper (she always has a notepad handy, to jot down ideas). But more important than organization is setting priorities. "You need to know what you feel is important, and map your schedule so the bigger chunks of time are meeting those high priorities," she says.

But Jan realizes that all the organization in the world can't prepare you for emergencies—like the time when her three children all caught the chicken pox one after the other and she had to miss six weeks' work. In cases like that, the key to survival is flexibility—and a positive attitude. "I've chosen to run my own business and work around the needs of my family, and I never apologize for that."

Another thing that keeps Jan stress-free is setting limits. While she will occasionally stay up until midnight to meet a deadline, there are certain areas of her life that are nonnegotiable. "I won't miss my children's soccer games or art shows, or cancel an anniversary dinner with my husband," she says.

A Care Taker

Nancy Kohler will do a lot for her family and her community, but she won't lose sleep over them. "I find that if I don't get my eight hours, all my problems become larger than life," says Nancy, a mother of four, part-time art teacher and active volunteer from Ossining, New York. That's why she has no qualms about rearranging her schedule to allow for a nap. "There's no point in doing anything if I'm not enjoying it," she says.

And enjoy herself she does—whether it's teaching, running a

From *Woman's Day* magazine, April 2, 1996, pp. 64, 66. © 1996 by Catherine Wald. Reprinted by permission.

Take It Easy: How to Live It Up By Calming Down

According to Ruth Luban, author of *101 Ways to Beat Burnout* and *Keeping the Fire: From Burnout to Balance* (audio series), stress-free women:

Accept their limitations. They give themselves the right to set boundaries and to say no when they feel they have to.

Put their own needs on their to-do lists. "You'll have tons more efficiency and energy to give to others," Luban says, "if you take care of yourself."

Establish regular self-care activities—including exercise, rest and periods of silence—that they incorporate into their daily schedules. "Spending a few minutes of simply being silent and letting your mind wander is a key to creative problem-solving," says Luban.

Know how to play.

Adapt to new situations, instead of holding to rigid beliefs of who they are and how things should be done.

Express their feelings in an assertive, confident way.

Use "decompression rituals" to switch gears from one activity to another—such as drinking a cup of herbal tea after the kids leave for school or taking a walk on the way home from work.

Have a strong sense of self. "Stress-free women have an identity that is inner-derived, an identity that is not based only on their careers or on roles such as parent, homemaker or wife," Luban says.

Provide good role models for their children. Instead of raising overscheduled, Type A kids, stress-free women value taking time out—and they encourage their children to do the same.

house or spending time with her children. Fellow members of a local volunteer arts council often compliment Nancy on her stress-free demeanor and sense of humor even in trying times. Part of her secret is avoiding the temptation to spread herself too thin. Instead of joining every single committee that wants her, Nancy agrees to be available on an as-needed basis. "I get a lot of calls, but I can say no when I need to."

Nancy adds that having good friends to talk to is an important stress-reliever. "The other day, three friends stopped by for coffee. It was only an hour, but it was such a nice hour."

Even seemingly stress-free women like Nancy can get overwhelmed by events that are out of their control. During times of crisis, she has sought help from a therapist. "To me, that's just

another part of taking good care of yourself," she says.

A Lemonade Maker

What could be more stressful than moving to a new state, giving up a successful career, and living in a cramped apartment with your husband and two children while looking for a house? For Louise Kursmark, whose husband was recently transferred to Cincinnati from Boston, the key is taking everything one day at a time.

"I don't believe in worrying, because I don't think it's constructive," Louise explains. "I'm just trying to let this be an interesting experience that some day we'll all look back on. Otherwise, by the time we get to the next step, I'll be such a nervous wreck that it will spoil *that* experience too."

To keep herself on an even keel during stressful times, Louise forces herself to slow down and enjoy life's little pleasures, whether it's watching a movie with her kids or talking with an old friend on the phone. "I like to stop and think to myself what a wonderful life I have," she says.

Her optimistic nature is also a big help. "I really do believe that things generally turn out well and that life is good," Louise says. According to Dr. Raskin, that kind of attitude is a hallmark of stress-free women. "Instead of feeling sorry for themselves, they focus on solutions. They figure out how to make lemonade from lemons."

A Life Lover

Benefits specialist Stacy Dye of Paris, Missouri, is another busy woman who still takes time out to count her blessings. That's because last December, Stacy almost lost her life when her third child was born prematurely. "I went to the hospital in an ambulance, hemorrhaging, and I didn't know if I was going to make it," she recalls. "Once you go through something like that, you really appreciate every day, and you don't sweat the little things any more."

Stacy has stopped trying to have a perfect house—and has begun to ask her husband and children to pitch in with the chores. "I was brought up that it was the woman's job to take care of the house, so when I first got married, I tried to be super-everything. Now I've learned to say, 'I need help.'"

To get through a busy work and family schedule, Stacy prepares for each morning the night before—making lists, laying out clothes and even putting things in the car. She also gets up at least a half hour before the rest of the family to allow herself time to bathe, fix her hair, put on makeup, and enjoy a soothing cup of coffee "without everyone climbing on me."

She also works fun into her schedule—occasional dates with her husband or a big shopping trip with her girlfriends. "I don't feel guilty about these indulgences because I know that I'm a better mother, wife and person if I take a little time to enjoy myself."

The Myth of the Miserable Working Woman

*She's Tired, She's Stressed Out, She's Unhealthy, She Can't Go Full Speed
at Work or Home. Right? Wrong.*

Rosalind C. Barnett and Caryl Rivers

Rosalind C. Barnett is a psychologist and a senior research associate at the Wellesley College Center for Research on Women. Caryl Rivers is a professor of journalism at Boston University and the author of More Joy Than Rage: Crossing Generations With the New Feminism.

"You Can't Do Everything," announced a 1989 USA Today *headline on a story suggesting that a slower career track for women might be a good idea. "Mommy Career Track Sets Off a Furor," declaimed the* New York Times *on March 8, 1989, reporting that women cost companies more than men. "Pressed for Success, Women Careerists Are Cheating Themselves," sighed a 1989 headline in the* Washington Post, *going on to cite a book about the "unhappy personal lives" of women graduates of the Harvard Business School. "Women Discovering They're at Risk for Heart Attacks," Gannett News Service reported with alarm in 1991. "Can Your Career Hurt Your Kids? Yes, Say Many Experts," blared a* Fortune *cover just last May, adding in a chirpy yet soothing fashion, "But smart parents—and flexible companies—won't let it happen."*

If you believe what you read, working women are in big trouble—stressed out, depressed, sick, risking an early death from heart attacks, and so overcome with problems at home that they make inefficient employees at work.

In fact, just the opposite is true. As a research psychologist whose career has focused on women and a journalist-critic who has studied the behavior of the media, we have extensively surveyed the latest data and research and concluded that the public is being engulfed by a tidal wave of disinformation that has serious consequences for the life and health of every American woman. Since large numbers of women began moving into the work force in the 1970s, scores of studies on their emotional and physical health have painted a very clear picture: Paid employment provides substantial health *benefits* for women. These benefits cut across income and class lines; even women who are working because they have to—not because they want to—share in them.

There is a curious gap, however, between what these studies say and what is generally reported on television, radio, and in newspapers and magazines. The more the research shows work is good for women, the bleaker the media reports seem to become. Whether this bizarre state of affairs is the result of a backlash against women, as *Wall Street Journal* reporter Susan Faludi contends in her new book, *Backlash: The Undeclared War Against American Women,* or of well-meaning ignorance, the effect is the same: Both the shape of national policy and the lives of women are at risk.

Too often, legislation is written and policies are drafted not on the basis of the facts but on the basis of what those in power believe to be the facts. Even the much discussed *Workforce 2000* report, issued by the Department of Labor under the Reagan administration—hardly a hotbed of feminism—admitted that "most current policies were designed for a society in which men worked and women stayed home." If policies are skewed toward solutions that are aimed at reducing women's commitment to work, they will do more than harm women—they will damage companies, managers and the productivity of the American economy.

THE CORONARY THAT WASN'T

One reason the "bad news" about working women jumps to page one is that we're all too willing to believe it. Many adults today grew up at a time when soldiers were returning home from World War II and a way had to be found to get the women who replaced them in industry back into the kitchen. The result was a barrage of propaganda that turned at-home moms into saints and backyard barbecues and station wagons into cultural icons. Many of us still have that outdated postwar map inside our heads, and it leaves us more willing to believe the horror stories than the good news that paid employment is an emotional and medical plus.

In the 19th century it was accepted medical dogma that women should not be educated because the brain and the ovaries could not develop at the same time. Today it's PMS, the wrong math genes or rampaging hormones. Hardly anyone points out the dire predictions that didn't come true.

You may remember the prediction that career women would start having more heart attacks, just like men. But the Framingham Heart Study—a federally funded cardiac project that has been studying 10,000 men and women since 1948—reveals that working women are not having more heart attacks. They're not dying any earlier, either. Not only are women not losing their health advantages; the lifespan gap is actually widening. Only one group of working women suffers more heart attacks than other women: those in low-paying clerical jobs with many demands on them and little control over their work pace, who also have several children and little or no support at home.

As for the recent publicity about women having more problems with heart disease, much of it skims over the important underlying reasons for the increase: namely, that by the time they have a heart attack, women tend to be a good deal older (an average of 67, six years older than the average age for men), and thus frailer, than males who have one. Also, statistics from the National Institutes of Health show that coronary symptoms are treated less aggressively in women—fewer coronary bypasses, for example. In addition, most heart research is done on men, so doctors do not know as much about the causes—and treatment—of heart disease in women. None of these factors have anything to do with work.

But doesn't working put women at greater risk for stress-related illnesses? No. Paid work is actually associated with *reduced* anxiety and depression. In the early 1980s we reported in our book, *Lifeprints* (based on a National Science Foundation–funded study of 300 women), that working women were significantly higher in psychological well-being than those not employed. Working gave them a sense of mastery and control that homemaking didn't provide. More recent studies echo our findings. For example:

• A 1989 report by psychologist Ingrid Waldron and sociologist Jerry Jacobs of Temple University on nationwide surveys of 2,392 white and 892 black women,

conducted from 1977 to 1982, found that women who held both work and family roles reported better physical and mental health than homemakers.

• According to sociologists Elaine Wethington of Cornell University and Ronald Kessler of the University of Michigan, data from three years (1985 to 1988) of a continuing federally funded study of 745 married women in Detroit "clearly suggests that employment benefits women emotionally." Women who increase their participation in the labor force report lower levels of psychological distress; those who lessen their commitment to work suffer from higher distress.

• A University of California at Berkeley study published in 1990 followed 140 women for 22 years. At age 43, those who were homemakers had more chronic conditions than the working women and seemed more disillusioned and frustrated. The working mothers were in good health and seemed to be juggling their roles with success.

In sum, paid work offers women heightened self-esteem and enhanced mental and physical health. It's unemployment that's a major risk factor for depression in women.

DOING IT ALL–AND DOING FINE

This isn't true only for affluent women in good jobs; working-class women share the benefits of work, according to psychologists Sandra Scarr and Deborah Phillips of the University of Virginia and Kathleen McCartney of the University of New Hampshire. In reviewing 80 studies on this subject, they reported that working-class women with children say they would not leave work even if they didn't need the money. Work offers not only income but adult companionship, social contact and a connection with the wider world that they cannot get at home.

Doing it all may be tough, but it doesn't wipe out the health benefits of working.

Looking at survey data from around the world, Scarr and Phillips wrote that the lives of mothers who work are not more stressful than the lives of those who are at home. So what about the second shift we've heard so much about? It certainly exists: In industrialized countries, researchers found, fathers work an average of 50 hours a week on the job and doing household chores; mothers work an average of 80 hours. Wethington and Kessler found that in daily "stress diaries" kept by husbands and wives, the women report more stress than the men do. But they also handle it better. In short, doing it all may be tough, but it doesn't wipe out the health benefits of working.

THE ADVANTAGES FOR FAMILIES

What about the kids? Many working parents feel they want more time with their kids, and they say so. But does maternal employment harm children? In 1989 University of Michigan psychologist Lois Hoffman reviewed 50 years of research and found that the expected negative effects never materialized. Most often, children of employed and unemployed mothers didn't differ on measures of child development. But children of both sexes with working mothers have a less sex-stereotyped view of the world because fathers in two-income families tend to do more child care.

However, when mothers work, the quality of non-parental child care is a legitimate worry. Scarr, Phillips and McCartney say there is "near consensus among developmental psychologists and early-childhood experts that child care per se does not constitute a risk factor in children's lives." What causes problems, they report, is poor-quality care and a troubled family life. The need for good child care in this country has been obvious for some time.

What's more, children in two-job families generally don't lose out on one-to-one time with their parents. New studies, such as S. L. Nock and P. W. Kingston's *Time with Children: The Impact of Couples' Work-Time Commitments,* show that when both parents of pre-schoolers are working, they spend as much time in direct interaction with their children as families in which only the fathers work. The difference is that working parents spend more time with their kids on weekends. When only the husband works, parents spend more leisure time with each other. There is a cost to two-income families—the couples lose personal time—but the kids don't seem to pay it.

One question we never used to ask is whether having a working mother could be *good* for children. Hoffman, reflecting on the finding that employed women—both blue-collar and professional—register higher life-satisfaction scores than housewives, thinks it can be. She cites studies involving infants and older children, showing that a mother's satisfaction with her employment status relates positively both to "the quality of the mother-child interaction and to various indexes of the child's adjustment and abilities." For example, psychologists J. Guidubaldi and B. K. Nastasi of Kent State University reported in a 1987 paper that a mother's satisfaction with her job was a good predictor of her child's positive adjustment in school.

Again, this isn't true only for women in high-status jobs. In a 1982 study of sources of stress for children in low-income families, psychologists Cynthia Longfellow and Deborah Belle of the Harvard University School of Education found that employed women were generally less depressed than unemployed women. What's more, their children had fewer behavioral problems.

But the real point about working women and children is that work *isn't* the point at all. There are good mothers and not-so-good mothers, and some work and some don't. When a National Academy of Sciences panel reviewed the previous 50 years of research and dozens of studies in 1982, it found no consistent effects on children from a mother's working. Work is only one of many variables, the panel concluded in *Families That Work,* and not the definitive one.

What is the effect of women's working on their marriages? Having a working wife can increase psychological stress for men, especially older men, who grew up in a world where it was not normal for a wife to work. But men's expectations that they will—and must—be the only provider may be changing. Wethington and Kessler found that a wife's employment could be a significant buffer *against* depression for men born after 1945. Still, the picture of men's psychological well-being is very mixed, and class and expectations clearly play a role. Faludi cites polls showing that young blue-collar men are especially angry at women for invading what they see as their turf as breadwinners, even though a woman with such a job could help protect her husband from economic hardship. But in highly educated, dual-career couples, both partners say the wife's career has enhanced the marriage.

THE FIRST SHIFT: WOMEN AT WORK

While women's own health and the well-being of their families aren't harmed by their working, what effect does this dual role have on their job performance? It's assumed that men can compartmentalize work and home lives but women will bring their home worries with them to work, making them distracted and inefficient employees.

Perhaps the most dangerous myth is that the solution is for women to drop back—or drop out.

The only spillover went in the other direction: The women brought their good feelings about their work home with them and left a bad day at home behind when they came to work. In fact, Wethington and Kessler found that it was the *men* who brought the family stresses with them to work. "Women are able to avoid bringing the contagion of home stress into the workplace," the researchers write, "whereas the inability of men to prevent this kind of contagion is pervasive." The researchers speculate that perhaps women get the message early on that they can handle the home front, while men are taking on chores they aren't trained for and didn't expect.

THE PERILS OF PART-TIME

Perhaps the most dangerous myth is that the solution to most problems women suffer is for them to drop back—or drop out. What studies actually show is a significant connection between a reduced commitment to work and increased psychological stress. In their Detroit study, Wethington and Kessler noted that women who went from being full-time employees to full-time housewives reported increased symptoms of distress, such as depression and anxiety attacks; the longer a woman worked and the more committed she was to the job, the greater her risk for psychological distress when she stopped.

What about part-time work, that oft-touted solution for weary women? Women who work fewer than 20 hours per week, it turns out, do not get the mental-health work benefit, probably because they "operate under the fiction that they can retain full responsibility for child care and home maintenance," wrote Wethington and Kessler. The result: Some part-timers wind up more stressed-out than women working full-time. Part-time employment also provides less money, fewer or no benefits and, often, less interesting work and a more arduous road to promotion.

That doesn't mean that a woman shouldn't cut down on her work hours or arrange a more flexible schedule. But it does mean she should be careful about jumping on a poorly designed mommy track that may make her a second-class citizen at work.

Many women think that when they have a baby, the best thing for their mental health would be to stay home. Wrong once more. According to Wethington and Kessler, having a baby does not increase psychological distress for working women—*unless* the birth results in their dropping out of the labor force. This doesn't mean that any woman who stays home to care for a child is going to be a wreck. But leaving the work force means opting out of the benefits of being in it, and women should be aware of that.

As soon as a woman has any kind of difficulty—emotional, family, medical—the knee-jerk reaction is to get her off the job. No such solution is offered to men, despite the very real correlation for men between job stress and heart attacks.

What the myth of the miserable working woman obscures is the need to focus on how the *quality* of a woman's job affects her health. Media stories warn of the alleged dangers of fast-track jobs. But our *Lifeprints* study found that married women in high-prestige jobs were highest in mental well-being; another study of life stress in women reported that married career women with children suffered the least from stress. Meanwhile, few media tears are shed for the women most at risk: those in the word-processing room who have no control at work, low pay and little support at home.

Women don't need help getting out of the work force; they need help staying in it. As long as much of the media continues to capitalize on national ignorance, that help will have to come from somewhere else. (Not that an occasional letter to the editor isn't useful.) Men need to recognize that they are not just occasional helpers but vital to the success of the family unit. The corporate culture has to be reshaped so that it doesn't run totally according to patterns set by the white male workaholic. This will be good for men *and* women. The government can guarantee parental leave and affordable, available child care. (It did so in the '40s, when women were needed in the factories.) Given that Congress couldn't even get a bill guaranteeing *unpaid* family leave passed last year, this may take some doing. But hey, this is an election year.

Stressed Out—and Sick from It

The Ultimate Prevention Guide

When you feel your life spinning out of control, you may also find yourself coming down with an assortment of common ills. But the right relaxation techniques, new research shows, can keep disease at bay.

SUSAN GILBERT

Susan Gilbert writes the "Ob/Gyn" column for Redbook.

FOR THE LAST MONTH, YOU'VE BEEN WORKING NIGHTS AND weekends on a report that your temperamental boss keeps criticizing. Meanwhile, your husband is irritated that you are spending so much time away from the family, and you're worried you'll never find the time to shop for your son's upcoming birthday party. Suddenly you begin to feel draggy, feverish, achy. It's not in your head—you've got the flu.

Did the stress make you sick? For years, doctors have written off any number of symptoms as "just nerves"—and we've resented them for not taking our complaints seriously. But recently, the stress-illness connection has been elevated from a touchy-feely concept to an area of serious research, with scientists making tremendous progress in nailing down the mechanisms of the link. When you're under stress, it seems, your body releases certain hormones, like cortisol, which in turn suppress immune-system cells, says Norman B. Anderson, Ph.D., director of the Office of Behavioral and Social Sciences Research at the National Institutes of Health. Lowered immunity, in turn, makes you more vulnerable to an assortment of illnesses.

Not all stress is harmful, fortunately. Routine hassles—car trouble, a tiff with a neighbor over garbage cans, an all-nighter with a teething baby—may leave you feeling strung out, but they won't make a blip on your overall well-being. The kind of stress that has been linked to illness, explains Curt A. Sandman, Ph.D., vice-chairman of psychiatry at the University of California at Irvine, falls into two categories: One is a major distressing change in your life, such as the death of a loved one, a divorce, or a job loss. The second category is the stress that accompanies extreme and ongoing anxiety, anger, or depression. These may be linked to sad events (worry about a parent's illness, for example) or to ongoing discord at home or work, but even so-called "good" stress (a promotion or move to a new home) can be bad for you if it makes you exceedingly anxious or depressed, says Dr. Sandman.

The illnesses linked to emotional turmoil are surprisingly common, the new research suggests. Indeed, it has been estimated that two-thirds of all visits to family doctors are—to some degree—stress-related, reports Dr. Anderson. But research is also showing that the number could be lower if we understand how stress makes us sick . . . and what steps we can take to offset its assault.

COLDS AND FLU

Six years ago, Sheldon Cohen, Ph.D., a professor of psychology at Carnegie Mellon University, conducted the pioneering studies that showed the connection between stress and colds. First, using standard psychological tests, he measured the stress levels of 394 women and men, then exposed them to one of five cold viruses. The results: 47 percent of those under the most stress became sick, compared to only 27 percent of the least beleaguered participants. The kind of stress associated with the greatest probability of developing a cold, Dr. Cohen found in a different study, stemmed from prolonged dis-

From *Redbook*, March 1997, pp. 110, 112, 128. © 1997 by Susan Gilbert. Reprinted by permission.

cord in personal relationships. This means six months or more of such troubled relations as ongoing fights with your spouse or constant and severe criticism from your boss.

Stress doesn't cause the cold, of course, but researchers believe that it makes us more susceptible to cold viruses by depressing the immune system. The same seems to happen with flu viruses: Studies at Ohio State University College of Medicine have found that women who are under a great deal of stress (they're caring for seriously ill relatives) have a weaker immune response to an influenza vaccine than women dealing with more routine pressures (long lines at the supermarket, for example). The weaker response to the vaccine, says Janice Kiecolt-Glaser, Ph.D., director of the division of health psychology at the college, indicates that the women may also be more vulnerable to the flu itself.

STOMACHACHES

Half of healthy adults say they get abdominal pain when they're stressed out, according to a survey done at the University of North Carolina at Chapel Hill. What seems to happen, says William E. Whitehead, Ph.D., a psychologist and physiologist at the university, is that the stress causes increased contractions of the gastrointestinal tract, resulting in cramps in the lower abdomen.

In addition, if when you're feeling edgy, you overeat (as many of us do), it puts extra pressure on the esophageal sphincter, the valve that separates the esophagus and the stomach. Under such pressure, explains Dr. Whitehead, acid backs up from the stomach into the esophagus, causing heartburn. And how you eat can distress your gut too. Tension can cause you to wolf down your food, filling your stomach with too much air, which leaves you feeling bloated and nauseated.

HEADACHES

You're stuck in traffic when you've got to pick up your child from day care and you're hit with that predictable dull, throbbing pain in your head. Stress is the most common cause of the aptly named tension headache, according to Seymour Diamond, M.D., director of the Diamond Headache Clinic in Chicago.

What happens, he explains, is that stress hormones cause muscle contractions in the face, scalp, neck, and jaw (as well as elsewhere throughout the body). Then muscles contract, they're deprived of blood; this deprivation initiates a chemical chain reaction culminating in the production of prostaglandins, hormonelike substances that enhance the sensation of pain.

IRREGULAR PERIODS

Stress hormones can delay or prevent the release of follicle-stimulating hormone and luteinizing hormone, chemicals that are essential to ovulation, says Machelle M. Seibel, M.D., medical director at the Faulkner Centre for Reproductive Medicine in Boston. As a result, during times of stress you may stop ovulating or ovulate erratically. Your period may be late, or it may not come at all for months. Fortunately, the effect is temporary, says Dr. Seibel. When the stress and its emotional fallout pass, your menstrual cycle usually returns to normal within a few months.

Surprisingly, however, tension doesn't cause PMS. When in a 1990 study Joseph F. Mortola, M.D., director of the division of reproductive endocrinology at Cook County Hospital in Chicago, asked women to list the stressful events in their lives for 90 days, he found no correlation between their stress level and the severity of their PMS.

INFERTILITY

Stress won't absolutely prevent pregnancy, but "in women whose fertility is compromised, the addition of substantial stress may be sufficient to prevent pregnancy from happening," reports Dr. Seibel. One way is by interfering with ovulation. If you're not ovulating, you can't get pregnant. And if your ovulation schedule is unpredictable, you have no way of knowing when you're fertile and may miss opportunities to conceive. Stress can also reduce your husband's fertility by lowering his sperm count.

PREGNANCY COMPLICATIONS

For a long time, many ob/gyns have believed that the amount of stress you're under while pregnant could influence the size of your baby, says Dr. Sandman of the University of California at Irvine. Recently, though, he adds, "we've been able to pinpoint that gestational age appears to be influenced by stress too." In a study of pregnant women, he has found that every point the mothers-to-be score on a 15-point stress scale (which measures the spectrum of turmoil—from daily hassles to anxiety about the baby's health) predicts a three-day decrease in the length of pregnancy.

Even if a pregnancy goes full term, other research suggests, stress can make labor more difficult. In a 1991 study, John Kennell, M.D., professor of pediatrics at Case Western Reserve University, compared the labor and delivery of two groups of women: those who had a doula (a woman specially trained to give emotional, physical, and informational support during labor) and women who had doctors and nurses only. Only 7.8 percent of the women in the doula group needed an epidural, compared to 55 percent of the others. What's more, just 8

Rx FOR STRESS: WHAT WORKS BEST

There's growing scientific evidence that relieving stress can keep you healthy or help you get well once you are sick. Any number of techniques may help; the trick is to pick one that suits your personality and lifestyle. Ordinary aerobic exercise—running, bicycling, swimming—reduces muscle tension *and* improves anxiety and coping skills, studies have shown. Meditation (see the classic *Relaxation Response*, by Herbert Benson, M.D., for a clear description), relaxation tapes, yoga (classes available at private studios, gyms, and Ys), or biofeedback (available at hospitals, clinics, and in psychologists' offices) work well for many women.

And when you feel tension creeping up, quick relaxation techniques can defuse the physiological responses. You might try closing your eyes for a few moments and imagining a beautiful scene (really focus on the details, counting the trees or ripples of water on the lake) or closing your eyes, taking a deep breath and then, on each exhale, slowly counting backward from 10 or 20, visualizing yourself slowing walking downstairs. In terms of specific illnesses, researchers have found that stress reduction alleviates the following:

HEADACHES Biofeedback to reduce emotional distress or psychotherapy to improve your ability to cope cuts down both on the number of tension headaches and their severity, reports headache specialist Seymour Diamond, M.D.

INFERTILITY In a 1990 study, infertility expert Machelle M. Seibel, M.D., and Herbert Benson, M.D., founding president of the Mind/Body Institute at New England Deaconess Hospital, found that 34 percent of infertile women who added relaxation training to their treatment regimens became pregnant. Since there was no control group, the researchers can't say exactly how much the training improved fertility rates, but "it was certainly higher than expected," reports Dr. Seibel.

ASTHMA Hypnosis and psychotherapy can actually halt the stress-induced biological response that makes the airways tighten, says David A. Mrazek, M.D., of Children's National Medical Center. Relaxation doesn't provide a quick fix, but decreases the number of attacks over the long run.

percent of the women supported by doulas ended up having C-sections, against 18 percent of the control group.

Dr. Kennell doesn't know exactly how the doulas helped, but it's a good bet, he speculates, that their support reduced the women's anxiety, which is associated with stress hormones. These hormones can make uterine contractions less effective, so it's possible that lowering the stress levels will result in more effective contractions, thereby shortening labor and delivery.

SKIN DISORDERS

Ever wonder why you break out just before an important dinner party? Emotional distress may cause flare-ups of acne, herpes, and psoriasis, preliminary research suggests. The mechanism seems to be the same as the one that makes you less resistant to colds: "Stress hormones go up and then immune function is suppressed," says Dr. Kiecolt-Glaser.

Emotional turmoil can also slow down the process of wound healing, she and coresearcher Ronald Glaser, Ph.D., a virologist at Ohio State University College of Medicine, have found. Compared to less-stressed women, the caregivers in their studies took an average of 24 percent longer—47 days compared with 38 days—to recover from small puncture wounds.

ASTHMA

Years ago children's asthma was blamed on their mothers' anxiety-providing personalities. While that notion has been laid to rest, research has found that stress can induce asthma in people who are genetically predisposed to it, says David A. Mrazek, M.D., chairman of psychiatry and behavioral sciences at Children's National Medical Center in Washington, D.C. High-anxiety situations can trigger asthma by stimulating the production of neurotransmitters, which in turn may "switch on" genes responsible for the condition, speculates Dr. Mrazek.

Thereafter, he says, a stressful event or negative emotion like anger can induce an asthmatic attack; the airways are assaulted with nerve impulses that cause the airways to constrict. "Half of the asthmatics out there have an attack from stress," says Dr. Mrazek.

These are only a few of the areas where researchers are pursuing links between illness and emotional distress. One big unknown: whether stress can cause cancer. Studies suggest a connection, but aren't yet definitive. As scientists figure out more sophisticated ways to research these mind-body connections, they should be able to pinpoint exactly which illnesses can be traced to stress and—even better—how we can use mind-calming techniques to cure ills or prevent them from taking root in the first place.

Depression

Way Beyond the Blues

Sandra Arbetter

Maria hasn't smiled in a month. Not even when her terrier rushes around in circles trying to bite his tail. Not even when her boyfriend lip-synchs to the Spin Doctors. Either of those things used to set her to howling, but lately she just wants to stay in her room and sleep, and it's a struggle for her to get up in the morning and go to school.

Andy, on the other hand, is always smiling. He talks nonstop, and his energy is endless. He jumps into things without a second thought—he drives too fast, drinks alcohol, and can't wait to bungee jump. At night his mind races over the next day's activities, until he finally falls into a restless sleep.

Which of these two may be depressed? If you say Maria, you're right. And if you say Andy, you're right, too. Even though they act very differently, they both are in the midst of a long period of depression. If you say that's confusing, you're right again. Depression is a murky pool of feelings and actions that scientists have been trying to plumb since the days of Hippocrates, who called it a "black bile."

To further muddy the waters, feelings of depression come and go in most of us from time to time. But short periods of sadness or hyperactivity don't mean clinical depression.

Clinical depression is severe enough to require treatment. It lasts a longer time than the blues—at least two weeks—and it interferes with daily life—school, friends, family. It's considered a medical disorder and can affect thoughts, feelings, physical health, and behaviors. Here's what it's not: It's NOT a personality weakness or a moral lapse. And it's NOT the fault of the person who is depressed.

Diagnosing depression in a teenager is not easy, says Dr. Richard Marohn, past president of the American Society of Adolescent Psychiatry. That's because it's normal for teens to have mood swings—within limits.

It's a confusing time of life, says Marohn. For one thing, the teen's body is changing. Teenagers have little control over those changes. Secondly, their relationship with parents is changing, and teens are pulled between

---

Science Whips Up a Moral Dilemma

Ron was a pleasant, quiet boy who liked to spend time by himself, mostly with his computer. His mother said he "moved at his own pace," which was a bit slower than the rest of the family.

When Ron was 17, he withdrew further from others, stopped showering and shampooing, and even lost his interest in computers. His parents arranged for him to see a psychiatrist, who prescribed an antidepressant medication.

To say he responded well would be an understatement. He was peppier than ever before, moved faster, laughed more readily, liked being with people, went from being a B to an A student, and got a girlfriend.

His doctor was pleased—but puzzled. Now that Ron was no longer depressed, should he go off medication

and return to his former quiet self? Or should he stay on medication and retain his livelier, more confident personality? Did the medication uncover the "real" Ron who had lived a lifetime beneath a cover of chronic, mild depression? Or did it create a false self?

Antidepressants are designed to relieve the symptoms of depression. But is it OK to use them as what one doctor called "mood brighteners"? That's the question posed by author Peter Kramer, M.D.

Mental health experts express the concern that we will look to a pill to make us feel better and we'll ignore the external problems in our world. Some fear that antidepressants interfere with reality by making things look more positive. Or could it be that depression distorts reality by making things look more grim?

---

the security of home and the challenge of testing out their own beliefs.

So how do you tell if it's depression? Time tells, says Marohn. If your feelings affect your schoolwork, your activities, your relationship with family and friends, then it's beyond normal.

Suicidal urges and plans are also a warning sign. But even that's not surefire, because lots of teens have transient thoughts of suicide.

Finally, adolescent depression is difficult to diagnose because adolescents don't necessarily look sad and depressed. To be a teen means to externalize feelings and deal with the world through action. So depression may show up as truancy, running away, violent behavior, or substance abuse. Teens may self-medicate with alcohol or other drugs to try to feel better.

WHAT IS DEPRESSION?

Lots of people assume they know what depression is because they've had at least a touch of it. It's natural to feel sad when you're hit by one of life's inevitable losses. It's a loss when you start kindergarten and give up the safety of home. It's a loss when you move to a new house and leave the old one behind. It's a loss to break up with a boyfriend or girlfriend, and it's even worse when he or she is doing the breaking up.

The sadness that comes with events like these can be intense at first, but usually mellows in a short while. If you get back to a relatively normal state in a week or so, there's nothing to worry about. But if feelings of great sadness or agitation last for much more than two weeks, it may be depression.

Depressed feelings after a major loss, such as the death of a loved one, last much longer, and no one expects recovery in a week or two. Experts won't make a diagnosis of depression (at least, not right away) if a person has had a recent major loss. They'll also hold off if a person is taking certain medications or has certain illnesses that bring on depression-like symptoms.

How Antidepressants Work

Antidepressants help people feel better by affecting neurotransmitters and, in turn, brain function. Neurotransmitters are brain chemicals that help nerve cells communicate with each other. Certain ones are thought to control feelings of security and alertness.

Although the specific effects have not been worked out, it is though that antidepressants work by helping to regulate the dysfunction in the brain that is causing a person to feel depressed.

CHECK THESE SYMPTOMS

Changes in habits and personality are clues to depression. Here are some specifics:
1. There's no interest in school and grades fall.
2. Being with friends holds absolutely no appeal.
3. Sleep problems are common—either not being able to fall asleep at night or wanting to sleep all day.
4. Appetite is out of whack. There's either no desire for food, or the person seems to be eating all the time.
5. The person is obsessed with thoughts of death, maybe suicide. It's estimated that 15 percent of people with major depression commit suicide, and many more attempt it. There are 6,000 suicides by adolescents each year, and depression is the biggest risk factor.
6. Everything seems hopeless, and there's the feeling it will never get better.
7. Headaches, stomachaches, or other aches and pains appear.
8. It's impossible to concentrate or make a decision.

WHAT IT FEELS LIKE

Anyone who's ever felt sad has only the barest clue as to what major depression is like, according to one 16-year-old who recently spent three weeks in a hospital after taking an overdose of pills.

"I had this buzzing in my head all the time," says Emmy, a small, dark-haired girl with large brown eyes. "And I felt tired. I didn't want to do anything except lie on my bed and listen to tapes. When my friends called, I didn't feel like talking to them. I knew they were getting mad, and sometimes I'd try to talk on the phone, but I couldn't push the words up out of my throat."

Emmy had always been a good student and had managed a B+ average while holding a job at a discount store and swimming in competition. Her father was a building contractor, and her mother was a secretary.

"My mother never liked her job, and she kept telling me that I needed to get into a good college so I could be a lawyer and have a happier life than she had. I know now that she was struggling with her own problems, but I used to worry all the time that I was disappointing her. I wanted so badly to be an A student, but no matter how hard I studied, I couldn't pull it off.

"Then I just started not caring. Nothing special happened; I just shut down. I felt so alone, like I was living in a bubble and couldn't punch my way out. I felt like screaming so someone would notice me.

"And I was so tired all the time. Nobody can understand that. I wasn't tired physically like after a swim meet or staying up late. I was tired in every cell of my body, so that I couldn't think straight, and it was too much of an effort to eat. Finally, one day I decided it was too much of an effort to live. That's when I took the pills."

The doctor prescribed an antidepressant drug for Emmy for about six months, and she and her parents were in family therapy for more than a year. She's a junior now and planning to go to college to study environmental sciences. Her mother is in law school.

DEPRESSION IS A MIXED BAG

For a long time, people who were feeling depressed were told to "snap out of it," and, if they didn't, people said they had a flaw in their personality. That's simply not true and only added guilt to the heavy burden these people were already carrying.

Research in the last decade or two has shown, first of all, that there are several kinds of depression and a multitude of causes.

•Major depression: More than one episode of clinical depression is considered major depression, an illness marked by hopeless feelings, inability to feel pleasure, physical changes or complaints, thoughts of death and suicide. The Public Health Service estimates that 11 million people in this country have episodes of major depression, women outnumbering men more than 2 to 1.

•Bipolar disorder (also known as manic-depressive disorder): A person with this illness alternates between periods of high activity, or mania, and periods of hopelessness or depression.

In the manic phase, people may talk a lot—and fast. They have feelings of greatness and think nothing is beyond them. They've been known to go days without sleeping. They've got lots of thoughts racing through their mind at once. They often act on these thoughts and get into trouble because of their behaviors. So, if you have a friend who is in the manic phase of this illness, don't be surprised if you get a call at three in the morning about his or her plans to save the earth.

Bipolar disorder occurs in about 1 percent of the population, or about 2 million people, equally in men and women. Bipolar disorder can take years to develop into its classic form. When a bipolar disorder emerges during adolescence, it's sometimes hard to distinguish it from the normal emotional ups and downs associated with that age.

•Seasonal Affective Disorder, or SAD: It's not exactly a news flash that most people feel better when the weather is sunny and bright than when it's gloomy. But for some people, wintry weather brings on feelings of depression. Here's one explanation: Many of the body's functions operate on circadian cycles, which are about 24 hours in length. Lack of light puts these cycles out of whack. One treatment is to have patients sit under bright lights for a few hours each day.

•Dysthymia: This is low-level chronic depression. It's usually not severe enough to put someone in the hospital, or to prompt suicide, but it robs a person of the capacity to take pleasure in living.

WHY, OH, WHY?

Experts don't completely understand the causes of depression, but there seems to be an important interplay of two factors: environmental and biological.

Environmental factors include such events as death of a parent, parents' divorce, physical or emotional abuse, family violence, and other difficult family relationships. A depressive episode can be triggered by moving, graduating, losing a job, winning an award, or a hundred other life changes. It can be related to emotional conflicts within the person, such as a past experience that was not resolved. It's been described as "anger turned inward." Or it can come on for no apparent reason.

Biological factors, primarily changes in brain function, are an important aspect of depression. It is not known whether the observed changes in the function cause depression, or whether depression from some other cause accounts for the changes in brain function.

There seems to be a genetic factor involved, too. A child whose parent has suffered from depression has a greater chance of developing the illness than a child with no family history of depression.

TREATMENT

Major approaches to helping depression are medication and psychotherapy, or counseling. Experts say upward of 80 percent of people with depression can be helped.

Medications affect brain function and reduce the symptoms of depression but do not provide a cure. All antidepressants have side effects. Experts worry that people will think of them as magic potions and not accept responsibility for their own behaviors. (See "Science Whips Up a Moral Dilemma".) Finally, parents are cautious about allowing medications for their children.

Psychiatrist Richard Marohn says that many experts view adolescent depression as short-lived and say treatment should deal with underlying issues rather than the symptoms themselves. Therefore, "talk therapy" is preferable and "most of us working with adolescents tend to stay away from medication." Exceptions are suicidal behaviors and depression that's been going on since childhood.

Dr. Marohn says he is concerned about the increasing lack of mental health services. "Kids wind up in prison," he says, rather than in hospitals where treatment is available and they may get some help.

TALKING IT OUT

Some experts say the most effective treatment for severe depression is a combination of medication and counseling. Counseling can help by making people aware of negative thought patterns, such as: "If I'm not perfect, people will think less of me." Or, "If I fail this test, it means I'll always be a failure." It can improve a person's ability to get along with others and to understand him- or herself better. It can bolster self-esteem.

What's more, there are lots of things people can do on their own to help themselves feel better. Michael Maloney and Rachel Kranz, authors of *Straight Talk About Anxiety and Depression*, suggest these:
• Try to focus on the positives about yourself rather than the negatives.
• Accept the fact that others aren't perfect. Then you won't be disappointed when they act human.
• Accept that you aren't perfect, either.

• Enjoy the present moment. Stop regretting the past and worrying about the future.
• Take care of yourself physically. Eat well, exercise, get plenty of sleep.
• Do something nice for yourself.
• Improve your surroundings. Clean your closet. Get a new poster. Surround yourself with things you like to look at.
• Talk to someone. Call up a friend you trust, or start a conversation with a neighbor to prove you *can* connect.
• Indulge your feelings. Let yourself cry and wallow in sad songs. But only for a little while.

Depression is one of the most common mental illnesses of our era and responds well to treatment. So while people don't do anything to make themselves feel bad, they *can* do something to make themselves feel better. A generation ago, there was a comic strip character named Arthur, who walked everywhere with a cloud over his head. If he knew then what you know now, he'd reach up and pull out a silver lining.

How to Help a Friend Who Is Depressed

Sometimes it's more difficult to help others than to help yourself. But here are some things to think about if a friend seems depressed.

1. Make an effort to be with your friend, even though it might not be easy. Depressed people tend to feel isolated.

2. Don't use false cheerfulness. Your friend may feel you aren't taking the problem seriously.

3. Don't blame. Depression is no one's fault.

4. Don't get angry. It's nothing personal if your friend doesn't respond to your help.

5. Express your own feelings. If you don't want to listen to your friend's woes again, just say so. Go out and have fun and don't feel guilty.

6. Get adult help. If your friend talks about suicide, or you're worried for any other reason, talk to your parents, your friend's parents, your school counselor. It's not a breach of loyalty to save a friend's life.

FOR MORE INFORMATION

American Psychiatric Association
1400 K St. NW
Washington, DC 20005
  Pamphlets: "Depression," "Manic-Depressive Disorder," "Teen Suicide," single copy of each free. Booklet: "Let's Talk About It," $1 per copy. Also available in Spanish.

S. James
Consumer Information Center-3C
P.O. Box 100
Pueblo, CO 81002
  Pamphlets: #564z "What To Do When A Friend Is Depressed—A Guide For Teenagers," #566z "You Are Not Alone," single copy of each free.

National Mental Health Association
1021 Prince St.
Alexandria, VA 22314-2971
  Pamphlets: "Adolescent Depression," "Adolescent Suicide," single copy of each free with self-addressed, stamped business-size envelope.

American Academy of Pediatrics
Dept. C-Depression
P.O. Box 927
Elk Grove Village, IL 60009-0927
  Pamphlet: "Surviving: Coping With Adolescent Depression/Suicide," single copy free with self-addressed, stamped business-size envelope.

Treating Eating Disorders

Few of us have a truly healthy relationship with food. We want to experience the pleasure of eating but fear becoming fat. For a growing number of women, this normally manageable conflict develops into a painful, destructive, and sometimes life-threatening eating disorder.

Two eating disorders — anorexia nervosa, a condition characterized by deliberate food restriction and severe weight loss, and bulimia nervosa, one involving frequent bouts of binge eating followed by self-induced vomiting, laxative abuse, or excessive exercise — are listed in the *Diagnostic and Statistical Manual of Mental Disorders (DSM)*. Some experts have proposed that binge-eating disorder be added to the *DSM*, the reference in which the criteria for all recognized psychiatric conditions are listed. Because there weren't enough data to warrant its inclusion as a diagnosis in the manual's fourth and most recent edition, it was listed as a proposed condition. According to the proposed criteria, the symptoms of binge-eating disorder are similar to those of bulimia, except that people who suffer from it do not purge and are usually significantly overweight.

The criteria for anorexia and bulimia are listed in the box on the next page. In the United States, more than eight million people, 90% of whom are women, are now believed to meet the criteria for one of the two.

These statistics don't tell the whole story: many more women may be unduly preoccupied with food and suffer from "subclinical" eating disorders. These abnormal eating patterns and attitudes do not meet all the diagnostic criteria for an eating disorder but are nonetheless disruptive enough to daily life to warrant treatment.

Possible causes

The term "eating disorder" is something of a misnomer, since these conditions may have more to do with how we perceive our bodies than how we feel about eating. As most of us know, the disorders are far more prevalent in industrialized countries where there is a strong cultural bias toward thinness. Sometimes, however, eating is the issue, particularly for anorectics, who may feel a strong need to control some aspect of their lives by denying themselves the pleasure of food.

Women with anorexia or bulimia have traditionally come from white, middle- or upper-middle class families in which there is an undue emphasis on achievement, body weight, and appearance. However, both seem to be increasingly independent of socioeconomic status. Although some experts once theorized that women with a history of sexual abuse were more likely to develop eating disorders, research has not substantiated this belief.

Some studies have shown that identical twin sisters of women with anorexia are more likely than fraternal twins to have the condition, suggesting that it may also have a genetic basis. A high proportion of people with eating disorders also have a mother or sister with an eating disorder or a family or personal history of major depressive disease, other mood disorders, or substance abuse. In fact, about half of those in treatment for anorexia or bulimia are clinically depressed; a quarter — particularly those with bulimia or bulimic symptoms — are alcoholics or have other addictions like compulsive stealing.

Because anorexia and bulimia so often coexist with mood disorders, many researchers have theorized that the conditions may be partly the result of faulty regulation of the neurotransmitter serotonin, which is believed to elevate mood and produce feelings of satiety, or fullness. The fact that selective serotonin reuptake inhibitors (SSRIs), such as fluoxetine (Prozac), sertraline (Zoloft), and paroxetine (Paxil) — which increase the amount of serotonin in the brain — may improve some of the symptoms of these conditions lends some credence to this theory.

Treatment approaches

For many people, eating disorders are essentially chronic conditions that can wax and wane over the course of a lifetime. Thus, once any health crises that have arisen from the condition are brought under control, treatment is directed at helping the patient understand the psychological, social, and physiological factors that may have contributed to her illness and develop strategies for managing them.

It isn't necessary to go to a specialized — and expensive — eating disorders "center" for treatment, but it is important to find a therapist who understands the chronic nature of the disorder and who has had experience treating people who have it.

Women with bulimia can recognize that they are ill and may seek treatment on their own, but because anorectic women deny that they are sick, they are more often brought for treatment by a family member or friend.

The first step in treatment is an evaluation by a psychiatrist or other mental-health clinician. During the initial meeting, the therapist will discuss the diagnosis and propose a treatment plan, which will most likely include a referral to an internist for a medical evaluation and to a nutritionist who has worked with people with eating disorders.

Some anorectic patients are already suffering the physical effects of starvation, including emaciation, drying and yellowing of the skin, the growth of fine downy hair over the face and arms, anemia, elevated serum cholesterol, decreased metabolic rate, decreased muscle mass, irregular heart rhythms, and osteoporosis. In extreme cases, women with anorexia may require hospitalization until they can regain at least some of their lost weight; rarely, some may need to be force-fed through a nasogastric tube or intravenous catheter.

By contrast, women with bulimia are usually of normal weight or slightly overweight. Those who induce vomiting often have tell-tale scrapes or abrasions on their knuckles, and their teeth may have lost enamel from repeated contact with stomach acids. Women who abuse laxatives may have chronic, watery diarrhea, and rectocele, in which the walls of the rectum protrude against the wall of the vagina. In extreme cases, bulimics may be dehydrated, have gastric bleeding, and suffer from life-threatening electrolyte imbalances. In general, however, women with bulimia are less likely to require hospitalization than those with anorexia.

The most successful treatment plans usually involve a well-coordinated team: a primary-care clinician to monitor the patient's physical condition, a nutritionist to provide counseling and instruction in developing acceptable eating habits, and a psychotherapist to help reverse destructive patterns and develop practical substitutions for them.

If the patient is depressed or has compulsive symptoms, she may also receive an SSRI, like fluoxetine (Prozac), or a tricyclic antidepressant such as desipramine (Norpramin). These medications are intended to treat only such symptoms, not the eating disorder itself.

No single method of psychological counseling has been shown to be universally effective for all of the eating disorders. However, some studies have found that women with bulimia often benefit from individual cognitive-behavioral therapy, in which the patient and her therapist examine distorted thinking about weight and food and come up with practical strategies for changing it. These programs may include keeping a journal of binge-eating and purging episodes and using it to identify feelings or situations that trigger binges. The patient and therapist can then work out more productive strategies for coping with these situations when they arise.

Psychotherapy, in which the patient sorts out family and personal issues that may have precipitated her illness, may be used alone or in conjunction with cognitive-behavioral therapy. Other family members are likely to benefit from counseling, both to help to break the patterns that contribute to the disorder and to learn to live with a person who has a complex and disruptive illness.

Group therapy led by a trained professional is often effective in addressing the sense of isolation that characterizes eating disorders, particularly anorexia. One of the more successful approaches is a three-step program in which patients learn about eating disorders and connect with other women in similar situations, work together with a therapist to understand the issues underlying their illness, and learn to use creative relaxation strategies to respond to the stresses that trigger the disorder.

For further information: Eating Disorders Awareness and Prevention, (206) 382-3587; American Anorexia/Bulimia Association, (212) 501-8351

EATING DISORDER CRITERIA

Anorexia

According to the DSM-IV, people who meet the criteria for anorexia nervosa experience all of the following symptoms:

- Refusal to maintain the minimum body weight for one's height and age.
- Intense fear of gaining weight even though underweight.
- Disturbed perception of one's body weight or size.
- In post-pubescent women, the absence of at least three consecutive menstrual cycles. (In some women, the loss of periods precedes any significant weight loss.)

Bulimia

People with bulimia experience all of the following:

- Recurrent episodes of consuming a much larger amount of food than most people would during a similar time period (this is usually about two hours) and a sense of loss of control over eating during each episode.
- Accompanying attemps to compensate for eating binges by vomiting, abusing laxatives or other drugs or by fasting or excessive exercise
- Both the binge eating and purging occur at least twice a week for three months.
- A negative perception of one's shape and weight.

Childless by Choice

Can I live a rich, balanced life without joining the parenthood procession?

By Katherine Griffin

SEVEN YEARS AGO, soon after my grandmother died, my mother handed me a packet of faded letters, kept tied up with a pink ribbon for more than 60 years. My grandfather had written them to my grandmother during their courtship, while he was away at college during the 1920s. The night I opened the packet and began to read, I had an odd sense of being propelled both backward and forward in time. As the letters grew more intimate, with talk of Latin class and football games giving way to reminiscences of kisses that left face powder on my grandfather's coat, I could feel the seed of my existence beginning to take form, buried deep in those long-ago years. And so I began to wonder what might be taking shape in my life that would come to fruition many years in the future.

Most especially, reading the letters made me think again about my longstanding ambivalence toward having children. I lived out my own childhood against a backdrop of warmth and love and care, but I was always aware of the unceasing struggle and sacrifice required of my parents to make it that way. Since I was the only girl, I got a closer look at the trade-offs my mother had to make. College-educated and a

teacher for several years before her marriage, she was one of those rare Catholic women for whom the rhythm method really did prevent pregnancy, at least for the crucial first three years of the marriage. That allowed her to continue teaching long enough to earn her lifetime credential. I came along soon after, followed during the next five years by two brothers.

Very quickly, my mother went from being an independent woman with a paycheck and career to a full-time homemaker whose days were filled with carpooling and coupon-clipping. I remember her struggles to carve out time for herself, and how refreshed and happy she seemed after she'd managed to squeeze in a class in calligraphy or guitar. I never doubted that she loved us, but the work of child rearing didn't look like a lot of fun. For as long as I can remember, the idea of having children brought images of doors closing, not opening. And when I married my husband, King, 20 years older than I and with a grown daughter, I knew that he had no great desire for a second family.

Still, if I don't have children, who will be there for me as I grow older? I think about the traditional transitions of a woman's life as she shifts from single woman

to wife to mother to grandmother, and I wonder what milestones will mark the years of my life. Who will pore over the traces of my days, searching for meaning and a sense of connection? In a world where ancestors are universal, what will it mean to be a woman without descendants?

These questions have become more urgent for me in the past few years, as it's seemed that nearly everyone I know has been having children or announcing their intention to do so. My 23-year-old cousin. My 44-year-old cousin. Lesbian friends, who have approached one woman's brother about donating sperm. My 51-year-old single friend who's adopted a baby boy from Vietnam. And, of course, dozens of thirtysomething friends and acquaintances. As I attend their showers and watch them unwrap tiny dresses and toys, the differences among these people blur to insignificance. All I see is that they're stepping together into another stage of life, a stage I won't share.

A friend who is infertile and chooses not to adopt said recently, "Every time I hear about someone else who is having a baby, it feels like, There goes one more person who used to be like me who isn't anymore."

When I think about not joining the parade, I get scared. Maybe the uncharted territory would seem less daunting if I liked to think of myself as a bold pioneer, happily striking out to create an unconventional life. But the truth is, I like the comfort of road maps. And in this culture, there are none for childless women. Sure, setting off without a map gives me the opportunity to find the path that suits me best. But every time I stumble over some unforeseen obstacle, there's that voice in my head saying that if I'd just taken the path that was good enough for all the other women, I wouldn't be in this fix.

In the middle of my 35th year, I still

Leslie Lafayette, a former teacher from Sacramento, California. "Not everybody needs children to have a full life."

That message has never been popular in America. But these days, it's in danger of being drowned out entirely by the din of millions of babies. My friends are not the only ones procreating like mad. All across America, the women of the baby boom, many of whom delayed childbearing until they had educated themselves and established careers, have been rushing to make up for lost time. Each year since 1988, some 4 mil-

married women who didn't have children were likely to be accused of witchcraft if they did not seem properly virtuous. At the turn of this century, as immigrants were having large numbers of children, President Theodore Roosevelt chastised white women for not doing their part to create future generations of Americans. In 1903, he sternly lectured the citizenry that " . . . willful sterility is, from the standpoint of the nation . . . a sin for which there is no atonement. No man, no woman can shirk the primary duties of life . . . and retain his or her self-respect."

The old stereotypes are still going strong. At the very least, judging from stories that Network members told, childless women these days can expect frequent encounters with insensitivity. "We just bought a video camera," says 45-year-old Vicki Braun, a stocky, blue-eyed marketing representative from Dayton, Ohio. "The saleslady asked how many children we have. I said, 'None.' She looked at me and said, 'Then why would you need a video camera?'"

It was easy to see why Network members felt the need to band together. It was a relief to me, too, to be in a roomful of adults and not be the only one without children. But many of the sessions at the conference were marked by a shrill, hostile tone. One speaker proposed child-free zones in airplanes and restaurants. Others

The number of baby boom women who are childless—by choice or circumstance—will reach 20 percent.

don't feel drawn to having children, but I have no idea what it will mean to create a life without them.

O N A WARM SPRING EVEning in Las Vegas, an excited hubbub animates a crowded hotel room high above the blinking neon of the Strip. Several dozen men and women, mostly in their thirties and forties, munch canapés, sip drinks, and swap stories. Down below, the once-seedy Strip has been made family-friendly, and on the edge of town, rows of tract houses designed for nuclear families march endlessly out into the desert. But in this room, at least, everyone is childless, and you can almost hear the whoosh of hair being let down.

The gathering is part of the ChildFree Network's annual meeting, where I've come to find out more about living without children. The Network is a 2,500-member national group started in 1993 to give childless people their own sense of belonging. "I want to make this kind of life more acceptable," says founder

lion babies have been born, creating a demographic spike almost as big as the boom that lasted from 1946 to 1964.

Along with the boomlet has come a new glorification of parenthood and the widespread assumption that everyone is a parent. Dewy-eyed images of children abound, advertising everything from car parts ("There's a lot riding on your tires") to perfume ("Reality," says a slinky brunette in the tub with a toddler, "is the best fantasy of all"). Politicians speak of a "middle-class" tax cut that turns out to be exclusively for people with kids. Movie after movie (*Parenthood, Baby Boom, Nine Months*) extolls the joys of child rearing. Childless women are largely invisible, and when they do show up, it's as characters like Alex Forrest, the bunny-killing psychopath in *Fatal Attraction*.

America has a long tradition of pushing childless women to the margins. University of Minnesota historian Elaine Tyler May, in her book *Barren in the Promised Land*, describes how for most of this country's history, women without children have been seen as deviant, pathetic, or dangerous. In colonial times,

---

Childless by choice or circumstance:

Barbara Mikulski, U.S. senator; Ann Beattie, novelist; Camille Paglia, literary scholar and essayist; Katharine Hepburn, actor.

Bonnie Raitt, musician and songwriter; Gloria Steinem, activist and author; Barbara Harris, Episcopal bishop; Joni Mitchell, musician and songwriter.

Dolly Parton, musician and songwriter; Janet Reno, U.S. attorney general; Oprah Winfrey, talk show host and producer; Lauren Hutton, model and actor.

Diane Sawyer, television journalist; Teri Garr, actor; Gertrude Elion, Nobel prize-winning biochemist; Amy Tan, novelist.

criticized mothers who breastfeed in public. Some said bluntly that the childless lifestyle was better—not just better for them, but better, period. I seemed to be seeing the flip side of the "pronatalism" so prevalent in the culture at large. It made me uneasy, not least because it fueled the stereotype that people without children just plain don't like kids. Which isn't true of me at all. I need goofiness in my life, and silly games, and startling questions that come out of nowhere—things you don't get often enough from grownups. Just because I don't have kids doesn't mean I want to stay out of the playground.

MY QUEST FOR CHILDLESS women who were creating rich, full lives for themselves soon brought me to the doorstep of Tess Gallagher. She's a writer of poetry, fiction, and essays who lives in Port Angeles, Washington, in a whimsical, many-windowed aerie overlooking Puget Sound. I'd first come to know Tess through a beautiful and heartbreaking essay that she'd written about her life with her husband, the writer Raymond Carver.

Ray had been a boyhood friend of my husband's; the essay served as the introduction to *A New Path to the Waterfall*, a book of poetry that was his last work before he died of cancer in 1988. I read Tess's essay when I was struggling with the decision of whether to marry King. I never questioned my love for him, but making my life with someone so much older meant opening myself to the likelihood of early loss. Ray's death had taken Tess where I feared to tread. Reading her essay, in which their joy together so clearly outweighed even the crushing sorrow of his death, helped me to see that the only answer I could make to King was yes.

When King and I finally met Tess a couple of years after Ray's death, I filed away for future reference the fact that she had no children. Like my husband, Raymond Carver had raised a family when he was young. When he and Tess met, he had just begun to recover from alcoholism and regain his strength as a writer. Although he would have been willing to have a child with Tess, she chose against it in favor of their relationship and their work. On my 34th birthday, weepy and wrestling with my own decision, I wrote Tess a letter asking if, at 52, she now had any regrets.

"Maybe if I hadn't run into Ray," Tess wrote, "that would be the case, but I think I did exactly the right thing for both of us, and that did mean some sacrifice on my side of the ledger."

She has had the occasional pang, Tess says. But she also recognizes that not having children has allowed her great freedom to develop herself as an artist, giving her space for reading, writing, creating, dreaming. "When one, as a young woman, begins to read the lives of male artists and to notice how often they needed to get away from their family environments in order to do work," she says, "it's easy to see the handwriting on the wall. If one is mainly in charge of rearing the children, as women still tend to be, you won't be getting your thinking and your writing done."

For Tess, not having children of her own hasn't meant being cut off from younger people. She and Ray's grown son, Vance, have drawn close since Ray's death, and she has built strong connections to her nieces and nephews. "When I haven't spoken to one of the family children for a while, I call them up," she says. "When I don't like something, I let them or their parents know. I also give them a lot of encouragement and praise."

Her role as aunt has not always been easy or clear, and sometimes has gotten her in trouble with her siblings. "It is definitely a pioneer enterprise," she says. "One must be ever mindful of being on borrowed territory, dependent on the graciousness and wisdom of the parents." Still, Tess says, "It's an effort I'm glad to be making. Those times with the children are precious for me.

"I often wish there were another way to put it," she adds, "instead of 'women without children.' I really don't go around thinking of myself as a woman without."

WHEN I READ TESS'S LETTER, it was as though a hand had reached out and hauled me up to a place where, finally, I could begin to see the outlines of a path for myself. Here was someone I admired, whose work struck a deep chord within me, saying that choosing against having children doesn't mean settling for an empty life.

And it's not just a handful of artists like Tess for whom the childless choice is rewarding, as I discovered when I started reading what researchers have learned.

Take the area of marital satisfaction. For parents, it tends to follow a U-shaped curve, starting out high, dropping when children are young, and climbing again after they are grown and gone. The marriages of the childless are less likely to experience that dip, and more likely to improve steadily over time. Of course, that's not to say that being a parent isn't rewarding, or that, for people who want children, the tradeoffs aren't worth it. But it does suggest that the marriage relationship is one arena in which childless women may reap the benefits of their choice earlier than mothers.

Even in coping with the losses and difficulties of old age, childless women do just as well as mothers. True, the social networks of the childless tend to be smaller, because they have neither children nor grandchildren, but they do not report feeling more lonely and isolated than parents.

In a study of 90 childless women over age 50, anthropologist Robert L. Rubinstein, of the Philadelphia Geriatric Center, found that some women did express regret at their childless state, especially those who believed strongly that a woman's primary duty is to raise children. Even so, Rubinstein says, "We didn't find any women who said, 'Woe is me, my life is nothing because I didn't have children.' People came up with satisfying alternatives for whatever nurturings urges they had." Like Tess, many had forged strong connections with younger people: nieces and nephews, fellow church members, or long-time neighbors.

Moreover, most of the older childless women in studies like Rubinstein's had not chosen their state. It stands to reason that the childless by choice are happier that those made childless by circumstance, yet until recently, researchers had made no distinction between the two groups. When sociologists Ingrid Connidis and Julie McMullin, of the University of Western Ontario, studied nearly 700 Canadian men and women over age 55, they found that those who chose childlessness were just as happy as parents who had good relationships with their children. And they were happier than those parents who described their relationships with their children as distant.

All in all, the research added up to a pretty positive picture. Why, I wondered, didn't I know this before? For that matter, why have I felt so isolated, when in fact the number of childless women is higher now than it's been for much of this century? That's right: Among women aged 40 to 44 (assumed by demographers to be past childbearing age), the proportion who are childless rose from 9 percent in 1975 to 16 percent in 1993. The National Center for Health Statistics has projected

Two years of tests later, the doctors told the couple that the problem was "unexplained infertility," a fancy way of saying "Who knows what's wrong?"

By that time, Jean's work had become a daily agony. "There was nowhere I could go to get a break from pregnant ladies," she says. She briefly considered training for a different medical specialty, then de-

to take shape. The room the Carters had hoped would be a nursery became a music room. Dolls they'd bought for future daughters were given to their nieces. A college fund turned into money for travel. Instead of focusing on being without, they looked to the things they could have.

When motherhood seems an increasingly unlikely prospect, says psychologist Mardy Ireland, it's crucial to make a conscious choice, rather than drifting for years in ambivalence. The result is often the freeing up of the psychic space set aside for motherhood. That, in turn, allows a new adult identity to emerge. In Ireland's study of 100 childless women, she found that making this kind of conscious decision was most important for those she identified as "transitional"— women who, like me, grew up ambivalent about having kids and can easily see the pros and cons of either choice. Such women who made the decision to be childless in their thirties often discovered a wellspring of creative energy to channel into new projects: a career change, community work, art. Those who did not come to terms with childlessness until their mid-forties found it more difficult to create new identities.

Women without kids are assumed to be either sad, barren spinster types or career-crazed imitation men.

that among the entire group of baby boom women, the figure may climb as high as 20 percent—nearly as high as the peak reached during the years of the Depression, when a full 22 percent of women remained childless.

One reason for the resounding silence may be that childless women, by their very existence, raise uncomfortable questions about womanhood. "There's an implicit threat that these women pose to traditional ideas about what women and men are supposed to be," says Mardy Ireland, a psychologist in Berkeley, California, and author of *Reconceiving Womanhood: Separating Motherhood from Female Identity.*

Women who don't have children, Ireland says, are assumed to be either career-crazed imitation men or sad, barren spinster types. Neither stereotype acknowledges that women—even those who have longed to be mothers—can have rich and balanced lives without children of their own.

FORTY-FOUR-YEAR-OLD JEAN Carter is such a woman. A soft-spoken obstetrician-gynecologist married to an English professor in Raleigh, North Carolina, she had always wanted to have children. She and her husband, Michael, began trying to conceive when she was 29, and after a year, began seeing an infertility specialist.

cided that, instead, she had to get off the monthly cycle of hope and despair. She and Michael thought about adopting, but concluded that the biological aspects of parenthood were more important to them than they wished they were.

Finally, one rainy November afternoon in 1983, the couple made the decision not to have children.

"We decided not to base the rest of our lives on what we couldn't have," Jean says. "I had done some reading, and the bottom line is that happiness depends not on whether you have children, but on whether you have a rich external life: friends, family, interest in the world around you. And there was a big distinction between those who were childless by choice and not. I thought, If the people who are childless by choice live happier lives, I'm going to hop over and get into that category."

It wasn't a matter of simply resigning themselves to the direction their lives were taking anyway. They wanted to actively move toward a life without children, though they didn't know exactly how. After all, there's no such thing as a no-baby shower, no ceremonies to mark the stages of life as a non-parent.

"The first step was to tell people," Jean says. "Do the things you do when you make a major life decision." Some people just didn't get it. "They would give us the names of adoption agencies."

But very quickly, new possibilities began

Jean Carter's choice has been marked by a renewed commitment to her work. "I give a lot of nurturing to my patients," she says. "I observe what goes on between a man and a woman when they see that baby for the first time. This is my way of connecting with something terribly important for the world."

It hasn't all been rosy, of course. "I've lost many friends to parenthood," says Carter ruefully. "But they always come back, when the kids are in grade school, and even more when they're teenagers. In the meantime, you find somebody else to pal around with."

The couple often speak before meetings of the infertility support group Resolve. When asked whether they would choose to have a child if their fertility could be restored, they say no. "That part of our lives is over," Jean says. "We like who we are now, and our plans for our lives do not include children of our own."

NOT LONG AGO, I SAT UNDER a tree with a circle of women at yet another baby shower, this one for my friend Taly, soon to give birth to her second child. Looking around, I saw that I was one of only three women present without children. Most of the rest of the women already had a second child or hoped to conceive again soon. Some had brought their new babies along.

As I held one of the babies and listened to the talk of pregnancy, child care, and schools, I realized that what I had worried about had come to pass: Most of my friends are having children, and I'm not. But I also realized that this was the first shower in a long time at which I didn't feel left out, or defensive, or pitied. I could enjoy the baby's soft, sleeping weight on my shoulder, without feeling that the others assumed I wished she was my baby. Because, in fact, I didn't.

Slowly and imperceptiby over the past couple of years, I've come to feel that being childless is the right choice for me. But it's not quite right to say that I've resolved all the questions that have plagued me; it's more that I'm learning to live with them.

There's no single thing I've opted to do "instead" of raising children. Mostly, being childless opens me to a sense of possibility. It gives me the feeling that my own path can take zigs and zags, that since I'm not responsible for another human being maybe I can take risks and explore things that I otherwise wouldn't. When I hear about a friend's trip to Greece and my travel bug starts buzzing, I don't have to swat it aside and think, Maybe in 20 years. And kayacking on the Rogue River last summer, playing on rapids bigger and trickier than any I'd attempted before, it was if I'd discovered an entirely new personality—confident, daring, uninhibited. I want to give free rein to these parts of myself—and others that I don't even know about yet—in ways that would be difficult to do if I had children.

As we cleared away plates after the shower, a friend confided, "I was hoping the conversation would be a little broader." She's one of the more adventurous women I know, but lately, as the mother of a small daughter, she's had to stay closer to home. She says that having me in her life keeps her in touch with the part of herself that loves to ride rivers and travel the world. Her words bring reassurance that my friends value me for who I am, not simply the ways in which I am like them, and that there will be a place for me in my circle of friends for as long as I want to be there.

I'm realizing that I need to find other circles for myself, as well. It probably won't be as simple as finding a not-mother's group to parallel the mother's groups my friends are flocking to. But I need to keep reminding myself that there are lots of other women, like Tess and Jean, who have made the choice that I'm making.

Never knowing what it's like to mother a child *is* a loss. But understanding that isn't enough, for me, to tip the balance toward motherhood. So I hope to create close relationships with the nieces and nephews I expect to have before too long.

I'm starting to try out the aunt role already. A few weeks after the shower, when Taly went into labor, she asked me to take care of her three-year-old, Elijah. We played bulldozer, and made funny faces, and read some books. That night, after the baby was born, we drove to the hospital together, and I got to see his awed, beautiful face as he looked at his baby sister for the first time.

The truth is, I can't know ahead of time how my choice will turn out, if at the end of my life I'll look back wistfully at the road not traveled. But I think the same holds true for parents.

Either choice is a leap of faith. And so we leap.

Katherine Griffin is a staff writer.

THE NEW
RITE OF
PASSAGE

As young girls, many women
weren't encouraged to be
physically adventurous.
But embracing challenge
is one of the best ways
for a woman to
boost her confidence
and get
what she wants from life.

Susan V. Seligson

I can't. The others fall respectfully mute as my private struggle becomes public. I must be quite a sight: a quivering 41-year-old woman rising out of a crimson kayak, neckless in a bloated life vest, goggles misted with tears, shrieking in the ear of her tutor. I don't have to do this, I tell myself as I'm scooped upright to safety once more after grazing the murky water and crying, "No!" with the urgency of a condemned woman pleading for her life.

But I do have to do this. I don't expect to be the next Esther Williams, but I signed up for Outward Bound's kayaking course precisely because I want to get over my fear of the water—and flipping under while strapped to the boat is something every kayaker must learn.

My desire to feel confident under water is just the latest hurdle in a halting, decades-long journey toward physical competence. I can't count the times in my life when the words *I'm afraid* closed the book on even the most mundane challenge. As a child, I believed myself to be hopelessly uncoordinated. Though sociable, energetic, and forever surrounded by rambunctious peers, I never trusted my body to perform in a way that would keep me alive, much less win me medals. I learned to disguise my fear and shame as caution or lack of

interest, slipping away just when my friends were preparing to swing from some newly discovered tree limb. Whether it was a round of volleyball at the park, cartwheels on the soft grass, skiing, or chicken fights, the prospect of having to physically perform traumatized me, and before I knew it two words always flew out of my mouth.

"I can't," I blurted to the hunky water instructor as I struggled to swim the four laps that would enable me to graduate along with my ten-year-old bunk mates at Camp Woodstock. "I can't," I moaned at the top of the superslide in Coney Island's Steeplechase Park while kids much younger gleefully gave themselves over to gravity. "I can't!" I howled to my big sister as she tried for the zillionth time to coax me into the surf at Jones Beach.

My parents weren't concerned. Why would they be? Depression-reared, they lived by the credo Nothing ventured, nothing lost. An overachiever in school, I was destined to reach adulthood in one piece without so much as a sprained ankle. My parents' stock reaction to any endeavor involving risk was and still is "You're going to *what?*" When I visit them in Florida, they wince every time I head out the condo door in workout clothes. "You're not going out of the complex, are you?"

They drive me nuts, but recently my mother redeemed herself with a joke, one that summed up the pall over my youth. "Why do you always have to do things?" she asked. "Why can't you just stay out on the terrace strapped to a chair?"

I can't pinpoint exactly when I set out to demystify and unlearn my lexicon of festering fears. It's been a gradual process, this moving from "I can't" to "why can't I?" to "maybe I can." Sometime in my twenties I began to experience a sense of loss. It would have been different if I didn't care, but I did, deeply. What was I waiting for? I have always loved the outdoors, and after years of excuses I longed to get in on the fun, to ski, ice-skate, ride a horse, frolic in the surf. Ordinary mortals do these things all the time and live to tell about it. Out of a mixture of impatience and disgust, I decided—still frightened as ever—to fake it, to impersonate someone in command of her body.

It worked. The first time I tried cross-country skiing I was in the company of an acutely unsympathetic acquaintance. I fell, stumbled to my feet, fell again, then lay shivering in the snow, skis akimbo, and wept while my so-called friend disappeared among the pines and never looked back. It was a mis-

discovered—better late than never—the adrenaline-fed wonder of going fast.

Still, there are hurdles I've yet to clear. A lifelong fear of drowning has made me so squeamish about water that I have spent much of my adult life secretly avoiding what is for many people the very meaning of summer fun. As fate would have it, I am lucky enough to live on a narrow barrier spit with the tide swelling outside my window. But I venture into the bay only under the calmest conditions, never in water over my head. To the frustration of my friends, I refuse to paddle a canoe beyond the point where the marsh or seafloor is visible.

So I signed up with Outward Bound's kayaking course off the coast of Cape Canaveral in Florida to make friends with the water under the watchful eye of professionals who, I'm assuming, will not permit me to drown. The water is warm, and I'm among peers—mostly women in their forties. In the 56 years since it began as a competence-building regimen for young Royal Navy seamen, Outward Bound has expanded its wilderness programs to tamer civilians of all ages who want to boost self-esteem and self-reliance. If anyone can help me, they can.

I am a person who is secretly afraid of drowning in the shower, and I am steering a fiberglass sliver of boat away from shore in the dark of night.

erable experience, but when it was over and I waddled home with windburned cheeks and throbbing quadriceps, I was proud of myself beyond measure. I skied, I survived, it'll be better next time. And it was. Now I ski every chance I get. If the snow's right, you can't keep me away from the trails.

Several years later I went at my fear with a direct, almost clinical approach, deciding to enter the belly of the beast. I went rock climbing. It was profoundly un-fun, and I'll probably never do it again, but there is nothing like rappelling off a rock face. It is the ultimate metaphor, an entire education about trust, confidence, taking the plunge. After sitting paralyzed on a narrow ledge insisting to my climbing partner that I would rather grow old and die in that spot than step backward into thin air, I gave in (I had to pee, I was hungry, my dog was waiting in the car) and went, so swiftly, from feeling utterly inadequate to feeling like Wonder Woman.

My physical achievements have equipped me to venture into other unknowns—from dicey social encounters to the unforgiving professional world. I used to make myself ill with dread before meetings with important editors or pompous luminaries, as if my entire career and self-worth were hanging in the balance. Now these things don't weigh on me so much. I know how to recover from fumbles and falls; my God, I've even gotten myself off a mountain face by straddling a rope. I have grown intimate with failure and know it is a relative phenomenon, a passing rather than earth-shattering condition. But I have also come to know success and the giddy feeling that comes with defying my worst assumptions about myself. After binding myself to training wheels for most of my life, I have

MY NEW FRIENDS and I will paddle nearly 45 miles along and around the Intracoastal Waterway, from the ominously named Mosquito Lagoon south to Indian River and the boundaries of Merritt Island Wildlife Refuge, with the NASA space shuttle assembly complex looming surreally in the distance. We won't venture into open ocean, but winds in the lagoon can soar higher than 20 knots, and the wake from larger boats motoring along the Intracoastal can rock a kayak until it tips over. My main consolation after we meet is that these women look reassuringly human; there's not an Olympian along them.

One of our group arrives late, so it's after eight when we put in the first night. Under a full moon, we cram our gear into the narrow holds of two-man kayaks the color of M&M's, and try on our spray skirts, those dowdy neoprene tutus designed to stretch tautly around the oval lip of the paddler's seat, keeping her dry—and trapped. You don't just sit in a kayak, you wear it low in the water. And if it capsizes and if you cannot release the skirt, you could drown. After a cursory paddling demonstration (we still have to get to a small island and set up camp), our leaders, Avery Larned and Carol James, tell us not to bother attaching the skirts to the kayaks this evening. Tomorrow morning we'll learn how to release the things in an underwater escape drill called a wet exit. Just the words make me shudder.

I'm relieved about the skirt, and even joke that the things make us look like the Lollipop Kids in *The Wizard of Oz*. But my heart feels as if it's going to pop out of my personal flotation device as we slide the kayaks into the tepid water and hold them steady for one another. Each woman hoists herself up and stuffs her legs inside. In minutes we're slicing through the open expanse of Mosquito Lagoon.

I am a person who is secretly afraid of drowning in the shower, and I am steering a fiberglass sliver of boat away from shore in the dark of night. We all keep close, and I figure my companions assume I'm shaking from the cold. Mullet spring cartoonishly from the inky water as we make our way to the campsite, the first of many tiny uninhabited islands where we'll spend the night. In a cruel rain of mosquitoes and no-see-ums we stumble through what will become the evening ritual: We scramble for our mosquito repellent, unpack the gear, carry the boats above the tide line, put up the tents, dig the privy, rifle through the maddeningly identical food bags, scare up supper. Tomorrow, Avery and Carol tell us as we slurp down a dinner of ramen noodles, we'll flip the kayaks and perfect the wet exit. I fall into a fitful sleep and dream of frantically trying to break free of my capsized boat.

A terrible sleeper, I'm normally grateful for morning, but when it finally arrives I sip bitter camp coffee and wish I could beam myself to a time, several hours from now, when the wet exit is behind me. I steel myself, only to discover that we're to spend the morning seated in a circle and "sharing."

The revelations come haltingly, and from time to time the circle is broken when someone spots a pod of frolicking dolphins or the shadowy prehistoric outline of a manatee. The women tell why they are here. Fear is a recurring theme. Dusty, a Washington, D.C., executive who is, at 49, the oldest of our group, says she wasted years concocting reasons for not doing active things that scared her. "I quit drinking, I quit smoking, and six months ago I got off my couch and started to exercise," she says. "And here I am. I've waited years to get to this place." Jill, a North Carolina mother of three, says the trip is "my 45th birthday present to myself, my chance to be a woman apart from someone's wife, someone's mom." Jill's upbeat perspective reveals another side of female midlife moxie. "I gave birth to three kids," she says, dodging a burst of flames from the temperamental camp stove. "All this stuff is peanuts."

WHAT IS IT ABOUT APPROACHING middle age that has so many women venturing into the wilderness, rappelling down mountains, or donning in-line skates? Outward Bound offered two women-only courses in 1974; in 1996 there were 12. And while the early courses attracted women under 30 almost exclusively, "the number of women over 40 taking courses has increased dramatically in the last five years," says Outward Bound spokesperson Elizabeth Banwell. Springing up at the same time have been women-only adventure outfits such as Michigan-based Woodswomen and women-only sailing trips. Today, according to the United States Bureau of the Census, nearly as many women as men go camping and hiking for pleasure.

"Older women are really ready," says Karen Warren, an instructor at Hampshire College in Amherst, Massachusetts, who's led wilderness programs for 23 years. While as young girls we may not have been actively dissuaded from embracing physical challenges, it was certainly acceptable for us to cave in to our fears. Now we members of the immortal baby boom generation find ourselves sprouting gray hairs, losing our parents and even our contemporaries to illness, and being overcome with a certain urgency: Life is short, too short to allow the fear of looking foolish to paralyze us. "Women in their forties begin to look to themselves rather than others for direction and judgment," says Susan Schenkel, a Cambridge, Massachusetts, psychologist who helps women take dramatic action. And when they finally do something they've feared for years, "it's a great 'ah-ha!' moment," says Warren.

The resulting jolt of satisfaction seems to boost confidence—and competence—in a general and enduring way. Everett Harman, a physiologist with the U.S. Army Research Institute of Environmental Medicine in Natick, Massachusetts, has followed up on a group of 41 female civilian volunteers, aged 20 to 37, who'd undertaken 24 weeks, five to nearly eight hours a week, of physical training. Under the guidance of expert trainers, the women, who were in various states of physical fitness, lifted free weights, tramped five miles carrying 30- to 75-pound packs, and did a series of long jumps, vertical jumps, and two-mile runs. Not only did the women, as expected, become more fit, nearly three out of four said they had greater peace of mind. What's more, 83 percent said they liked themselves better, more than half said their social skills had improved, and the vast majority said that they had developed a more positive opinion of women's physical capabilities in general. One volunteer, a homemaker and mother of three, reported such a surge of self-assurance that she went from being "depressed and uninvolved to being a civic leader in her town," says Harman.

"Once the fear is demystified, women often make applications to other parts of their lives," says wilderness guide Karen Warren. "They say, 'I kayaked so many miles and never thought I could. Now I can go after that job promotion.'"

Because I have overcome fears in the past, even as I sit on the beach in queasy anticipation of the capsizing drill, I'm already envisioning the cathartic rush of victory to follow. I choose to go last, after the others flip, escape, and surface, one by one, to resounding cheers from the rest of us. But I can't do it.

In theory there's nothing to it. Avery, my quick-witted, self-effacing, and refreshingly rubenesque instructor, would guide my boat seaward. Then I'd tip the kayak over in one swift motion. Under water, I would tug on the skirt release—a strap like the ones you hold on a crowded subway train—and wriggle my legs out of the boat as if I were pulling off a pair of jeans. The whole ordeal would take about three seconds; in yoga class I've held my breath for a full minute.

I know all this, and yet Avery's gentle encouragement and infinite patience aren't enough. Each time I hit the water I freak out. "Nothing can happen to you," Avery says softly. "I'm right here, you're in four feet of water, and even if you forget to yank on the skirt you'll probably just fall out of the boat." Why don't I believe her? Why don't I trust myself? After about 20 minutes of floundering I'm so breathless and cold I decide it's unsafe to continue. "It's okay," says Avery. "We'll try again tomorrow." I stagger to shore, where some of the other women come over to rest a hand on my back.

But over the next morning and those that follow, the opportunity is lost. Avery doesn't mention it, and there is always breakfast to cook, navigational charts to consult, boats to pack. Each day when we set out I feel ashamed. Avery advises me not to fasten the spray skirt because it would be dangerous.

I try to make up for my deficiencies by paddling hard and

I'm already envisioning the rush of victory. I choose to go last, after the others flip their kayaks, escape, and surface, one by one, to resounding cheers.

steady, refusing to take a breather. And I console myself with other achievements. Pauline, a housewife from Florida, and I are the navigators on the day of our toughest route, a serpentine paddle through narrow tributaries, past mangroves rustling with snow egrets, blue herons, and pelicans. We guide the group right smack to the half-moon cove of our destination. I learn to tolerate and even enjoy the rocking of the kayak in the wake of passing yachts or a choppy wind.

But at night when I lie in the stuffy heat, my tent mates lost to their REM stupors beside me, I obsess over flipping that stupid kayak and repeat the drill like a prayer: Pull the strap, grab the boat, shimmy out, pop right up. It's unthinkable to go home without accomplishing this. I've watched these other determined women triumph over their own fears—of intimacy, of expressing anger, of appearing foolish, of being last. Pauline the trouper has never even been camping before. How can I return from a kayaking "adventure" without having put my head underwater?

It's our final morning, a morning so perfect I am up at dawn to make coffee while the other women sleep. Avery appears dangling the nose plugs. It's time. I gulp some coffee and find my life vest and spray skirt. The two of us push off Avery's one-man kayak, and I secure my nose plugs and climb in. "Tell me what you want me to do," says Avery. The morning is so still and quiet my fear seems a bit ridiculous. I realize I've grown weary of it. I take a few breaths, relieved the others aren't watching, and say, "Let's just do it."

Avery pushes the kayak down and over, and in a flash I'm underneath it. But before I have time to contemplate this, I feel for the strap, give a tug, grab the boat, free my legs . . . and I'm up. Avery and I throw our salty arms around each other and splash about in a kind of victory dance. That's when I hear the cheers and realize the others have come to watch.

On the flight home, after a night of communing with the tub and towels at the Orlando airport Hyatt, I'm seated next to two chatty Rhode Island matrons. "You did what?" they exclaim when I tell them that, no, I didn't get this tan at Disney World. "My, aren't you brave!" says one. "I could never, ever do anything like that," says the other. "You might be surprised," I hear myself saying. "I bet if you had to, you could."

Susan V. Seligson is a contributing editor.

Looking for Adventure?

DOZENS OF OUTFITTERS now cater to women seeking a challenge in the wild. Most keep the size of groups small, say ten to 12 women, and send along two instructors or guides. Here are HEALTH's best bets, based on the reviews of adventure-travel experts.

OUTWARD BOUND

This is the oldest of the adventure organizations. With five decades of experience, it offers more than 40 women's trips throughout the United States. Try sailing in the Florida Keys, dogsledding in Minnesota, or white-water canoeing down the Rio Grande.

EMPHASIS Rugged trips teach women how to summon the most from themselves both physically and mentally.

PRICE TAG Trips range from four days to three months and cost between $395 and $7,600. Call 800/243-8520.

WOODSWOMEN

Its 50 excursions cover the United States, Europe, South America, New Zealand, and Egypt. Consider biking through California's wine country, hiking around the Swiss Alps, or trekking in Nepal.

EMPHASIS Woodswomen designs trips to have distinctly different levels of challenge. You can choose from nearly a dozen indulgent adventure vacations, rugged wilderness journeys, tours designed to cultivate leadership, and expeditions geared to develop specific skills such as sailing.

PRICE TAG Some trips last a weekend, some two weeks; the price range is $150 to $3,500. Call 800/279-0555.

OUTDOOR VACATIONS FOR WOMEN OVER FORTY

Founder Marion Stoddart began this outfit for women who don't want to be pushed to Outward Bound's limits. She sets a more relaxed pace on these 22 trips throughout the United States, Mexico, and Europe. You can embark on a gentle walking tour of Tuscany, bike through Holland, or shoot the rapids in Massachusetts.

EMPHASIS All trips focus on the environment. A naturalist accompanies each tour to lend insight into the ecosystem.

PRICE TAG Vacations range from two to 11 days and cost between $280 and $3,000. Call 508/448-3331.

RAINBOW ADVENTURES

Women over 30 can choose among 21 comfortable expeditions throughout the American West, Europe, Asia, and Mexico. You can hike in the Greek islands, sail in the West Indies, or scout for whales off the Baja peninsula in Mexico.

EMPHASIS These are adventure vacations without the rough edges; you'll typically spend the night at a guest ranch or lodge.

PRICE TAG Tours last one to two weeks and cost $1,400 to $5,500. Call 800/804-8686. —*Paula Motte*

Chronic Diseases

Chronic diseases are those long-term problems that can be managed but not really cured. Often called diseases of lifestyle, these ailments frequently result from a lifelong disregard for our own health. Although it may be argued that certain risk factors for disease like age, gender, and genetics cannot be changed, a larger number of other risk factors are under our control. The more notorious of these risk factors include smoking, abuse of alcohol and other drugs, lack of exercise, and poor diet. Also of great importance in a discussion of disease prevention is the failure of many to take advantage of periodic medical screenings such as cholesterol and blood pressure; failure to obtain appropriate medical care if a problem is suspected; and, of course, failure to deal appropriately with the uncontrolled stress of modern life. Although this list is quite comprehensive, it is by no means complete. Keeping in mind the focus on prevention, the articles in this chapter were chosen because they not only represent a broad spectrum of chronic illnesses, but they place emphasis on personal responsibility and control—what the individual woman can and should do to prevent, identify, or alleviate major health problems. Often the necessary first step in gaining control over one's life and health is to gather appropriate information. It is hoped that this section will help to put the reader's feet on the path to personal empowerment regarding health and well-being.

In "Mending the Female Heart," Ann Japenga addresses the number-one killer of women in this country today, heart disease. Although previously considered to be a "man's disease," heart disease has proven to be an equal-opportunity killer in regard to gender. One difference, however, should be noted. The symptoms of heart disease in women are often different from those in men, and most doctors are trained to recognize and treat the classical male symptoms. Continuing in this vein, "Heart Disease in Women: Special Symptoms, Special Risks" identifies and discusses these differences in terms of both diagnosis and treatment.

Turning attention to the number-two cause of mortality in the United States, the chapter examines cancer. Since cancer is actually a family or constellation of diseases, several different forms of the disease commonly affecting women are examined. "Redesigning Women: Breast Cancer and Estrogen" takes a very avant-garde look at this well-recognized disease. First, author Rosie Mestel examines the sedentary lifestyle of women in affluent countries and links this factor to high levels of estrogen. Next she discusses high levels of estrogen in terms of increased incidence of breast cancer. Gary Goldenberg examines breast cancer from a different perspective. "Consensus: No Long-Term Link between the Pill and Breast Cancer" seeks to dispel this popular myth.

In "The Cancer Nobody Talks About" Janice Graham profiles the third-leading cause of death in women, colorectal cancer. Not only is prevention and detection discussed here, but the point is made that when it comes to certain organs or systems in the body, embarrassment and subsequent failure to seek treatment may very well prove fatal.

No discussion of cancer would be complete without a look at skin cancer. Katherine Greider, in "Mole Patrol," discusses how easily this disease may be detected. Advice is given on how to spot problems and what to do if you find them.

Susan Lang turns to another chronic condition. "A Silent Epidemic" looks at diabetes in women. Although it kills twice as many women each year as breast cancer, this disease simply does not get the attention it deserves.

Another chronic disease which is frequently not in the public consciousness is lupus. Lupus is a disease that for some unknown reason turns the body's own defense mechanisms against itself. Although it affects between 1.4 and 2 million people in the United States, it is often undiagnosed due to the vague, elusive nature of its symptoms. "Living with Lupus" profiles a young black woman who is suffering from this condition.

Adding to the list of chronic diseases with which women must contend is arthritis. By the age of 65, women are five times more likely to suffer from this disorder than are men. "When Arthritis Strikes," by Marie Savard, presents the symptoms and treatment for the most common form of the disease.

In "Running on Empty," Barbara Kelley sheds light on a problem that has been gaining considerable attention lately, thyroid disorders. The thyroid gland, located in the neck, is responsible for helping to regulate the body's

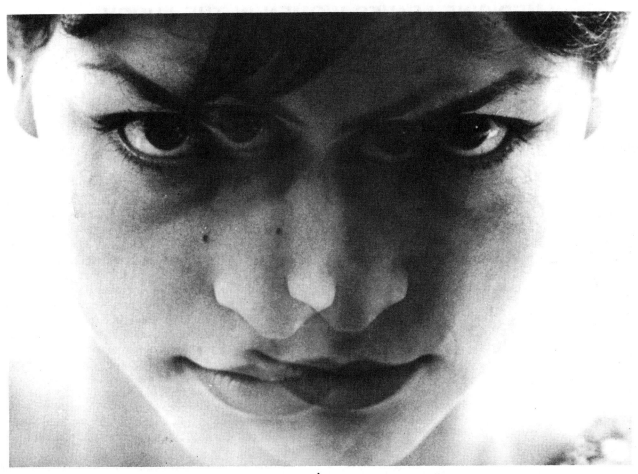

metabolism. If this gland is over- or understimulated, a number of uncomfortable and inconvenient symptoms occur. Since this condition is frequently misdiagnosed, the author recommends that all women experiencing the symptoms listed should go to the doctor and ask to be evaluated.

This unit's last article outlines two very common health problems experienced by women everywhere, UTIs or urinary tract infections and vaginal infections. "What to Do for Urinary-Tract and Vaginal Infections" takes a very straightforward approach to the problems. It presents a list of symptoms, self-help remedies and tips, and advice on when to see the doctor for each condition.

Looking Ahead: Challenge Questions

Why is heart disease in women often misdiagnosed?

Why do so many cancers remain undiagnosed and untreated in women?

After reading the articles on thyroid disease, lupus, diabetes, and arthritis, what conclusions can you draw about the health status and treatment of women in this country?

MENDING

THE FEMALE HEART

WHEN IT COMES TO HEART DISEASE, MAINSTREAM MEDICINE LEAVES WOMEN IN THE LURCH. DOES DEAN ORNISH HAVE THE ANSWER?

ANN JAPENGA

THERE'S A VALLEY in eastern Pennsylvania where they celebrate, just before Lent each year, something called Fasnacht Day: Doughnut Day. It wouldn't be surprising if a youngster who came of age here—among the butter-loving Pennsylvania Dutch in the valley of the doughnuts—developed a taste for rich food. That was certainly the case for Beverly Stolz.

Stolz, now 48, grew up to marry a New Jersey doctor who shared her gustatory passion. The couple spent their leisure time hopscotching across the country from famous deli to four-star restaurant, sampling the lobster in cream sauce at Angels in Manhattan, the sourdough bread slathered with butter at Boudin's in Chicago.

Stolz worked off the butter and sauces by living in constant motion. "From 6 A.M. to midnight," she says, "I just go." She has to: She works as a nurse anesthetist and also runs a jewelry business.

"She's a fireball," says her friend Eileen Borkenhagen. "She's just driven by this zest for life."

That driven nature is not always the best thing for a person's health, however. Stolz's pace left her little time for quiet, stress-reducing interludes, or for exercise. And eventually she began to put on pounds. She tried a Jenny Craig diet, Optifast, Weight Watchers, diving into each new effort with fervor. In each case, though, she'd lose motivation—too busy living to squander precious hours going nowhere on a treadmill.

Two years ago, at Christmas, a fluttering in her chest reminded Stolz that her health was begging for attention. Her doctor told her the heart palpitations were not serious, but her blood work was another matter. Her cholesterol level, at 230, was somewhat high. Her triglycerides were a frightening 720, more than four times normal.

Cholesterol, of course, is the fatty substance that can accumulate inside arteries, constricting blood flow and, sometimes, leading to a heart attack. But for women, triglycerides—another sort of fat found in the bloodstream—are thought to be important, too. Together with her 40 extra pounds and overabundance of stress, Stolz's triglyceride level put her in the high risk category for heart disease, stroke, or other problems.

The threat wasn't immediate, since women don't tend to get heart disease until after menopause, or beginning around age 55. Nevertheless, Stolz had enough medical background to know she might eventually need a heart bypass or other intervention.

Then something came along to really bolster Stolz's resolve to cut her risk. Last year, she and her husband assumed custody of their eight-year-old grandson, Julian. (The boy's mother was unable to care for him because of addiction problems.) "Before, I wanted to get back to a size 7," Stolz says. "And I still want to look good. But now, I want to stay around to take care of this little boy."

Around that time, Stolz began to notice a name cropping up on best-seller lists, in news magazines, and on the lips of friends. Dean Ornish had found fame after his 1990 study showed that heart disease can be reversed through rigorous lifestyle changes: a diet with less than 10 percent of calories from fat, a half hour a day of aerobic exercise and an hour of stress management, as well as regular group support sessions. But with the publication of his 1993 book, *Eat More, Weigh Less*, Ornish had broadened the audience he was trying to reach. The best-selling book recommended the Ornish regime not just for heart patients but for everyone. The internist had also begun offering week-long courses in his approach, open to the worried well. For a cost of $3,500 (a bargain compared to a $60,000 bypass operation), Stolz could

> MOST OF THE MEN
> IN THE PROGRAM
> HAVE WIVES WHO WILL
> COOK THEIR MEALS
> AND COACH THEM IN
> LIFESTYLE CHANGES.
> WHO WILL BE STOLZ'S
> CHEERLEADER?

change. On the other hand, she held a trump card: her drive and enthusiasm. She decided to sign up.

"I'm really planning to put 100 percent effort into this," Stolz said. "I think I can reverse . . . no, I *know* that I can reverse my blood work."

IT'S A SUNNY April morning at the Claremont Resort and Spa, in Oakland, California, a stately old hotel set in 22 acres of gardens overlooking San Francisco Bay. It may seem paradoxical that Stolz has come to such an opulent resort to learn to live more abstemiously. But a spa is the one place she might set aside concerns for her husband, her grandson, and her two jobs and simply focus on herself. "The only person I have to take care of here is me," says Stolz, "while at home, I'm usually the last person."

When Stolz has a chance to look around, it's clear that her challenge is not a common one here. For one thing, the other attendees are mostly affluent couples at or near retirement age, with time and means to experiment. More strikingly, almost all the heart patients in attendance are men, generally accompanied by wives avidly taking notes and jotting recipes.

Ann Girard is typical. Girard, 58, signed up along with her husband, Pascal, who had a bypass in 1982 and angioplasty in 1995. Ann Girard herself is overweight, with high blood pressure and a family history of heart problems. Yet, she says, "I'm doing this because of my husband. I don't think I would have come if it wasn't for him."

Women like Girard throw themselves into the program knowing they are the ones who will cook the meals and coach their husbands in their efforts to make lifestyle changes. Who will be Stolz's cook and cheerleader when she gets home?

Despite a touch of jet lag, Stolz enters a conference room looking bright-eyed and eager in head-to-toe black sweats and sequined socks. She takes a seat at a long table along with the other students, all awaiting the sad-eyed guru, Dean Ornish.

In a culture obsessed with longevity and health, the 42-year-old internist has become so well-known that tourists wandering the Claremont grounds ask about him as if there were a rock star in residence. "Is Dean Ornish really here? Where can I see him?"

When he walks onstage, the doctor has, in fact, not a glimmer of rock-and-roll about him. His delivery is mild; even when he goes for a joke, it's low-key. "I'm Doctor Dean Ornish. We call everyone by their first names here, so you can call me 'Doctor.'"

Stolz scribbles notes as a slide of a tabloid newspaper headline flashes on a screen: DEAD MAN'S HEART STARTED BY JUMPER CABLES. "This is how I was trained to deal with heart disease," Ornish says, with a sidelong glance at the screen. "I was trained to see the heart as a mechanical pump."

Rather than attack the underlying causes of heart disease, says Ornish, doctors typically bypass, or sidestep, the problem by splicing or reaming out arteries and by prescribing cholesterol-lowering drugs. The therapies have their place, yet in the long run they're frequently ineffective. Arteries routinely clog up again after bypass or angioplasty; and cholesterol-lowering drugs don't have the desired result in all people. The drugs also come with possible side effects such as liver damage and intestinal problems. As Ornish wrote in one of his books, *Dr. Dean Ornish's Program for Reversing Heart Disease*: "Treating only the physical manifestations of heart disease without addressing the more fundamental causes will provide only temporary relief."

What, then, are the bedrock causes? To understand where Or-

learn how to eat, exercise, and live the Ornish way. Most importantly, she'd learn ways to take the program home.

Of course, many women with Stolz's degree of risk might have elected to do nothing: While most of us would see a doctor about a suspicious mole or a lump in a breast, we might ignore chest pains, soaring cholesterol, or other warning signs of heart disease. The common belief is that women don't have heart attacks.

But in fact heart disease—not cancer—is the number one killer of women. If we have been slow to get that message, the medical profession is partly to blame. Doctors too often dismiss a woman's chest pains as harmless twinges of stress. Perhaps because of that, if a woman has a heart attack, she's nearly twice as likely as a man to die in the next few months. If she has bypass surgery, she is, again, about twice as likely to die in the aftermath. And, until recently, a woman undergoing angioplasty, in which a balloon is inflated inside a blocked artery to increase blood flow, had been ten times more likely to die from the procedure than a man. A new, smaller balloon has brought angioplasty's risk way down. Still, for a woman like Beverly Stolz, who is at high risk and wants to head off trouble, good advice is hard to come by. Virtually all the studies on preventing heart disease have ignored women.

From the small and admittedly preliminary studies that *have* been done, Ornish thinks that women may actually have an easier time than men in staving off heart attacks. "Whether it's through our lifestyle program, or even in studies of cholesterol-lowering drugs," he says, "women show more reversal of heart disease than men, and more women show reversal. I think women benefit as much as men, and maybe *more* than men, from our program."

Still, many experts aren't convinced his program will work for most people. "The concept is fine," says Mary Ann Malloy, a cardiologist and American Heart Association spokeswoman. "But the problem with the Ornish approach is, unless people are scared to death, they just won't stay on it. People can't deprive themselves all the time."

Stolz was nervous about her health problems, but certainly not scared to death. And she'd already tried without success to nish is coming from, recall every cliché you've ever heard regarding the heart—it's broken, battered, closed, and constricted, or it's full, whole, big, and open. Now, imagine that these are not just empty phrases but ways of explaining the effect our emotions have on the muscle pulsing in our chests.

Open your heart and your arteries relax and fill with life-giving blood; shut down in cynicism, anger, and isolation and the blood supply is squeezed off. Ornish says our closed hearts are killing us. The goal, then, is to prod them open by reaching out to others, as well as by opening to our deeper selves (and, perhaps, a higher power) through techniques like meditation, yoga, visualization, and breathing and relaxation exercises.

"It's easy to dismiss this as touchy-feely," says Ornish, "but we are touchy-feely creatures." For anyone who thinks the concepts sound airy, he backs up his recommendations with science. For instance, several massive studies—one in Alameda County, California, and another in Finland—have shown that socially isolated people had a three to five times increased risk of death from heart disease and other causes.

Of course, the part of the Ornish program that typically gives people pause is not all the deep breathing and connecting. No, the showstopper is the ultra-low-fat, low-cholesterol vegetarian diet. To many retreat participants, a diet getting only 10 percent of its calories from fat looks like ultra-deprivation.

Such a diet also goes well beyond what the American Heart Association and other authorities have been telling us for years: that we need to limit our fat consumption to 30 percent of daily calories. But several studies in the past few years have suggested that a 30 percent diet is not lean enough to halt the advance of heart disease. In Ornish's research, people in the control group followed a 30 percent–fat diet—and actually saw their coronary blockages worsen.

The jury is out on whether a 10 percent–fat diet is really necessary for healthy people. Ornish says people without heart disease may be able to liberalize the diet to 20 percent, or even more if their cholesterol is below 150. Still, he clearly believes 10 percent is best. "The closer people adhere to the program," he says, "the more improvement they show."

> TRADING HOPES
> AND FEARS IS VITAL
> TO OPENING HEARTS.
> STOLZ HAS NO
> TROUBLE SHARING
> HER EMOTIONS.
> IT'S THE EXERCISE
> AND DEMANDING DIET
> THAT WORRY HER.

Dean Ornish Wants You

Do You Need Him?

EVEN THE HEALTHIEST of us can probably feel better by making the changes proposed by Dean Ornish. That said, do you really need to exert the effort? Don't assume your doctor will alert you to an increased risk of heart disease. Health care providers often miss the signs in women.

You're considered to be at high risk of heart disease if you have two or more of the following risk factors: age over 54; HDL cholesterol under 35; diabetes or high blood pressure; a family history of premature heart disease; a smoking habit.

Age A woman's risk rises as she ages (but rises earlier if she experiences premature menopause and doesn't take estrogen replacement therapy). If you're postmenopausal, you are two or three times more likely than a young woman to develop heart disease.

Blood Cholesterol The general rule for men and women is that a red flag should go up if total cholesterol is above 200 milligrams per deciliter. But there is considerable controversy over just how significant these readings are for women. The ratio of total cholesterol to HDL ("good") cholesterol may be more important, and, indeed, experts recommend that in healthy adults, both levels should be tested every five years. The ratio should be less than 4 to 1. That is, HDLs should account for at least 25 percent of total cholesterol.

It's thought that a low level of HDL (less than 35 mg/dL) is a more significant predictor of heart disease in women than in men. Some experts believe that high levels (above 190 mg/dL) of the blood fats known as triglycerides are also especially bad news for women. One reason this may be true: High triglycerides tend to be accompanied by low HDL.

Diabetes The illness appears to increase the likelihood of heart disease more for women than for men, tripling the chance of dying from heart problems.

Blood Pressure If your blood pressure consistently measures above 140/90, you are at greater risk. Keep an eye on those numbers; as you age, you're more likely than a man to develop high blood pressure.

Family History If anyone in your immediate family was diagnosed with heart disease at an early age—before 65 for women and before 55 for men—you are at greater risk yourself.

Smoking A cigarette habit increases the odds of a heart attack by two to six times. —A.J.

MORE THAN PERCENTAGES, though, what participants really want to know is, What do I have to give up? Meat, poultry, fish, oils, fats, nuts, seeds, and egg yolks, as well as avocados, coconut, olives, and caffeine. What stays? Pasta, rice, vegetables, beans, and fruit, along with little dollops of nonfat dairy products, salt, sugar, and alcohol.

All pretty daunting to a lifelong lover of rich food. But when Stolz ducks into a cooking class, she finds that what seemed so spartan in theory looks much more appetizing in practice. Intent on proving that low-fat food can look and taste good, Ornish has hired French chef Jean-Marc Fullsack—formerly of L'Ermitage in Beverly Hills and Lutece in New York—to demonstrate cooking and prepare meals. Stolz watches him plop eggshells into a tureen of tomato consommé to bleed out the crimson, leaving the palest imaginable pink broth.

Fullsack's lessons are supplemented by Hank and Phyllis Ginsberg, graduates of the Ornish program, who cook up a huge pot of Ginsberg's Corn Soup. Several years ago, Hank Ginsberg had bypass surgery, then angioplasty, followed once again by new coronary artery blockages. On the Ornish regimen, his blockages have shrunk. The Ginsbergs' theme: Low-fat cooking can be as easy or as elaborate as you want to make it. (Ornish is even marketing a new line of microwave-ready frozen meals that meet all the program requirements.)

Stolz jots down cooking times and special ingredients; she samples the corn soup and the delicate broth—all the while knowing there's no way she'll ever have time at home for bleaching the crimson from consommé.

After cooking class comes lunch. Visits to the banquet room quickly turn out to be a highlight of each day. Stolz can hardly wait to see what new versions of a bean and vegetable diet the chefs have heaped on the groaning buffet table. Banana mango strudel. Roasted eggplant and pepper soup. Tofu stew with sweet potatoes. There are no cheers for the caffeine-free coffee, but then again, no one is complaining about caffeine withdrawal headaches. Nor do they complain about the intestinal ravages that come with the radical shift to a vegetarian diet. There seems to be an unspoken agreement: *We're going to be cheerful about this, no matter what.*

That evening, Stolz pulls a chair into a circle of retreat-goers at the first meeting of the social support group. The groups originally were meant as a place to trade practical tips: Where can I buy veggie pepperoni? What are the best walking shoes? But as they turned into a place for people to talk honestly to each other, Ornish came to realize that the ability to trade fears and hopes was vital to his goal of "opening hearts" and reversing coronary blockages.

When it's Stolz's turn, she speaks comfortably of her constant worry: that she just won't be able to make the changes stick. Stolz has no trouble sharing her emotions this way; at home, she gets on the phone every day to check in with her best friends, Eileen Borkenhagen and Karen Pitts. Ruth Marlin, an internist with the Ornish program, says that this part of the program tends to come more easily to women. Indeed, many studies have shown that women maintain connections more readily than do men. It's the other changes that Stolz worries about: the exercise, the demanding diet.

Back in her room, Stolz calls home. Julian tells her he had a steak for breakfast, just to taunt her. She ponders how different things

Recipes for a Change

DEAN ORNISH'S OWN *Eat More, Weigh Less* includes useful tips for cooking without fat. But the book's 250 recipes, while delicious, are often fussy and laborious. Fortunately, other cookbooks cater to a home cook's constraints. Two of these books are fat-free. The others call for minimal amounts of oil and occasional egg yolks, poultry, and even red meat. But by using the nutritional information that accompanies the recipes, you'll find many dishes that fit into a 10 percent diet—which, according to Ornish, can contain 18 grams of fat per day for a moderately active 120-pound woman, and 30 grams for an equally active woman of 180 pounds.

500 FAT-FREE RECIPES by SARAH SCHLESINGER (*1994, Villard Books, $23*)

When Schlesinger's husband was diagnosed with heart disease, she found few nonfat cookbooks, so she wrote her own. A helpful introduction gives suggestions for stocking a low-fat pantry and techniques for cutting back on fat. The recipes, generally vegetarian, cover every meal and are simple and easy to follow.

FAT FREE, FLAVOR FULL by DR. GABE MIRKIN AND DIANA RICH (*1996, Little, Brown, $12.95 paper*)

Pediatrician Gabe Mirkin has no cooking background; he began to develop recipes after cutting back on fat consumption for his own health. As a result, the recipes in this book are unpretentious and friendly for novice cooks. The recipes, for soups, appetizers, and salads, don't include nutritional information—a drawback if you want to count calories. But the dishes all have less than one gram of fat per serving, which means they fit easily into a 10 percent diet.

ALMOST VEGETARIAN by DIANA SHAW (*1994, Crown, $18 paper*)

A vegetarian diet is the most effective way to consume less fat, but if you love meat, it's not easy to cut it out. This book offers recipes to ease the transition. There are no red-meat dishes here, but plenty of chicken and seafood, along with vegetarian and "either/or" recipes. Shaw's instructions are clear and the recipes reliable. Most contain fewer than ten grams of fat per serving.

THE LIGHT TOUCH COOKBOOK by MARIE SIMMONS (*1992, Chapters, $19.95 paper*)

Simmons has taken classic recipes and made them significantly lower in fat. Meat loaf, for instance, is bulked up with low-fat lentils and spinach. Recipes for every course are delicious, and most contain fewer than ten grams of fat per serving. —*Lisë Stern*

5. CHRONIC DISEASES

will be when she returns. No French chefs in skyscraping hats, no yoga classes, no hand-holding. "This is like a fake world," she reminds herself before going to sleep. "A protected environment."

O N THE FLIGHT HOME, during a layover in the Chicago airport, Stolz strolls through the Mrs. Fields cookie store. She strolls out again, cookieless. At home that night, she sets her alarm clock for 5:15 A.M., a half hour earlier than usual. When the buzzer rings, she pads down the hall and manages 15 minutes of yoga and meditation before the day begins. That evening, after getting off work and picking up Julian from school, Stolz climbs on her stepper for 45 minutes of cardio, as she calls it, picking up the phone to call first Borkenhagen, then Pitts.

Day 7: The 5:15 bugle call is a thing of the past. "I had to draw the line somewhere," says Stolz.

Many people find the prescription of an hour a day of stress management at least as difficult to stick to as the diet. In fact, half of the folks who drop out of the program say it was this requirement that gave them trouble. During the retreat, Stolz attempted—through meditation and visualization—to make what the instructor called a healing journey into her heart. She got stuck somewhere en route, fidgeting. "I'm not a sitter," she explains.

But she's persevering with the diet and exercise. The chihuahua-sized chocolate bunny sitting on the hall table—a leftover from Easter—remains untouched. She rarely cooks dinner, but when she does, she finds herself dishing up lots of variations on vegetarian burgers. While her husband, Ralph, supports her attempt to change, the shopping, cooking, and planning of meals are up to Beverly. And like many retreat graduates, she finds that preparing Ornish-approved meals is just too time consuming. Besides, she hasn't been able to make her low-fat dishes taste as good as the ones at the retreat, and they haven't exactly met with unqualified approval from Ralph and Julian. She and her family eat out just about every night, at restaurants that offer low-fat fare.

After dinner each night, Beverly undergoes mild torture while she watches Ralph gobble down one or even two ice cream bars. "Ralph eats what he always did," says Stolz. "He still has low cholesterol."

Week 8: On a June morning, Stolz rushes into her husband's office, eager to see the results of her latest blood work. She is sure her diligence has paid off.

In fact, her cholesterol and triglyceride counts have actually gone *up* slightly. Triglyceride levels sometimes do rise in people on low-fat vegetarian diets, but the increase is generally offset by a greater dip in cholesterol levels. Stolz, though, may have a genetic disorder that leaves her slower to respond to dietary changes. "I just feel that I've been making such an effort and I'm not getting rewarded," she tells her husband.

Total rebellion is not in her nature, but Stolz stages a minor uprising. She samples forbidden foods—butter, ice cream, chocolate—and she lays off her stepper when she develops tendinitis. "I have all kinds of excuses," she says. "Just life in general throws me off."

That's Stolz at the two-month marker: discouraged. Ann Girard, of Rehoboth, Delaware, who altered her habits to help her husband, has had an easier time of it. "To do the yoga, stress management, and exercise takes two hours out of every day," says Girard. "So we sometimes alternate: yoga one morning, exercise the next.

"I still miss my daily six cups of coffee. All in all, though, we're doing really well."

Month 6: Stolz has bounced back from her rebellion, propelled by good news: Her blood tests are finally looking better. Much better. Her cholesterol is edging downward; her triglycerides have plummeted 200 points.

"She still pushes herself too hard," says her friend Karen Pitts, "but she doesn't go as long now without slowing down."

Stolz has been working out three times a week with a trainer. At a favorite restaurant, she routinely orders simple pastas. She's even managed to get Julian to notice the fat content in foods, though the second-grader still loves his toasted cheese sandwiches.

With her occasional splurges and halfhearted stress reduction efforts, Stolz's regimen might be called Ornish Lite. The fact is, the naysaying experts might be right: For those of us who haven't suffered a heart attack or other stark reminder of mortality, the full glory of Ornish's program may require more day-in, day-out discipline than we can muster. The good news is that even moderate success may well be enough to produce big improvements in health.

Stolz is happy with what she's been able to accomplish so far. A short time ago, she managed to pass a major hurdle: a return trip to Boudin's bakery in Chicago. She still reveled in the sourdough bread, but said no to the butter. For a native of the valley of the doughnuts, that just might be called victory.

Ann Japenga is a contributing editor.

122

Heart disease in women: Special symptoms, special risks

Coronary heart disease in women, often overlooked or undertreated, is finally getting its due.

The prevalence of risk factors for coronary heart disease and the death rate from the disease itself have both been dropping steadily in the U.S. for several decades. But those declines have been much less impressive in women than in men. One major reason: Physicians have traditionally regarded coronary disease as mainly a man's disease. So they've diagnosed and treated it less aggressively in women, and they haven't pushed women as hard as men to reduce their risk of the disease by changing their health habits.

Equally important, researchers have traditionally studied coronary disease mainly in men. That has obscured significant differences between the sexes concerning both the symptoms and the causes of the disease—and may have further hindered efforts to prevent or diagnose the disease in women.

The box on the next page focuses on symptoms; here, we tell how the traditional risk factors—and risk-reducing factors—differ in women.

The differences in risk

The female hormone estrogen, abundant in premenopausal women, may protect the heart in at least four ways: It helps lower the "bad" LDL cholesterol, elevate the "good" HDL cholesterol, increase blood flow to the heart, and distribute body fat favorably. That protection helps explain why heart attack rarely strikes women before age 50, the average age of menopause, while it often strikes men in their forties. After menopause, when estrogen levels fall, the protective benefits generally start to fade, and coronary risk starts to rise; by age 60 or so, coronary disease becomes the leading cause of death in women.

Estrogen's benefits may contribute to at least some of the following differences between women's and men's coronary risk factors:

■ **Low HDL cholesterol.** Average levels of the "good" HDL are significantly higher in women than in men. (For unknown reasons, that gap shrinks only slightly after menopause.) So a low HDL level—less than 35 mg/dl—increases a woman's risk more than a man's, possibly because it represents a greater deviation from the norm in women. Further, a North Carolina study suggests that women may be able to raise their HDL level more than men can. The study found that aerobic exercise increased HDL by 20 percent in female coronary patients but by only 5 percent in male patients. (Other steps that can boost

> **Estrogen may protect the heart in at least four ways.**

HDL include weight loss, smoking cessation, moderate alcohol consumption, and medications that not only lower LDL but also raise HDL, provided the patient needs both benefits.)

■ **High blood pressure.** Women tend to develop hypertension later in life than men do, so the elevated pressure typically has less time to damage a woman's heart. That difference has led some doctors to treat hypertension less aggressively in all women. But when a woman does develop hypertension, it's just as harmful as in a man of the same age.

In addition, women are more likely than men to develop isolated systolic hypertension, or elevation of just the upper blood-pressure number. While doctors used to consider that condition relatively harmless, research has shown that reducing elevated systolic pressure reduces substantially the risk of both coronary disease and stroke. (To lower blood pressure: Lose weight, exercise regularly, don't drink alcohol excessively, reduce stress, restrict sodium intake, and, if necessary, take medication.)

■ **Diabetes.** Diabetes is more likely to damage the arteries, raise blood pressure, and worsen cholesterol levels in women than in men. Further, it can blunt the protective effects of estrogen. Indeed, diabetes multiplies the chance of developing coronary disease substantially more in women than in men.

So it's particularly important for female diabetics to reduce their alterable risk factors for coronary disease, including the ones listed in this story as well as obesity, inactivity, and high levels of the "bad" LDL cholesterol. In addition, postmenopausal women with diabetes should strongly consider hormone replacement therapy and regular aspirin use to further protect the heart.

Women who have had gestational diabetes—high blood sugar during pregnancy—are at high risk for eventually developing type II diabetes, the most common kind; that, in turn, increases their coronary risk. So they need to take protective steps against both diseases, particularly losing excess weight, exercising regularly, and not smoking.

■ **Body-fat distribution.** Fat tends to accumulate around the hips in women, the belly in men. The male pattern poses greater coronary risk; that's mainly because belly fat breaks down more readily than hip fat, causing metabolic changes that push up the "bad" LDL cholesterol, lower the "good" HDL cholesterol, and increase blood pressure.

Reprinted with permission from *Consumer Reports on Health*, May 1997, pp. 54-56. © 1997 by Consumers Union of U.S., Inc., Yonkers, NY 10703-1057.

But when women do develop that typically male pattern, it may be even more worrisome than when men do, since it often reflects a disorder dubbed "syndrome X." The disorder involves insulin resistance, probably the underlying cause of diabetes; that resistance leads to increased insulin levels, which may contribute to hypertension. Women with syndrome X also tend to have increased male-hormone levels, which reduce the protective benefits of estrogen.

The waist should be considerably smaller than the hips in women; in men, the waist and hips should be about the same size. Fortunately, the instability that helps make belly fat more dangerous also makes it easier to eliminate than hip fat. (Take the same steps you would to lose weight anywhere in your body: Do regular aerobic and strengthening exercise, and follow a low-fat, moderately low-calorie diet.)

■ **Smoking.** Some women incorrectly believe that smoking is less dangerous to a woman's heart than to a man's heart. Smoking not only damages the lining of the arteries but also lowers levels of the protective HDL and can speed the onset of menopause. Smoking may be particularly bad for the heart in women who take birth-control pills.

How the risk reducers differ

Exercising regularly and eating a low-fat diet can provide broad coronary protection by reducing several risk factors at once. Here are three other broadly protective steps that women may want to consider.

■ **Hormone replacement therapy.** Taking female hormones sharply reduces the risk of coronary disease by restoring the protection that women had before menopause. It also eases menopausal symptoms, slashes the risk of osteoporosis, and may decrease the chance of colon cancer, tooth loss, and possibly osteoarthritis and Alzheimer's disease. For most women, those benefits clearly outweigh the treatment's main drawbacks—renewed menstrual bleeding with some regimens, and possibly a slight increase in the risk of breast cancer and blood clots in the legs and lungs. Potential exceptions include women who have a personal or family history of breast cancer; a low risk of coronary disease and osteoporosis; or large uterine fibroids, active liver disease, or a history of blood clots.

■ **Aspirin.** Regular use of low-dose aspirin clearly lowers the risk of heart attack in men by lowering the risk of blood clots. The available evidence suggests that aspirin may have the same effect in women. However, aspirin can also cause gastrointestinal bleeding and may increase the chance of hemorrhagic stroke, the kind caused by bleeding.

So an aspirin regimen is worth considering only by people who are at increased risk of having a heart attack. That includes anyone with coronary disease; postmenopausal women under age 60 or so who have at least two risk factors for the disease; and postmenopausal women over age 60, as well as men, who have at least one risk factor. (Risk factors include the

---

Diagnosis in women: Why the delay?

Heart attacks are twice as deadly in women as in men. That's partly because the attacks typically strike women when they're older and in poorer health than men. But it's also because doctors often diagnose and treat the underlying coronary disease in women at a later, more advanced stage.

One reason for the later diagnosis is that women's coronary complaints may be harder to interpret than the usually unmistakable symptoms in men. For coronary disease, the hallmark in men is angina, or central-chest pain that comes on with exertion and subsides with rest; for heart attack, it's crushing chest pain, often spreading to the shoulders, neck, jaw, arms, or upper back.

The same symptoms often signal coronary disease or heart attack in women. But female coronary patients tend to be less physically active than male patients, partly due to age and poorer general health. And the disease is often diagnosed at a later, more advanced stage in women. For both reasons, women are more likely than men to develop chest pain when they're resting.

Further, women with coronary disease are more likely to report vague symptoms that can be caused by many other ailments or even medications. Those symptoms include breathlessness, heartburn, nausea, and severe fatigue for coronary disease; and mild chest pain accompanied by breathlessness, dizziness, heartburn, or nausea for heart attack. Researchers theorize that advanced age, diabetes (which is far more prevalent in female than male coronary patients), and unknown causes may all help produce vaguer coronary symptoms in women.

But vaguer symptoms may not be the only reason for the delayed diagnosis: Some evidence suggests that doctors may take coronary disease less seriously in women. For example, a recent study found that when women come to the emergency room with essentially the same coronary symptoms as men do, they're less likely to receive heart medications, and more likely to be handed drugs for an "anxiety attack." Other studies have shown that even when women have *worse* coronary symptoms than men or are actually having a heart attack, they're less likely to undergo angiography, the definitive diagnostic test.

So if you're a woman, you need to know all the symptoms listed above—the classic complaints as well as the vague ones. And you need to take those symptoms seriously, and make sure that your doctor does the same.

items listed in the preceding section, plus high LDL-cholesterol levels, physical inactivity, and a family history of coronary disease before age 60.)

But those guidelines consider only the general risks of aspirin. Many specific conditions and medications can make aspirin excessively dangerous (see *Consumer Reports on Health* March 1997 issue). So it's essential to consult your doctor before starting to take aspirin regularly.

■ **Alcohol.** Moderate drinking may reduce the risk of coronary disease by up to 40 percent, mainly because it boosts HDL cholesterol and fights blood clots. But even moderate drinking has significant risks, such as an increased chance of alcoholism, auto accidents, falls, and breast cancer. In men, the benefits start to outweigh the risks by age 40 or so. In women, that shift doesn't start until after menopause. However, the same precaution about taking aspirin applies even more strongly to drinking alcohol: Talk with your doctor first.

Note that the definition of moderate drinking differs between the sexes, too: no more than two drinks per day for men, one per day for women. That's because women tend to have smaller amounts of a certain stomach enzyme as well as a smaller liver, both of which help break down the alcohol.

Summing up

The following measures are even more important for women than for men—or apply to women only:

■ Try to boost low HDL, stop smoking, and lose abdominal fat.

■ Be particularly diligent about reducing your overall coronary risk if you have diabetes.

■ Make sure your doctor is aware of—and takes seriously—any coronary risk factors you may have, including isolated systolic hypertension.

■ If you're postmenopausal, talk to your doctor about estrogen therapy and possibly moderate drinking. If you're postmenopausal *and* at increased coronary risk, talk about aspirin therapy as well.

CONSENSUS: NO LONG-TERM LINK BETWEEN the Pill and Breast Cancer

By Gary Goldenberg

MR. GOLDENBERG IS A FREELANCE SCIENCE WRITER.

Experts worldwide on oral contraceptives and cancer collaborated recently on a study designed to settle a long-standing issue: Does taking the Pill increase a woman's long-term risk of breast cancer? Their consensus is no.

"This study answers the major outstanding question we had about the Pill: Does it have any persistent effect on breast cancer long after women stop taking it? We now know that more than ten years after stopping the Pill, women are not at increased risk." So says Dr. Valerie Beral, chief of the Cancer Epidemiology Unit at Oxford University, who led the multinational effort.

"The absence of any increase ten or more years after stopping is found consistently for all groups of women studied—young women, older women, women with a history of breast cancer, women of different ethnic origin, from developed or developing countries," adds Beral. "It was also true regardless of how old women were when they began taking the Pill, how long they took it and what type of Pill they took."

The Imperial Cancer Research Fund in the United Kingdom underwrote the four-year study, which *The Lancet* published in June 1996. The complete paper constitutes a special supplement to the September 1996 issue of *Contraception*.

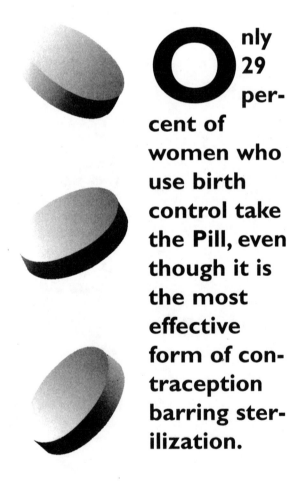

Only 29 percent of women who use birth control take the Pill, even though it is the most effective form of contraception barring sterilization.

The researchers did observe a very small rise in breast cancer among current and recent users of the Pill. But according to Oxford University researcher Dr. Gillian Reeves, who helped interpret

Good News Is No News?

The news media seriously neglected the Pill/breast cancer study, even though it had all the hallmarks of a major story: The study was the most authoritative investigation of its kind; it was published in a prestigious medical journal; it purported to settle a controversial public-health question; and it had the potential to affect tens of millions of American women.

Only after a public-relations effort by Columbia-Presbyterian Medical Center and Elsevier Science (which publishes *Contraception*) did the study receive wide coverage. (*NBC Nightly News* covered the study in 15 seconds, during which it alluded to scientists who disagreed with the findings.) To be sure, public-relations offices are a major means of getting news to the public. Still, one wonders why this study generated so little coverage directly. Is it simply that good news is no news?

"This is something that I come up against all the time," says Joshua M. Peck, a former reporter for Gannett newspapers who works for Jaffe Associates, a national marketing and public-relations firm. "If something isn't alarming or threatening to the reader, the chances of it being covered by the media moves down several notches and sometimes reaches zero. . . . The heart of this story is, 'You were worried about something, [but]

there's nothing to worry about,' and to most journalistic ears that doesn't sound like a story. Give them something to worry about and you've got the front page."

Dr. Scott Ratzan, director of the Emerson-Tufts Program in Health Communication and editor of the *Journal of Health Communication*, evidently agrees.

Reporters and editors, he says, typically look for something "that upsets the status quo, where it knocks the train off the track, and that's a major problem [with] the way that health and medical news is covered." The opposite problem, he says, is making something out of nothing. "A year ago in Britain, [reporters] blew things out of proportion when they talked about [the link between] oral contraceptives and deep venous thrombosis [blood clot formation in the heart]. Well, the risk went up from 1 in 10,000 to 2 in 10,000," Ratzan notes. The misleading media coverage lead to an excess of 5,000 pregnancies, 3,000 of which ended in abortions and 2,000 of which ended in births.

The *London Sunday Times* secretly obtained a prepublication copy of the Pill/breast cancer article before its publication in *The Lancet*—and ran the story under the banner, "Pill Users Face a 10-Year Tumour Risk."

the study data, "After women come off the Pill, this excess declines, disappearing completely after ten years."

"The Pill Causes 'Diagnosis'"

"This finding does not mean that the Pill causes cancer," emphasizes Dr. Carolyn Westhoff, a birth-control specialist at New York's Columbia-Presby-

terian Medical Center, who reviewed the paper for *Contraception* and wrote an accompanying editorial. "What it probably means is that the Pill causes 'diagnosis.' It may be that doctors who prescribe the Pill feel more compelled to do more breast exams, or that the sort of women who ask for the Pill are more likely to ask for mammograms. Cancer is a disease that develops over many years. If the Pill actually caused cancer, you would see a delayed effect, not an immediate one."

The finding that the cancers discovered in Pill users were less likely to have spread outside the breast than the cancers discovered in nonusers lends credence to Westhoff's hypothesis. "Women on the Pill are probably benefiting by getting diagnosed sooner, before their cancers become metastatic," she states.

Feeling the Whole Elephant

For years researchers have been giving women mixed signals about the link between the Pill and breast cancer. According to Westhoff, this inconsistency is not due to "shoddy science" but rather to the difficulties inherent in analyzing small risks and in studying a drug whose patterns of use have changed over three decades. "It has not been possible to get all the situations in a single study," she adds. "Any one of those studies will get only a little piece of the answer. It's like the [fable of the] blind men feeling the elephant." Ultimately, researchers agreed that the only way to "feel the whole elephant" was to combine and reconsider data from as many existing studies as possible. Thus, in 1992 more than 200 scientists from around the world joined to form the Collaborating Group on Hormonal Factors in Breast Cancer. The researchers combined data on more than 150,000 women from 54 studies conducted in 26 countries.

"The data presented here represent about 90% of the worldwide epidemiological evidence on breast cancer risk and use of hormonal contraceptives. What is known about the 12 studies for which data were not included would have been consistent with the main findings," Beral and her colleagues stated in *The Lancet.*

"Everybody put their egos aside and submitted all their data for this combined analysis, which has taken years to do. It's very rare that controversial areas in medicine get resolved in such a fashion," says Westhoff.

What Will the Public Believe?

The question remains: How will women react to this study? "There have been all these conflicting studies saying it depends on which Pill you're taking, what age you were when you took it, family history, length of time on the Pill, and so on," says Westhoff. "It has raised people's level of anxiety. At the very least, it has given them the idea, where there's smoke there's fire. The average person doesn't understand that science progresses by two steps forward, one step back, and 18 steps sideways. The whole issue has been bad for trust of the Pill and bad for trust of science."

Because of such confusion, only 29 percent of women who use birth control take the Pill, even though it is the most effective form of contraception barring sterilization. Most women who take the Pill are below age 26. Very few women in their later childbearing years take the Pill, apparently because they fear that doing so will lead to breast cancer and blood clots. The risk of blood clots leading to a heart attack or stroke has been limited largely to smokers over age 35; this risk has diminished with the introduction of lower-dose oral contraceptives.

"This anxiety has driven women from a highly effective form of contraception, with devastating consequences," says Westhoff, who reports that half of all pregnancies in the United States are unintentional. The unplanned pregnancy rate is even higher—77 percent—in women in their 40s. "Women need to know that we now have enough data to say that the Pill does not cause breast cancer," she says.

Women should also know that there are many reported benefits to taking the Pill, Westhoff adds. Studies show that Pill-taking decreases the risk of ovarian, uterine, and endometrial cancer; endometriosis (the extrauterine growth of mucosal tissue native to the uterus); ovarian cysts; pelvic inflammatory disease; benign breast disease; ectopic (extrauterine) pregnancy; and excessive menstruation. Taking the Pill reportedly also increases bone density.

So why didn't the media jump on this story?

REDESIGNING WOMEN

Breast Cancer & Estrogen

Women in rich countries like ours are at a greater risk of breast cancer than women in poor societies. Some scientists think they now know the reason why—and they're proposing a radical solution.

Rosie Mestel

TIME AFTER TIME it happened during the nine months he spent in Zaire: Peter Ellison would be earnestly explaining his theories to a Lese villager, a slash-and-burn farmer eking out a living planting cassavas, plantains, rice, peanuts, and maize in the hot, humid rain forests. A woman's body, Ellison would say, is cleverly designed to assess whether it is a promising time to carry a baby based on how much food the woman is getting to eat and how many calories she's burning. In seasons of plenty she'll be extra-fertile, since her body has what it needs to bring a new life into the world. In times of want—such as the famines the Lese endure each year when their harvest gives out—fertility will plummet. As Ellison jabbed at his explanatory charts, sooner or later the villager would pipe up. "Oh, that's well known. No one gets pregnant in the hunger season."

Well known to the Lese it may be, but Ellison's work has some startling implications for the rest of us. The evolutionary biologist has directed research in Africa, Asia, Europe, and North and South America, sampling spittle from the mouths of indulgent farmers, animal herders, weight watchers, and joggers. From that saliva he measures estrogen, a hormone that nudges eggs in the ovary to mature, and progesterone, another key sex hormone. In every culture hormone levels seem perfectly in line with the amount of energy women have available—essentially, the calories they gain in food minus those burned in work. In the Lese, for instance, Ellison found that the estrogen in samples from the lean months was about half that in spit from the bountiful months, enough of a drop to pretty much render the women temporarily infertile.

No prizes, of course, for guessing which of the groups studied by Ellison produced the most estrogen. A quick cruise through a U.S. supermarket—with all of its steak and eggs, cheese and chips—provides a clue, as does that propensity we Westerners have for loafing on a couch with the TV remote. Our plentiful diet and easygoing lifestyle have prompted our bodies to produce unusually high levels of estrogen. And that's bad news.

It's true that we need the hormone to be fertile, to protect our bones, and to keep our bad cholesterol in check. We may even need it to help ward off Alzheimer's disease. Yet estrogen—too much of it—carries a high price: It significantly increases the risk of developing breast cancer. American women have the highest rate of breast cancer in the world; more than 184,000 of them will be diagnosed with it this year and another 44,000 will die of it. The breast cancer rate has been climbing steadily for decades, fast enough to have entirely canceled out the progress in treatment over the past 60 years. It's a sad fact that as many women per 100,000 die of breast cancer today as did in 1930.

Sloth and gluttony aren't the only reasons we're overdosing on hormones. Contraception has freed us from lifelong cycles of pregnancy and breast-feeding—both of which quash estrogen production—so we ovulate much more often and churn out estrogen for much longer periods of time. Consider the life history of a typical professional woman in the United States: puberty on average at age 12; childbirth often postponed until her thirties or even early forties while she slogs through grad school or gets her career up and running; just a couple of kids, when she finally gets around to having them, followed by a few months of breast-feeding at best.

Then consider the life that our hunter-gatherer ancestors likely lived. Girls were not as well nourished and thus hit puberty later, probably around the age of 16—similar to young women in groups like the farming Lese and the Kalahari Desert's hunter-gatherer !Kung today (and even among the rural Chinese and Japanese until recently). Pregnancy wasn't far behind, followed by breast-feeding for as long as four years and of an intensity that would boggle most Western women's minds. (The !Kung, even today, carry their babies everywhere and suckle them two to four times an hour through the day.) After weaning would come another pregnancy.

"PIKE'S PILL" WOULD BE A NEW KIND OF BIRTH CONTROL PILL, ONE THAT ARTIFICIALLY KICKS OUR HORMONE LEVELS BACK TO WHAT THEY USED TO BE.

In fact, if you were to do all the number crunching, you'd find that our typical female ancestor probably had as few as 50 fertile menstrual periods in her life. By the time *we* start worrying about hot flashes, that number is more like 450.

In other words, we're living a very different life from the one evolution fashioned our bodies for, with some very unfortunate consequences. The dismal breast cancer statistics, together with the work of evolutionary biologists, are prompting some strong measures. Malcolm Pike, head of the preventive medicine department at the University of Southern California, is proposing a drastic remedy indeed: He wants to put women on a regimen of drugs that would shut down their ovaries—and hence estrogen production—from puberty until death, with occasional time-outs for childbirth. Darcy Spicer, a breast cancer specialist at USC, has joined Pike's campaign. Their idea is to offer "Pike's Pill" as a new kind of birth control pill—one that would artificially kick our hormone levels, if not our lifestyles, back to something more akin to the way things used to be. The approach may sound shockingly heavy handed, but breast cancer specialists are taking it seriously.

"You're not going to get women to forgo college and opt for early childbearing simply so that they can decrease their breast cancer risk," says Spicer. "It's not about to happen. Especially with career-oriented women, who are if anything delaying childbearing even further. Instead, we want to create new ways to go back to the way our physiology evolved to be."

A lifelong regimen of chemicals, say Pike and Spicer, may offer modern women the most natural way to live.

FORTY-THREE-YEAR-OLD Jackie DeHay has had a taste of this new kind of life. Her history, more than any sheaf of statistics, has told her what the breast cancer stakes really are. Her grandmother had breast cancer.

When DeHay was in her twenties she watched her mother die of the disease. "It was a horrifying experience, watching the cancer destroy her body," she says.

DeHay was left to deal with the knowledge that she's at high risk herself. Her sister once thought about having her breasts removed before cancer could have a chance to grow in them. DeHay says she'd consider that herself if a genetic test were to show she carries a mutation in the gene BRCA1 or BRCA2, which can raise the lifetime risk of breast cancer to as high as 85 percent. (She hasn't yet decided whether to be tested.) But DeHay is fond of her breasts and would much prefer to keep them. Even more, she'd like some gentler preventive measure for her daughter, who at 26 is full of verve and still, her mom says, feeling immortal.

So DeHay barely hesitated in 1990 when she was asked to participate in a study at Spicer's clinic. Once a month for two and a half years she would jump into her car outsider her desert home in Palmdale and fight her way 70 miles down commuter-packed freeways to the clinic in downtown Los Angeles. There she'd get a checkup and an injection of a synthetic hormone with the decidedly unwieldy designation of "gonadotropin-releasing hormone agonist." (Call it the ovary regulator, because that's what it is.) Between visits DeHay would swallow an assortment of pills containing other hormones. She rarely got her period—and she loved it.

"I never felt better in my whole life," she says. "I always thought women who complained of PMS were weak women who needed an excuse. I never realized I had the symptoms myself." Suddenly she found herself free of those crabby, tearful moments (until she came off the regimen, that is, and her husband remarked on her mood swings). She was free, too, of monthly breast tenderness, also part and parcel of monthly estrogen cycles. "If I could I'd go back on those drugs in a heartbeat," she says.

But DeHay can't go back. The trial is over. It was just a preliminary test of the idea behind Pike's Pill: If you stop the division of breast cells that occurs naturally each month, you'll cut the risk of cancer.

Here's how a normal bodily function can lead to cancer: Every month a surge of estrogen, followed by a surge of progesterone, courses through the bloodstream to the breasts. "Go on," say the hormones to the breast's epithelial cells. "Divide—just on the outside chance you're soon going to suckle a baby." The cells duly divide, beginning the development of glands and ducts that will deliver milk to the nipple if the woman becomes pregnant. She usually doesn't, and the cells die off at the end of the cycle. "The breast is going up and down like a yo-yo," says reproductive biologist Roger Short of Melbourne University in Australia, who's long believed that modern reproductive patterns damage women's health. "It gets all excited, gets ready to start enlarging during pregnancy, and then there's no pregnancy. So hormone levels fall, and the breast says, 'I'll try again next month.'

Well, it really wasn't meant to keep trying month after month, year after year."

All of that trying carries a risk. In the normal course of things, DNA in cells is constantly being injured, mostly by free radicals produced as by-products of metabolism. That damage is usually repaired quickly, but if the cell divides first the mistake is set in stone. And mistakes in DNA can beget cancer. The more menstrual cycles, then, the higher the breast cancer risk. It makes sense that nuns have exceptionally high breast cancer rates—a phenomenon noted as far back as the 18th century—and that childless women generally have higher rates than those who have given birth. Childless women, after all, have periods each month until menopause, with nary a break for pregnancy. Moreover, breast cells don't completely mature until they're exposed to hormones released only during the late stages of pregnancy; once cells have fully developed, they are forever less vulnerable to chemicals or other agents that can damage DNA. So the earlier in her life a woman carriers a child to term—and the more often—the better.

"We've got to abandon this concept that if you don't ovulate every 28 days from age 11 to 45 there's something wrong with you," Spicer says. And the last thing the world needs is for every woman to have six kids, says Emory University radiologist Boyd Eaton, who coauthored an article with Pike and others about cancer and evolution. But how to mimic the protective effect of pregnancy in women who have few children or none?

The best bet, says Spicer, is the ovary-regulating hormone that was injected into DeHay once a month. It's actually a synthetic version of a hormone our bodies naturally produce, a small protein generated in a part of the brain called the hypothalamus. This ovary regulator is key to setting our monthly cycles in motion. Pulses of the hormone trigger puberty in girls; in a roundabout way, the pulses also command our ovaries to produce estrogen and progesterone. If it's produced in the right set of pulses, the ovary regulator makes our 28-day menstrual cycles tick by, regular as clockwork. But if you give the body a steady dose of the regulator, the system gets confused. The ovaries shut down, halting the production of estrogen, progesterone, and the small amounts of the male hormone testosterone women also require. Used this way, the ovary regulator is a contraceptive, plain and simple.

As it happens, chemicals similar to the one used by Spicer and Pike were considered for contraceptive use in the 1970s and early 1980s. Nasty side effects such as hot flashes and bone loss—the same problems some estrogen-deficient menopausal women suffer—persuaded scientists to look elsewhere. Today's birth control pills are a mix of synthetic progesterone and estrogen, or some type of progesterone alone. These may be fine as contraceptives since they, like Pike's Pill, shut down the ovaries when taken regularly, but they don't reduce cancer risk because they prompt breast cells to divide. The hormone

Cutting Risk Without Pills

Until there's a drug to prevent breast cancer, lifestyle changes offer the only hope of improving your odds. The most effective are unpalatable; A woman who is pregnant and then breast-feeding continually from puberty to menopause has a very low risk, for instance. But less extreme measures might help.

Exercise

Three to four hours of exercise a week throughout a woman's reproductive life may cut risk—possibly by as much as half, says Leslie Bernstein, an epidemiologist at the University of Southern California. Strenuous activity may delay puberty in girls, decreasing their lifetime estrogen exposure. And a number of studies indicate that women who exercise even moderately ovulate less regularly, reducing estrogen production.

Weight Control

Obesity can lower a young woman's chances of breast cancer slightly because it makes her ovulate irregularly. But carrying a lot of extra pounds after menopause can raise the risk, because fat cells produce estrogen, albeit a fraction of the amount put out in earlier years by the ovaries.

Alcohol

Drinking almost certainly raises the chances of developing breast cancer, most likely by interfering with enzymes that break estrogen down. Researchers say two alcoholic drinks a day can hike breast cancer risk by as much as 30 percent.

Dietary Fat

Breast cancer rates are highest in the countries with the richest diets—for example, the United States, where on average 35 percent of calories come from fat. But rigorous studies show the link is weak, if it exists at all. The Women's Health Initiative may provide a definitive answer; the study will track thousands of women on high- and low-fat diets for nine years. However, results are at least a decade away.

Other Dietary Changes

Compounds in soy protein may prevent estrogen from attaching to breast cells and ordering them to divide. Soy may also lengthen menstrual cycles, which would reduce estrogen exposure. Oat and wheat bran contain chemicals that may bind to estrogen and take it out of circulation. And cruciferous vegetables, such as broccoli and cabbage, contain a chemical that may lower levels of one type of estrogen. Scientists say it's not yet clear whether these foods really cut breast cancer risk. But a diet rich in fruits and vegetables can't hurt.—R.M.

in Pike's Pill, however, doesn't send a go-forth-and-multiply message to cells, and therein lies its hope. By Pike's calculations, if a woman stayed on his regimen for ten years, her breast cancer risk would fall by 50 percent. If she took it for 15 years, the decrease would be 75 percent.

That's the theory, anyway. But before forging ahead with the development of a brave new contraceptive, Pike and Spicer had to know if their regimen really cut the number of cell divisions in the breast. That's where De-Hay—and 17 other women at high risk for breast cancer—came in.

Twelve of these guinea pigs got a monthly shot of the regulator to "turn off" their ovaries. (The other six women were controls who received no medication.) There was more to the regimen than that, though. Each day DeHay swallowed a pill containing a smidgen of synthetic estrogen—far less than a premenopausal woman normally produces—to ward off hot flashes and to ensure that her bones stayed strong, her cholesterol levels low, and her mood chipper. She also took testosterone to limit bone loss and maintain libido. And every four months, just in case the estrogen pills were stimulating the uterine lining to grow excessively, she took synthetic progesterone tablets to trigger a period.

DOES IT REALLY MAKE SENSE TO TINKER WITH YOUR HORMONES THROUGHOUT LIFE IN HOPES OF WARDING OFF A DISEASE YOU MIGHT NEVER GET?

At the study's outset and again at its end, DeHay and her cohorts had mammograms. Comparing the two X-rays taken of each woman on the ovary-regulator regimen, radiologists found an encouraging difference: The breast tissue in the later films was less dense. Meanwhile, the mammograms of the women who'd received neither injections nor pills showed no change. Spicer and Pike think a less-dense breast is one in which cells are dividing less rapidly. If they're right, there's powerful reason to believe Pike's Pill does just what theory says it should: slash the risk of breast cancer.

AS PROMISING AS THIS SEEMS, don't expect your doctor to wax enthusiastic about "the brand-new anti-cancer birth control pill" anytime soon. For one thing, the regime is complicated and impractical right now. It's hard enough to remember to take vitamins once

a day, never mind all those pills and injections. For another, Pike and Spicer can't be certain that the changes apparent on the mammograms truly reflect a decrease in cell division. They recently tried to recruit women to take the drug for a few months and then give up a small sample of breast tissue, so that the dividing cells could actually be counted. Not surprisingly, they had such trouble finding volunteers that they abandoned the attempt.

There are other concerns as well, such as whether Pike's Pill might pose risks that outweigh its benefits. After all, no matter how much fear breast cancer engenders, no one is fated to get the disease. The fact that one in nine American women falls victim means that the average lifetime risk—calculated as the chance of developing breast cancer by age 90—is 11 percent. Does it really make sense to tinker with your body's natural hormonal fluxes throughout life in hopes of warding off a disease you might never get?

So far the ovary regulator seems to be quite safe; it's been tested in animals and used for up to six months at a stretch to treat women with a variety of conditions, including endometriosis and advanced breast cancer. But long-term risks haven't been studied. "There's no free lunch," says Susan Love, breast cancer surgeon and author of *Dr. Susan Love's Breast Book*. "There's no way you can take drugs for a long time and not have consequences, even though we might not know immediately what they will be."

Pike and Spicer are well aware that it's hard to get the Food and Drug Administration to approve drugs meant to be taken by healthy people, who have less to gain in compensation for any side effects. It's much easier to win approval for a new therapy to treat a disease than for, say, a new contraceptive. That's why the current round of testing for Pike's Pill is on a group of women who suffer from fibroids, noncancerous uterine growths that are spurred on by estrogen. (The standard treatment for fibroids is surgery, sometimes performed after the patient has spent a few months on the ovary regulator to shrink the tissue.) The hormones are easier to take now than they were for DeHay: Most are delivered by nasal spray, although the women may still have to swallow progesterone pills every few months. It will be at least several years before the results are known.

Pike and Spicer aren't the only ones hoping for the success of that experiment and those that will follow. There isn't exactly a plethora of guaranteed-safe ways to fend off breast cancer—a fact that puts the concerns about side effects into perspective. "I think most people in this field realize that we don't know enough—and I suspect will never know enough—to prevent most breast cancer," says Walter Willett, an epidemiologist at the Harvard School of Public Health. "And I say that having spent 20 years looking at risk factors. Actually we *do* know how to prevent almost all breast cancer, but the risk is so embedded in what we regard as a desirable lifestyle that we'd never get anyone to sign on. So we're probably going to have to do something partly artificial. I think Pike's Pill needs to be pursued."

If everything goes well, says Spicer, the regime will probably be offered first to the women with the most at stake, those with a high risk for breast cancer. Experts generally agree that it makes sense to focus on these women. "I could see that if you had a gene predisposing you to breast cancer and you were 20, still wanted to have a family someday, and needed contraception, this would be a reasonable way to go," says Love. "It certainly makes more sense than something like a preventive mastectomy."

Meanwhile, Pike's Pill isn't the only remedy with an evolutionary twist to it. Several crafty chemicals might con the body into thinking it's back in the good, old hunter-gatherer days. Scientists are studying other artificial hormones, especially those known as antiestrogens, which retain estrogen's benefits for the heart and bones without triggering cell division in the breast.

One of these, tamoxifen, is currently used to treat breast cancer and lower the risk of the tumor's return, but it may eventually do more than that. Early studies to see whether the hormone could prevent recurrence found that the rate of cancer in the unaffected breast dropped 40 percent. In other words, it seemed to be warding off new tumors as well. Several large clinical trials are exploring tamoxifen's potential as a breast cancer preventive for women at high risk. Still, the rest of us are unlikely to ever use it. Tamoxifen brings on hot flashes in 20 percent of the women who take it; worse, it seems to increase the likelihood of uterine cancer. The chance may be worth taking if you know your chromosomes carry some nasty baggage. But if you have no special reason to worry, the trade-off may not seem so reasonable.

Another antiestrogen may prove to be a safer alternative to postmenopausal estrogen replacement therapy. Raloxifene appears to maintain bone density and lower cholesterol without increasing the chances of breast cancer. The hormone is under development by Eli Lilly, which hopes to obtain FDA approval within a couple of years.

Pike's Pill is at least five years away from large-scale, long-term trials, says Spicer, and a decade or more from reaching the market. If and when it finally arrives, no doubt some people will feel squeamish or even outraged about such major manipulation of women's bodies. But,

argues Emory radiologist Eaton, look at a drug we already take: the Pill. It's a synthetic hormone. We swallow it day in, day out, for decades. It interferes with our physiology, throwing our normal hormonal cycles completely out of whack. "I remember when people first brought out birth control pills there was a big dispute over whether it was ethically or biologically appropriate to do this," he says. "Well, if you think about the things we're proposing now, they're not so different from birth control pills. They're altering reproductive experience for an expected benefit."

SOME MIGHT BE LEERY OF MANIPULATING THE BODY SO DRASTICALLY. BUT WOMEN AT HIGH RISK FEEL THEY CAN'T TRUST THEIR BODIES ANYWAY.

Spicer certainly understands why people might be leery of the kind of hormonal tinkering he and Pike are proposing, regardless of whether those worries are rooted in fears about unforeseen consequences or simply in philosophy. But as a physician he cannot forget what's at stake. Every day he treats women who are dying of breast cancer and women who, like DeHay, have reason to feel particularly scared of one day finding a telltale lump. These women, he says, need more than lifestyle changes, and they aren't likely to be put off by the notion of altering a body they feel they can't trust to begin with.

"When I first started in oncology about 20 years ago, I came on board with enormous optimism that breast cancer would be the next curable malignancy," Spicer says. "I was young, and I wanted to be involved in something that was immediately likely to be successful. Well, in medicine, we're generally far more successful at preventing something than we are at treating it. I think we actually can develop something that will make people feel not just normal but better than normal."

Rosie Mestel is a contributing editor.

The **Cancer** Nobody Talks About

Last year, when Beth Moore was thirty-seven, she began to have gas pains and found blood in her stool—symptoms she knew all too well can signal colorectal cancer. "I was alarmed because both my father and grandmother died from it," she says.

When Moore, a mother of three in Birmingham, Alabama, consulted her doctor, he strongly recommended that she undergo a diagnostic test for colorectal cancer. But he also told her that the gas might be related to lactose intolerance, the inability to digest milk and milk products.

As soon as Moore began to avoid dairy products, her gas and bleeding stopped. She decided to put off scheduling the test. "I had lots of excuses," she says. "But I think the truth was, I was a little scared. I had heard the test was quite unpleasant."

It took Moore six months to overcome her reluctance. To her surprise, the colonoscopy, a procedure in which a thin scope is inserted through the anus to view the colon walls, was much easier to undergo than she expected (it's done while a patient is sedated). Even better, no malignant growths were found.

Unfortunately, many other young women aren't as lucky as Moore. Contrary to a widely believed myth, colorectal cancer is not primarily a male problem: The disease ranks third after lung and breast cancer as a leading killer of women. And, unfortunately, young women are not spared. A recent study published in *The New England Journal of Medicine*

It's the third leading cancer killer of women, yet most of us know little about it. Could you be at risk? Here, how to protect yourself from colorectal cancer

By Janis Graham

revealed that women between ages thirty and forty-four with a family history of colorectal cancer (defined as a mother, father or sibling with the disease) have a threefold greater risk for developing it than women over age fifty-five with a similar background.

Despite the prevalence of the disease, many young women are not aware of their risk or familiar with the early-warning signs. The good news is that early symptoms are easy to recognize, and simple screening and diagnostic tests are widely available. Plus, there are steps women can take right now—

while in their twenties, thirties and forties—to reduce their risk.

How trouble starts

The colon, also referred to as the large intestine, is a five- to six-foot pipeline. The uppermost section connects to the small intestine, which helps digest and remove nutrients from food. After digestion, food moves into the colon, where any remaining water is absorbed into the body and solid waste (stool) is produced. Stool is pushed into the last six to eight inches of the colon—the rectum—and exits through the inch-long anus.

When healthy, both the colon and the rectum have a smooth inner lining that helps process wastes. But as many as 20 to 35 percent of all adults over fifty have an overgrowth of cells in the colon's lining, which leads to the formation of precancerous growths called polyps. These can also develop in the rectum (5 to 10 percent of all colorectal cancers arise in the rectal-wall tissue). While many polyps remain harmless, over the years some may grow and undergo an array of cell changes that lead to a malignancy.

These potentially cancerous polyps tend to run in families. A study published last January in *The New England Journal of Medicine* found that siblings, children and parents of people with adenomas, one type of benign polyp, have nearly twice the risk of a person with no family history of developing colorectal cancer. But with proper screening, these polyps can be detected early and removed—effectively staving off cancer.

Your best defense

Watch for any of the following early-warning signs: persistent diarrhea or constipation (occasional bouts may be nothing to worry about); blood in the stool; frequent gas pain, bloating or cramps; a feeling of incomplete emptying after bowel movements; a frequently urgent and painful need to defecate; change in stool size; unusual fatigue; anemia.

Developing any one of these signs rarely means you have advanced colorectal cancer, according to Sidney J. Winawer, M.D., chief of gastroenterology and nutrition at Memorial Sloan-Kettering Cancer Center, in New York City. "In fact, they could be signs of other unrelated conditions, like hemorrhoids or ulcers," he explains. "But no one, no matter what age, should ever neglect suspicious symptoms. These things always warrant a visit to the doctor."

Because the disease sometimes produces no symptoms, your best level of defense is to be screened regularly, based on your age and family history (see "Colon Health Checks," right). Genetics plays a large role in determining who develops the disease, as does what you eat: A high-fat, low-fiber diet slows the movement of fecal content through the colon—and thus increases exposure to toxic substances. Popcorn (minus the oil and butter), fiber and fresh fruits and vegetables, on the other hand, speed digestion. So, the final defensive tactic is to eat a healthy diet, but also be sure to get lots of exercise and limit your alcohol intake. In addition:

● **Get enough calcium and wheat bran**. A diet high in these nutrients may lower the risk of colorectal cancer by reducing the level of acids that may promote tumor growth. In a small study published last January in *The Journal of the National Cancer Institute*, people at high risk for colorectal cancer who ate 13.5 g of wheat bran supplements daily for nine months produced 52 percent

Colon Health Checks

*b*ecause of better screening tests, about 60 percent of colon cancers are now caught in their earliest stages, when the cure rate is about 91 percent.

In fact, if everyone followed early-detection screening guidelines, the number of deaths from colon cancer could easily be slashed in half, say the experts. The American Cancer Society recommends the following three tests:

Fecal occult blood test This is a safe, simple and inexpensive (under $20) screen for hidden blood in the feces. The patient smears a sample of stool on a card, then sends it to her doctor or a lab for analysis. Its usefulness is hotly debated, but women at average risk for colorectal cancer—anyone with no symptoms whatsoever and no family history of the disease—should have a fecal occult blood test annually, beginning at age fifty. Women with a family history of colorectal cancer should begin to have the fecal occult blood test annually at age thirty-five.

Digital rectal examination Less than 10 percent of rectal cancers are detected this way, but this should be part of any routine exam for women over forty.

Sigmoidoscopy The sigmoidoscope is a thin, flexible, lighted tubular instrument that is inserted into the colon through the anus, enabling a physician to view the walls of the bottom third of the colon. It is done in a doctor's office, takes less than ten minutes, requires no sedation or anesthesia and costs less than $200. The chief drawback is that sigmoidoscopy detects cancers only in the lower third of the colon (called the sigmoid), and approximately half of all malignancies occur in the upper part.

Women at average risk should have sigmoidoscopy performed every three to five years, beginning at age fifty. For women at higher risk, sigmoidoscopy is often recommended every three to five years, starting at age thirty-five.

If you have a family history of colon cancer or have symptoms of the disease, these diagnostic and screening tests may be recommended:

Colonoscopy A colonoscope is similar to a sigmoidoscope, but it is longer and capable of examining the entire five- to six-foot length of the colon. The other advantage is that polyps can be removed during the procedure. It is more expensive, however—about $1,000—and it requires sedation.

For those at high risk, this test is performed every five years, starting at age thirty-five.

Double-contrast barium enema After you are given an enema containing barium, a white, chalky solution, X rays are taken. The barium outlines the colon and rectum on the X rays, highlighting any polyps. This test is often combined with sigmoidoscopy.

Like colonoscopy, the barium enema allows examination of the entire colon, but it is less expensive (about $300) and requires no sedation.

This test is for those with no known risk factors who are experiencing symptoms.

Genetic testing A blood test can now reveal whether you carry the familial polyposis gene, which, when mutated, can cause hundreds to thousands of polyps to develop throughout the colon. (In all, at least eight genes involved in the origin of colon cancer have been identified.) The gene is inherited by just 1 percent of people whose families carry it, and the gene is deadly: Carriers will almost definitely develop colon cancer by age fifty-five. Anyone with a first-degree relative who died from or was diagnosed with colon cancer at a young age is a likely candidate for testing.

Virtual colonoscopy On the horizon is another test, which combines X-ray and computer technology for a three-dimensional view of the colon. Currently being tested as a substitute for barium enemas and traditional colonoscopy, this technique requires the patient to hold her breath for thirty seconds while air is inserted in the colon and 400 or 500 images are gathered, fed into a computer and combined onscreen. The examination would last less than one minute.

Treatment Breakthroughs

many women fear colon-cancer surgery because they link it to the need for a colostomy—a procedure in which a surgeon removes the colon and creates an opening in the abdominal wall so wastes can be excreted into an exterior collection bag. Today, however, because of advances in surgery, permanent colostomies are necessary less than 2 percent of the time.

Early colon cancers (which make up about 50 percent of all cases) often can be removed entirely through the colonoscope. When abdominal surgery is required, the diseased tissue is removed and healthy segments of the bowel are reconnected. Although colon cancers that have spread outside the bowel wall require radiation and/or chemotherapy, more than 61 percent of all patients treated for colon cancer are disease-free five years later.

Surprisingly, surgical techniques have become so advanced that the entire colon can be removed without the need for a permanent colostomy. Once the colon is taken out, the small intestine is reconstructed so that it connects to the anal muscles. The result: Bowel movements tend to be more frequent.

Researchers are making even more progress. They are testing a vaccine that would stimulate the body's immune system to fight the disease. The trial will include twelve to fifty men and women who have had colon cancer. "The vaccine would help reduce the colon-cancer recurrence rate," explains the study's principal investigator, Albert F. LoBuglio, M.D., director of the University of Alabama at Birmingham Comprehensive Cancer Center. Results are expected in a year.

less bile acid than those who had low fiber intakes; those who consumed 1,500 mg of calcium daily had a 35 percent reduction.

Further research needs to be done, but in the meantime, the National Institutes of Health recommends that women between ages twenty-five and fifty get 1,000 mg of calcium a day and 20 to 35 g of fiber.

● **Ask your doctor about taking aspirin regularly.** The research so far is impressive: A large study of almost 90,000 women published in *The New England Journal of Medicine* last September, for instance, indicated a 44 percent reduced risk for those who took four to six tablets a week over a period of ten or more consecutive years. Aspirin may slow tumor growth by blocking the formation of prostaglandins, substances that regulate pain, fever, and cell and tumor growth. But it is too soon to recommend universal use, cautions Robert S. Sandler, M.D., professor of gastroenterology at the University of North Carolina School of Medicine, in Chapel Hill. "We don't know what dose is best or whether aspirin increases the risk for some other diseases, such as strokes," he says. Consult your physician.

● **Don't smoke.** A recent study published in *The Journal of the National Cancer Institute* showed that women who started smoking before age thirty and continued to smoke a pack a day for more than ten years doubled their colorectal-cancer risk.

● **Consider postmenopausal estrogen replacement therapy (ERT).** Among women who had been using ERT for more than ten years, there was a 55 percent reduction in colorectal-cancer risk, according to a new study published in *The Journal of the National Cancer Institute*. The longer their use, the lower their risk. A possible explanation: Estrogen has been shown to reduce the concentration of tumor-friendly bile acids in the colon.

Experts consider colon cancer highly preventable. In fact, the biggest risk factor for the disease may be unwillingness to address the topic. In other words, as long as women aren't too embarrassed or fearful to practice preventive health habits, to get properly screened and to see their doctors about any early-warning signs, most will find that their odds of developing colon cancer will remain low.

Janis Graham is a health writer who lives in Ithaca, New York. She has written for Fitness, Shape and Self.

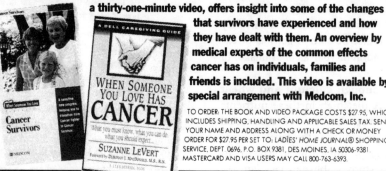

Mole Patrol

Are you ready for body mapping? You will need one totally naked body (your own), a hand mirror, and a blowdryer.

Katharine Greider

Oh, dear, we've made it sound like fun. It's not, unless you get a kick out of getting intimately acquainted with the various spots on your skin. But do it. Once you know them, you can check yourself regularly for changes that might presage a skin cancer. Dermatologists recommend you do this every few months.

The first time can be an exercise in paranoia (*"Tumors,"* comes the cry from the bathroom). It's true that malignant melanoma, the most deadly of the skin cancers, can resemble a mole, or can develop from an existing one. But the vast majority of moles are benign. The average young adult has 20 to 30, which can be raised or flat, hairy or not, dark or light. An evenly colored, distinctly round or oval mole—your run-of-the-mill mole—has probably been there for years and means you no harm.

ABCD is a handy mnemonic device for detecting the warning signs of melanoma. *A* is for asymmetry. One side of a melanoma may not match the other. *B* is for border, which may be ragged, with satellites of color spreading beyond the growth. Pictures of malignant melanoma call to mind the word *splotch*. *C* is for color. Mottled pigmentation, with a mixture of black, brown, tan, or even a bluish or reddish color, is a warning sign. *D* is for diameter—anything bigger than a pencil eraser is worth noticing.

Any change in a mole—it suddenly gets bigger, changes color, becomes irritated and crusty, or bleeds—also warrants immediate attention. Hugh Greenway, MD, a skin cancer expert at the Scripps Clinic and Research Foundation in La Jolla, CA, recommends watching for two signs: a mole that itches, or one that you suddenly become aware of for no apparent reason.

Women tend to get melanoma on the legs, possibly because that's where they tan most often. Men are more likely to get it on the head. Melanomas also commonly develop on the back and torso. Scorching childhood sunburns raise your risk, as does intermittent, intense sun exposure—tunneling around indoors all year, then frying under an equatorial sun while on holiday.

Heredity also plays a role. People with a family history of melanoma, those for whom atypical, or dysplastic, moles (which are usually large and irregularly shaped) run in the family, and those who just happen to have multiple moles are more likely to get melanoma, and should see a dermatologist. Anything suspicious will be biopsied.

Surgical excision—cutting out a mole along with a slender border of normal tissue—is the most accepted way to remove a melanoma. If caught while it's still thin, it's almost always curable.

If what you've got is a mole that's benign in all respects but for the cosmetic, you can have it excised or shaved flush to the skin to minimize any indentation. Shaving a mole (or over it) won't make it cancerous, nor will plucking a hair from it. Dermatologists often recommend the removal of moles in chafed areas, where recognizing changes may be difficult.

While you're at it, you should check for two forms of skin cancer that are less dangerous but far more common than melanoma. Basal cell cancer looks like a pimple—a pearly, translucent nodule—but it doesn't go away. Worse, it may erode, bleed, and (very slowly) grow. Squamous cell cancer looks like a red, scaly growth. Both forms can be removed using various outpatient procedures, including Moh's surgery, a tissue-sparing technique that removes the tumor with the help of a microscope.

Happy mole hunting. By the way, the blowdryer is for searching your scalp. The hand mirror speaks for itself, no?

For a brochure with self-examination tips and photos of moles, send a SASE to the American Academy of Dermatology, P.O. Box 681069, Schaumburg, IL 60168-1069.

A SILENT EPIDEMIC

Could you be one of the more than 4 million women who have diabetes and don't know it? How to spot the symptoms—and take advantage of new treatments.

by Susan S. Lang

Barbara Clayton just didn't feel right last year. At first, the 43-year-old teacher from Westminster, CO, was fatigued and constantly thirsty. When her vision became blurry, she finally saw her doctor, who said her symptoms—including a sudden and effortless weight loss—pointed to diabetes. "I never once suspected," says Clayton, even though her sister and two aunts also had the condition. Clayton's story is far from unique. Approximately 16 million Americans have diabetes, and roughly half of them don't know it. Below, answers to the most frequently asked questions about this chronic and potentially fatal disease:

What exactly is it?

Diabetes affects the body's ability to produce or respond to insulin—a crucial hormone made by the pancreas that enables blood sugar (glucose) to cross from the bloodstream into the cells where it's used for energy. Without adequate insulin, glucose builds up and eventually damages small blood vessels and causes complications in the heart, kidneys, eyes, and nerves. Diabetes is the sixth leading cause of death in the United States and a leading cause of blindness, kidney failure, and amputations. The disease also increases the risk for heart disease two to four times and more than doubles the risk for stroke.

There are two types of diabetes: Non-insulin-dependent (type II or adult onset) is far more common—accounting for roughly 90 to 95 percent of all cases. It occurs when the body can't use the insulin it produces and usually doesn't develop until after age 40. Insulin-dependent (also known as type I or

juvenile) diabetes occurs when the body doesn't produce *any* insulin, and generally strikes children and young adults.

Type I is more serious and harder to manage because all patients must receive daily insulin shots in order to survive. Fifty years ago, many type I diabetics faced much shorter life expectancies because of the life-threatening complications. Today, thanks mainly to advances

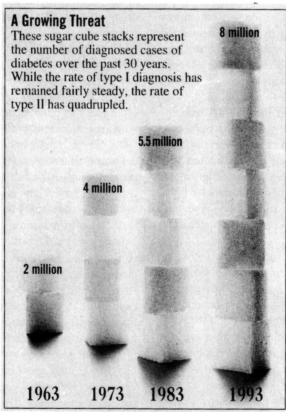

A Growing Threat
These sugar cube stacks represent the number of diagnosed cases of diabetes over the past 30 years. While the rate of type I diagnosis has remained fairly steady, the rate of type II has quadrupled.

8 million

5.5 million

4 million

2 million

1963　1973　1983　1993

in insulin therapy and blood-glucose control, individuals with type I diabetes have a good chance of living into their 60s and 70s.

But managing the disease in children is complicated and time-consuming, and all kinds of events that most families take for granted—such as sleep-overs, vacations, and growth spurts—can trigger the need for adjustments in insulin levels. And some teenage girls (knowing

that weight loss is one side effect of getting too little insulin) will intentionally skip their insulin injections.

What are the symptoms?

In addition to those mentioned above, other signs of diabetes include frequent urination, extreme hunger, recurrent skin and vaginal infections, and tingling or numbing sensations in the hands or feet. Doctors say one reason so many people don't realize they have the disease is that the symptoms often develop gradually and are either overlooked or mistakenly attributed to other medical causes or to the normal aging process.

Who's at risk?

Although both forms of diabetes tend to run in families, researchers believe that only about a quarter of us are genetically predisposed, and we don't yet know who these people are. "Until we identify the genes linked to diabetes, everybody's considered at risk," says Richard Eastman, M.D., director of the division of diabetes, endocrinology, and metabolic diseases at the National Institute of Diabetes and Digestive and Kidney Diseases (NIDDK) in Bethesda, MD.

For reasons that are unknown, African-Americans and Hispanics are one and a half to two times more likely to develop diabetes than whites, and Native-Americans are at an even higher risk. Type II diabetes is particularly common among the obese, but *where* fat is stored is also important. "Those who gain weight in the abdomen are more susceptible than those who gain weight in the buttocks and thighs," says F. Xavier Pi-Sunyer, M.D., director of the Obesity Research Center and chief of endocrinology, diabetes, and nutrition at St. Luke's-Roosevelt Hospital Center in New York

City. One possible reason for this phenomenon is that abdominal fat seems to be more resistant to the effects of insulin. Other risk factors for type II include having a close relative with diabetes, being over 45, being sedentary, and having high blood pressure.

Are women at higher risk?

Yes. They comprise 55 to 60 percent of all diabetics, and every year, more than twice as many American women die from the disease than from breast cancer. "Diabetes in women wipes out the protective effect that estrogen might have for heart disease," says endocrinologist David Brillon, M.D., the associate director of The Diabetes Center at New York Hospital–Cornell University Medical Center in New York City. Diabetic women are also more prone to vaginitis, urinary tract infections, and endometrial cancer.

Another risk factor for type II is giving birth to a baby weighing more than nine pounds, which is a sign that gestational diabetes may have been present. Like type II diabetes, gestational diabetes—which occurs in about 3 percent of pregnancies—is more common in older, heavier, and minority women. "Pregnancy is a kind of stress test," says Dr. Eastman. "Hormones produced at this time tend to bring out a diabetic condition in women who have the genetic tendency in the first place."

What's the treatment?

Right now, there's no cure for diabetes, but with the proper care, it can be well managed. People with type I diabetes must take insulin every day. Sometimes type II can be kept under control with diet and exercise alone. That's because when you're closer to your ideal weight and exercising regularly, cells become more sensitive to insulin and more efficient in taking glucose from the blood. But about 85 percent of type II diabetics aren't able to adequately control their blood-sugar levels with these methods alone, and so must also take oral medication and, sometimes, daily insulin injections.

One of the most important advances in recent years was a landmark NIDDK study that found that diabetics can maintain close to normal blood-sugar levels by using a home blood-glucose monitor several times a day and adjusting their diets, exercise, and medication doses as needed. By practicing such tight control, patients were able to reduce their risk of complications anywhere from 35 to 76 percent.

IS A CURE IN SIGHT?

Type I
Prevention:
● Scientists are investigating whether injecting daily low doses of insulin in children at very high risk for type I diabetes (because of a family history of the disease) acts as a kind of immunization. The hope is that this might allow the beta (insulin-producing) cells to rest, or alter the immune system.
● Researchers are looking into whether feeding or injecting oral insulin or other proteins would stimulate high-risk patients to produce immune cells.
Cures:
● Being tested: specially packaged beta cells that allow insulin out but don't let attacking immune cells in.
● Pancreas transplants are now rarely performed because of the cost and high risks, but an artificial pancreas is being developed. "We have the pump and computer chip but we need a breakthrough in developing a glucose sensor," says Priscilla Hollander, M.D.

Type II
Prevention:
● The NIDDK recently launched a six-year study of 4,000 people to see if type II diabetes can be prevented or delayed in high-risk patients. For information on enrolling in the study, which will be completed in 2002, call 888-377-5646.
Treatments:
Although few cures are predicted, researchers are optimistic that more medications will become available. Now in trials or development:
● Antiobesity drugs to promote a feeling of being full, speed up the burning of calories, or block the absorption and digestion of some dietary fat. Researchers speculate that these medications might reduce the risk of developing diabetes or make the disease a lot easier to manage.
● Drugs that reduce insulin resistance so that cells take up more glucose from the blood.
● Glucose blockers might help reduce the devastating effects of chronic high blood sugar in the cells. The goal is to reduce diabetic complications.
● The hope is that genetic testing will eventually provide an inexpensive way to screen for the risk of type II. Genetic research could also pave the way for drugs that could boost insulin secretion and effectiveness, or prevent or treat obesity.

Do diabetics have to be on restricted diets?

Not anymore. In the past, diabetics were advised to stay away from candy, cakes, and other sweets. "But studies have found that the rise in blood-sugar levels after eating such simple sugars is no different from eating complex carbohydrates such as rice, pasta, and potatoes," says Dr. Brillon. But he adds that since these foods have little nutritional value and can be high in fat and calories, it's still best to limit or exchange them for other carbohydrates so you don't add calories to the day. Overall, recommendations for diabetics are similar to general dietary guidelines: Watch total calorie intake to prevent obesity or weight gain, limit fat to less than 30 percent of calories, and get 10 to 20 percent of calories from protein and 50 and 55 percent from carbohydrates.

Are there any new medications?

Until recently, medication options were limited to oral drugs that stimulate the pancreas to pump out more insulin. Over time, however, the pancreas can't produce as much insulin and the ensuing high levels of glucose in the blood make the body even more insulin resistant. "It's a vicious cycle and you become more and more dependent on large doses of insulin," explains Dr. Eastman. That's why roughly 70 percent of type II patients usually end up needing to take insulin injections after about 20 years.

But new drugs now on the market offer ways to help keep blood-sugar levels normal and may delay or possibly prevent the need for injections down the road, says Priscilla Hollander, M.D., Ph.D., an endocrinologist and medical director of the Ruth Collins Diabetes Center at Baylor University Medical Center in Dallas. One, called acarbose (Precose), slows starch digestion, which helps keep blood sugar from surging after eating. Another is metformin (Glucophage), which helps the liver function normally—mopping up glucose when blood sugar is high and not releasing it unless the blood sugar gets too low, says Dr. Hollander.

LIVING WITH LUPUS

*Everything you need to know to detect and manage a disease
that affects many Black women*

ZIBA KASHEF

In February 1984 Rosemary Graham, then a word processing specialist in Atlanta, came down with a bout of bronchitis. After several months of recurring symptoms, she felt better. But her recovery was short-lived: By September Graham found herself in the hospital with double pneumonia. After a week the doctors sent her home and promised, "You'll get better." She never did.

Graham's persistent problems with her lungs and lingering fatigue led her from her HMO internist to a pulmonary specialist, who, on the day before Thanksgiving, finally diagnosed her with lupus. Graham was 32.

Unlike many people, Graham had heard of lupus: Two members of her Seventh Day Adventist church had died of it—one women at the age of 19. Although lupus is rarely fatal, Black women tend to have more severe cases of it and higher mortality rates. When Graham was given her diagnosis, she believed she had only a few years to live. "As a strong Christian, I thought God would either deliver me or I would die."

Graham finally had a name for her mysterious ailment, but she nevertheless remained baffled and frustrated by the disease that allowed her to be fairly active one day and nearly incapacitated the next. Her mother pleaded with her to move back home to California, but Graham chose to stay in Atlanta and learn as much as she could about lupus. "I asked a lot of questions," she says. Unable to maintain a full-time job, Graham got involved with a local chapter of the Lupus Foundation and kept busy as a counselor for other women with the disease.

Today, at 43, she continues to have problems with her lungs and suffers from fatigue and joint pain. But despite her own initial prognosis, with the help of medication, regular doctor visits and an eye on her diet, Graham has lived with lupus now for 11 years.

Lupus, which has been referred to as a "women's disease" (nine out of ten patients are female), could just as easily be considered a "Black women's disease" as it strikes a far greater number of sisters than White women. "Most studies show lupus is three times more common in Black women than in White women," says Margaret

Fountain, M.D., an internist and rheumatologist in Maryland. "We don't know why."

While lupus raises many unanswered questions, it is no longer considered the death sentence that it was 20 or 30 years ago. Research into the disease, its causes and treatments is ongoing. Only a small percentage of patients will die of lupus. In fact, for most the outlook is good. "Patients can live a normal life by getting a diagnosis and becoming comfortable with it," says Fountain. "The women who fare the best are those who learn about the disease, stick with their follow-up care and make realistic choices about their lives."

WHAT IS LUPUS?

Lupus is an autoimmune disease—that is, one that causes the body's own immune system to turn against itself, attacking the skin, joints or internal organs. It has been called "America's least-known major disease," but it is more common than leukemia, multiple sclerosis, muscular dystrophy, cystic fibrosis and cerebral palsy.

In some patients lupus, Latin for *wolf*, causes a red rash across the bridge of the nose, which was thought to resemble a wolf's bite. Lupus occurs mainly in three forms: The most common, systemic lupus erythematosus (SLE), affects many parts of the body including joints, skin and vital organs such as the lungs, kidneys, heart and brain; discoid or cutaneous lupus targets the skin with its characteristic rash; and drug-induced lupus is caused by certain drugs used to treat heart problems, hypertension or seizure. The disease largely affects women in their childbearing years, ages 15 to 44. Today there are between 1.4 million and 2 million lupus patients in the United States.

Lupus can have debilitating effects, yet it is often hard to detect. Many people with lupus can look healthy but be very ill. In fact, it may take up to a year—and several doctor's visits—before a lupus patient knows what she has. "Lupus is difficult to diagnose because it looks different in each person who has the disease," says Fountain. Other factors may stand in the way of an early diagnosis. "It is known that Blacks have more limited access to health care," says Patricia A. Fraser, M.D., a rheumatologist at Brigham and Women's Hospital in Boston and an assistant professor of medicine at Harvard Medical School, "and this disparity affects one's ability to get diagnosed and get treatment."

When should a woman suspect she has lupus? Though doctors agree there is no typical lupus case, the following are common signs (a combination of symptoms more likely indicates lupus): •A red or brownish rash, sometimes raised and sensitive, and often in the shape of a butterfly, occurring across the bridge of the nose and cheeks. •Painful, swollen joints. •An unexplained low-grade fever. •Chest pain with breathing. •Unexplained hair loss or weight loss. •Pale or purple fingers or toes from cold temperatures or anxiety. •Photosensitivity (a rash or lesions may develop after exposure to the sun or to other light). •A low white-blood-cell or platelet count. •Sores or ulcers in the mouth or the nose. •Extreme fatigue or weakness.

Aside from assessing the symptoms, doctors usually perform blood tests to confirm a lupus diagnosis. There are no known causes of the disease, and it's not contagious. Some experts, however, point to genetic predisposition, hormonal factors and possible environmental triggers. Symptoms can range from mild to severe and require that many patients dramatically change their lifestyles, as did Mary W. Broussard in Minneapolis, a former nurse who was forced to quit her job when she nearly died of the disease in 1983.

MANAGING LUPUS

Early detection is crucial in controlling the disease and learning to live with it. If you suspect you have lupus, see a doctor, preferably a rheumatologist, and *ask questions.*

Because lupus is a very individual disease, a patient must know her own symptoms and what factors may bring about a lupus "flare-up" (a period in which symptoms reappear or worsen). Stress, sun exposure and certain foods can trigger a flare-up. "I have a three-day rule," says Broussard. "If something goes on for longer than three days, I make an appointment to see my doc-

tor." Depending on the severity of the disease, patients should visit their doctors regularly, at least once a year.

Doctors can prescribe medication to ease symptoms and reduce the frequency of flare-ups, though some, such as steroids and immunosuppressive drugs, have side effects. For patients who have sun sensitivity, avoiding the sun and using sunscreen on all exposed body parts are critical, says Fraser. Sufficient rest is also key. In addition, some experts advocate a high-fiber diet that's low in fat, salt and red meat, along with exercise and relaxation techniques such as yoga.

Doctors cannot recommend a way to prevent lupus, but they are learning more about the disease and the different drugs that can be used to manage it. "The outlook for lupus patients has improved," Fraser says, "and will continue to get better as we address access to health care and develop new treatment and regimens."

GETTING HELP

For some lupus patients, support groups can offer consolation and information. Contact the following organizations for a list of their chapters nationwide, in addition to medical referrals, pamphlets, programs, support groups and other resources: the Lupus Foundation of America, Inc., 4 Research Place, Ste. 180, Rockville MD 20850-3226, (800) 558-0121; and The American Lupus Society, 260 Maple Court, Ste. 123, Ventura CA 93003, (800) 331-1802. Another good source of information on lupus is *The Lupus Handbook for Women* (Fireside, paperback, $10) by Robin Dibner, M.D., and Carol Colman.

To launch a lupus-awareness campaign in your community, request a free copy of the booklet "What Black Women Should Know About Lupus." Write to the National Institute of Arthritis and Musculoskeletal and Skin Disease, 1 AMS Circle, Bethesda MD 20892-3675. Also contact your congressional representative and urge them to support the Lupus Research Amendments of 1995, a bill seeking to increase funding for lupus research and education.

Ziba Kashef is a freelance writer who lives in New York City.

When Arthritis Strikes

MARIE SAVARD, M.D.

Dr. Savard is director of the Center for Women's Health at Medical College of Pennsylvania Hospital.

By the time we reach middle age, most women have some arthritis, although we may not feel it yet. Osteoarthritis, the most common form of the disease, is one of the most frequent causes of illness and disability in aging women. I help care for a retirement community of nuns, and many of them suffer pain and difficulty in their daily routines. I struggle to help each one find the best and safest treatments. The good news is that doctors are learning ways to make life easier for women with arthritis.

What Happens?

The problem starts when the cartilage that covers the ends of the bones at the joints starts to wear away. The bones rub together and form growths or spurs—and that's what can hurt and inhibit movement. Often the first hint is some mild morning pain and stiffness.

Almost all people over age 60 have lost some cartilage. Trauma, such as ligament or tendon rupture, surgery or a twisted or sprained joint, may cause earlier damage, which explains why so many football players and other athletes get arthritis. Work that involves a lot of bending, such as housework, also can lead to problems. You're more likely to develop arthritis if it runs in your family, and by age 65, women are up to five times as likely as men to have it.

Problems affect mainly the lower back, hips, knees and toe joints. Osteoarthritis usually isn't sharply painful—it's more of a deep, dull ache. The stiffness may limit your activities, and you may have trouble slipping off your rings or putting on shoes due to swelling. (Rheumatoid arthritis, which is much less common, can cause severe pain, swelling and deformity.) Screenings such as MRIs can show damaged cartilage, but you do not need these unless you are considering surgery.

Finding Relief

There's no cure for arthritis, but you can do a great deal to feel better. See your doctor for specific advice on managing your case. Most women I work with try different things and end up with a combination of treatments.

Exercise. Women often tell me they "overdid" it in the days before a flare-up of stiffness and pain. It may feel better to do nothing, but if you stop using a joint the muscles around it stiffen and weaken. This puts more stress on the joint and ultimately destroys more cartilage.

Experiment—under your doctor's supervision as much as possible—to see what works best for you. Most people stick to gentle, non-pounding activities such as walking and swimming. Isometric strength exercises (in which the muscles work against resistance without moving) also help. Working with a physical therapist can be useful and your insurance may cover it.

Weight control. Getting your weight to within 10 percent of the ideal for your height can help prevent or lessen symptoms of arthritis, and it helps you feel better in general.

Drugs. No medication can stop or reverse the loss of cartilage—don't let anyone tell you differently. Talk to your doctor about pain-relief drugs. I usually recommend acetaminophen (Tylenol), which is just as effective as ibuprofen, aspirin or prescription-strength nonsteroidal anti-inflammatory medications, yet has fewer side effects. Using ibuprofen drugs for weeks on end can cause gastrointestina! problems and small increases in blood pressure in some people, and beware that overdoses of acetaminophen may cause liver and kidney problems. Make sure your doctor knows about any other medications you are taking.

Medical treatments. Capsaicin, a prescription skin cream made from pepper plants, may help control joint pain; other nonprescription gels and ointments may relieve pain temporarily. Steroids injected into a painful joint can help but should be given no more than three or four times a year. I've known of many cases of acupuncture relieving pain, and heat (either moist or dry) may calm muscle spasms.

Lifestyle changes. If you can, work with a physical therapist to help adjust your daily routines. Tools such as a phone headset or speakerphone and special neck pillow can relieve neck pain and stiffness; a raised toilet seat makes things easier on the knees.

Surgery. Joint replacement is a last resort when exercise, drugs and lifestyle changes are not enough. Most replacements are of the knee and hip, and the joints last 20 years or longer. Of course, you'll still want to keep your joints as healthy as possible after surgery.

For more information, contact the Arthritis Foundation, P.O. Box 7669, Atlanta, GA 30357; 800-283-7800.

running on empty

ONE IN FIVE WOMEN WILL DEVELOP A SIMPLE DISORDER THAT LEAVES THEM FEELING EXHAUSTED, DEPRESSED, OR JUST PLAIN STUPID: A THYROID THAT ISN'T UP TO SPEED. SO WHY HAVEN'T YOU BEEN TESTED?

BARBARA BAILEY KELLEY

ANYONE WHO HAS BEEN THERE WILL tell you: An underactive thyroid can send you on a slow boat to hell. You're too wiped out to get off the couch. You can't concentrate. You can't remember what you had for dinner yesterday or who you promised to meet for lunch today. You can't seem to please your boss, or connect with your husband, your friends, or your children.

And no one knows what's wrong with you.

You're under too much stress, your doctor tells you. You're suffering from depression. Try exercise. Try Prozac. Try to accept it: You're getting older.

A thyroid disorder is generally one of the easiest maladies to treat, but it's also one of the easiest to miss or misdiagnose. Nestled below the adam's apple, the thyroid is the body's accelerator, controlling the tempo of all its internal processes: heartbeat, digestion, even thought. When the gland doesn't work hard enough—or, for that matter, when it starts to work too hard—life goes haywire. Women are particularly vulnerable: At least one in five eventually develops a thyroid problem, and half of the sufferers don't know it.

Ignorance, in this case, can be agony. But there's a simple, inexpensive blood test that can spot a malfunctioning thyroid in no time flat. Thyroid experts recommend all women be checked; in fact, say the authors of a recent study, they should get their first test as early as age 35.

Just don't expect your doctor to tell you about it.

A TIMELY THYROID TEST would have saved Onley Cahill years of grief. Sales manager for a radio station in the Boston area, Cahill was in her fifties when she came down with what seemed like the flu and never bounced back.

The worst part was the way the fatigue hung on. Cahill would drive home from work and have to rest in her car before mustering the energy for the climb to her second-floor apartment. She was used to frequenting the theater and the opera; now she stopped going out at night, afraid she'd never make it back home. She'd spend entire weekends in bed, only to feel even more tired come Monday morning. At work she'd close her office door and collapse on the floor. At meetings, where she'd once been quick with statistics and suggestions, she was having trouble speaking. "I felt like an absolute idiot," she says. "I couldn't string two words together. I kept wondering if something was wrong with my mind."

It seemed clear to her that something was wrong with her body. A cluster of symptoms—constipation, constantly feeling cold, and difficulty swallowing, among others—had her hopping from doctor to doctor. None could identify a medical problem.

Finally, nearly three years after her symptoms appeared, Cahill checked into a hospital just north of Boston. A number of specialists, including an allergist, a heart specialist, and a psychiatrist, examined her; the latter wondered if her problems weren't rooted in depression. The suggestion gave her pause, though she felt too much of a physical mess for the problem to be entirely psychological. "I said, 'Listen, you'd be depressed too if you didn't have the energy to get out of bed,'" she recalls.

The doctors also gave her a battery of tests, among them something called a thyroid-stimulating hormone (TSH) assay. That was when Cahill learned that she had an underactive thyroid—indeed, that her thyroid had shut down almost entirely.

Hypothyroidism, as the disorder is called, is the most common thyroid problem, affecting 20 percent of all women over age 60. In most cases, it develops when for some unknown reason the immune system begins attacking the thyroid. (This autoimmune condition is known as Hashimoto's disease.) Surprisingly, what people often think of as a hallmark of an underactive thyroid—conspicuous weight gain—often doesn't materialize: While a sufferer is likely to get a bit heavier because of a slowdown in metabolism, the average gain is only five to ten pounds. But if untreated, an underactive thyroid can raise cholesterol levels and increase the risk of heart disease. Even a slightly sluggish thyroid can cause depression, mental fuzziness, and fatigue.

"People just don't interact," says endocrinologist Martin Surks of Albert Einstein College of Medicine in New York City. "Not with family, not at work. They're exhausted. And because all their body functions are slowed down, they can get into trouble if they're given any medicine for another illness. The right dose for someone with a healthy thyroid may be an overdose for them."

At the radio station where she worked, Cahill had been responsible for finding airtime for public service announcements about thyroid disorders but had never made the connection between her symptoms and the ones mentioned in the bulletins. Now everything began to make sense. She started taking synthetic thyroid hormone—a pill a day—to make up for her body's failing supply. In six months her aches and pains were gone, and her energy and quick wit were back—along with anger. "I spent all those years feeling rotten," she says, "when all it took was a little thyroid hormone to make me feel normal again."

THE MOST COMMON THING I hear from people with an underactive thyroid is that they thought they were just getting older," says Surks, who sees patients at Montefiore Hospital in the Bronx. "Fatigue, chilliness, constipation, muscle cramps—this is the stuff people associate with aging."

Primary care physicians are often fooled, too, in part because medical education puts little emphasis on endocrinology, the study of hormones. Relatively few endocrinologists teach at medical schools, says Sheldon Rubenfeld, medical director of the Thyroid Society for Education & Research in Houston. Moreover, thyroid patients rarely end up in the hospital, where young doctors get most of their hands-on training. Many doctors have little chance to practice the proper way to feel whether a thyroid gland is growing larger, often the first sign of malfunction, says Rubenfeld. They're likely to miss the more subtle clues altogether.

An overactive thyroid is harder to overlook, as it typically sends out dramatic signals. Even so, diagnosis may take time and a number of fruitless trips to the doctor's office. That's what happened to Wendy

> ONE DOCTOR SUGGESTED A SUFFERER'S PROBLEMS WERE ALL IN HER HEAD. SHE SAID, "LISTEN, YOU'D BE DEPRESSED TOO IF YOU DIDN'T HAVE THE ENERGY TO GET OUT OF BED."

Jacquemin, whose symptoms were anything but subtle. An administrator at a Los Angeles bank, Jacquemin began losing weight in May 1994, when she was 40. She was already lean: At 5 foot 7, she weighed 130 pounds. Soon she was down to 110. But neither the weight loss nor the pounding of her heart bothered her as much as the way she felt: jittery, ready to jump out of her skin.

She visited an internist, who ran a series of lab tests, then told her she was simply under a lot of stress. The diagnosis made sense to her at first. But the feelings escalated, and by mid-June she was frantic. Back in her doctor's office, she broke down crying. Once again, he suggested that she try some stress-reduction techniques or see a psychiatrist.

Instead, she went to visit her mother in Idaho. The visit was calming, but her heart pounded as she got off the plane back in Los Angeles. She'd become friendly with her seatmate on the trip; when she tried to exchange phone numbers, her hand was shaking so badly she couldn't write her name.

It was the constant churning in her stomach that spurred Jacquemin to seek a second opinion. She went to a gastroenterologist, who gave her a thorough workup, then called her at home a few nights later with a bad news–good news message: A TSH assay showed she had an overactive thyroid, but the condition was treatable.

If It's Not Your **Thyroid**

Enduring fatigue troubles one in four Americans, and they can't all blame it on a malfunctioning thyroid. It can be difficult to pinpoint the cause of exhaustion, which may be a clue that you're developing diabetes, that you're pregnant, or that you're simply not getting enough sleep. Here are some of the most likely suspects in a bad case of the blahs.

SLEEP PROBLEMS

Most Americans don't get the seven to nine hours of sleep they need each night, and even people who sleep a lot may not sleep well. In a condition called sleep apnea, the airway in the throat briefly but repeatedly collapses during sleep; a sufferer is apt to snore and gasp for breath, and may unknowingly wake hundreds of times a night. One person in 12 has sleep apnea. Mild cases can be helped by losing weight or sleeping on one side; severe cases may require wearing a dental device to bed or even undergoing surgery. Other common culprits in troubled sleep include too much caffeine or alcohol, irregular hours, and lack of exercise.

ANEMIA

Sometimes your very cells are tired, because they lack oxygen. That's what happens in anemia, a condition in which the blood doesn't have enough hemoglobin, the oxygen-carrying molecule. In this country one woman in five is anemic, many of them because of iron deficiency. But don't pop iron pills without consulting your doctor; some people are genetically prone to store iron, and for them supplements can be dangerous. A blood test will show whether you need to boost your iron intake by changing your diet or taking supplements.

DEPRESSION OR GRIEF

When doctors suggest a patient with an undiagnosed thyroid problem is simply depressed, they aren't being insensitive: Clinical depression is the explanation in up to half of the cases of fatigue that doctors see. Profound exhaustion can also be a symptom of grief, whether over the death of a loved one, a divorce, or the loss of a job. Support groups and time may be enough to ease grief; in cases of depression, talk therapy and antidepressants can be useful.

CHRONIC FATIGUE SYNDROME

Sometimes dismissed as "yuppie flu," chronic fatigue syndrome is real, although most experts think it afflicts only about ten out of 100,000 adults. The condition brings debilitating fatigue, often so intense that a sufferer feels unable even to read. Flu-like symptoms such as muscle aches may accompany the exhaustion. Antidepressants and pain medications can help, as can moderate exercise.

RECENT ILLNESS

Even when the fever has dropped, the sluggishness of the flu or another infection can linger for a month or more, because the immune cells that fight sickness can also make you tired. If you can't get up to speed after you've been ill, there's a simple cure: Take it easy.

Hyperthyroidism, in which the gland pumps out too much thyroid hormone, is almost always caused by Graves' disease—an autoimmune condition in which antibodies latch onto the thyroid, essentially jamming all control switches in the on position. Left in overdrive, the gland pushes the heart too hard, sometimes inducing an irregular heartbeat, occasionally to a life-threatening degree. Bone turnover speeds up, raising the risk of osteoporosis. The metabolic overload exhausts the body and stresses the psyche; a person may become so erratic and unreasonable that job and relationships suffer.

The extravagant symptoms of an overactive thyroid mean that, almost without exception, both patient and doctor know something is wrong. The problem is rarely a missed diagnosis; instead a doctor may make, at least temporarily, a misdiagnosis.

Looking back, Jacquemin wonders if her first doctor chalked up her weight loss to anorexia and her other symptoms to psychological imbalance. "I understand how people with thyroid disorders used to end up in mental institutions," she says. "I'm lucky I didn't wind up on Prozac."

JACQUEMIN AND CAHILL could have had their problems treated before their lives were disrupted at all. The TSH assay measures thyroid-stimulating hormone, made by the pituitary gland to keep the thyroid under control. Between about .35 and 5.5 microunits per milliliter of blood is normal. But if the pituitary senses things starting to slow down, it puts out more TSH to give the thyroid a kick; if the thyroid is working too hard, the pituitary stops manufacturing TSH for a while. Measure the TSH level, then, and you know just how well the thyroid is functioning.

Endocrinologists say every woman should periodically get a TSH assay, whether she has symptoms or not—just as she gets mammograms and Pap smears. It's an inexpensive test, costing $30 to $50, and easy to do, requiring only a little blood.

So why aren't women hearing about it? Most doctors take their cue from the U.S. Preventive Services Task Force, which has not endorsed regular screening. Its reasoning mainly has to do with the best way to use scarce health care dollars: Why test asymptomatic women, most of whom will prove not to have a thyroid problem? Since any procedure occasionally gives a false result, you'll unnecessarily worry some healthy women. Better to wait for signs to surface and test then, with no lasting harm done.

If only it worked that way. Too often people suffer debilitating symptoms for years before they or their doctors think of the thyroid. Besides, say thyroid experts, even if early signals reliably produced a prompt diagnosis, why wait? A malfunctioning thyroid can chip away at a woman's quality of life long before she can put her finger on what's wrong.

"Our recommendation is that all 'older' women should be screened for an underactive thyroid on a yearly basis," says Dallas endocrinologist Stanley Feld, past president of the American Association of Clinical Endocrinologists, which issued guidelines in 1995. "We didn't define the age. But really, it's 40."

Some endocrinologists would quibble with Feld, saying it's more practical to wait until a woman hits 50 or even 60, when the likelihood of thyroid disorders climbs sharply. On the other hand, when researchers at Johns Hopkins University recently did a cost-effectiveness analysis, they concluded that it makes sense from both an economic and a medical standpoint to screen women as young as 35.

According to endocrinologist Paul Ladenson, who led the Johns Hopkins study, doctors could simply piggyback the TSH assay on a cholesterol test. (The National Cholesterol Education Project advises men and women to have their cholesterol levels measured every five years starting at age 20.) With such a system, doctors could identify and treat thyroid problems before symptoms appear. "The benefits you would derive from early thyroid testing are greater per dollar spent than with many things we already do, like screening for high blood pressure or high cholesterol," Ladenson says.

Of course, if you're at high risk for thyroid prob-

lems, you shouldn't wait for experts to agree on the proper time to begin screening. Get checked now, specialists say, whatever your age.

And many women are at high risk. Most thyroid diseases run in families, so a family history of any such problem ought to prompt a request for a TSH test. If you have an immediate relative with an autoimmune condition—such as diabetes, pernicious anemia, or rheumatoid arthritis—you should also consider yourself at risk for thyroid problems. Even prematurely gray hair (appearing before age 30) seems to spring from an overactive immune system and has been linked to an increased vulnerability.

In addition, anyone suffering from a laundry list of symptoms for more than a month or two should ask for the test. "If you feel sluggish or depressed, if you tire easily, if you feel bloated or overweight, it's prudent to measure your TSH," says Boston thyroid expert Lawrence Wood, president of the Thyroid Foundation of America. "If someone in your family, or a friend who hasn't seen you for a while, says, 'You don't have the pep you had last year,' you should think about getting tested. Or if they say, 'Holy smokes, you never used to be this nervous.' A friend who hasn't seen you in a while is more likely to make the diagnosis than you are."

The bottom line, says Onley Cahill, is that women should be alert to the signals, since their doctors may not be. At 60, Cahill is now managing several musicians and writers, and she feels great. "A lot of 50-year-old women go to the doctor complaining of being cold and tired, and the doctor tells them they're just emotional because their kids are gone," says Cahill. "I want to tell them, a bit of thyroid hormone and they'll feel terrific again."

Barbara Bailey Kelley is a writer living in San Jose, California.

What to do for urinary-tract and vaginal infections

Genitourinary infections are among the most common of women's health problems. Here are the solutions for typical infections:

Urinary-tract infections

Causes. Bacteria can easily migrate from a woman's anal area to the opening of the urethra, and from there up into the bladder itself. Sexual intercourse and the use of spermicides can increase the risk of infection.

Symptoms. Bladder infections, or cystitis, usually cause frequent, burning urination and an intense urge to urinate, although little urine may be passed. If the infection spreads to the kidneys, symptoms can include chills, fever, nausea, vomiting, and kidney pain, usually felt on either side of the small of the back.

Prevention. To reduce your risk:
■ **Keep clean.** Wash genital and anal areas daily with soap and water, always wiping from front to back. Wipe in that same way after urination or a bowel movement.
■ **Drink up.** Make it a habit to drink a glass of water every few hours to flush out the bladder.
■ **Don't hold it in.** Urinate frequently and empty completely.
■ **Take steps after sex.** Urinate after sexual activity to wash away any bacteria transferred to the urethra. Then drink a glass of water so you'll urinate again soon.

Treatment. Appropriate treatment depends on proper diagnosis. Home test kits, such as *URI-TEST* and *UTI Home Screening Test Kit*, are of limited value, since you should consult a physician anyway—at least by phone.

Drinking cranberry juice as soon as symptoms appear may clear up an early bladder infection. But if symptoms worsen, or last for more than a day or two, see your doctor in person. Taking antibiotics for just a few days will quash most infections. A new antibiotic option, fosfomycin tromethamine (*Monurol*), requires just one dose, but may be a somewhat less reliable cure. Until antibiotics take effect, the nonprescription drug phenazopyridine (*Baridium, Uristat*) can relieve pain and burning.

Vaginal infections

Causes. The vagina's natural environment can be altered by many factors, such as diabetes, pregnancy, antibiotics, birth-control pills, douching, or being overweight. That can leave the vagina susceptible to overgrowth of normal bacteria and yeast cells. Another type of vaginal infection, trichomoniasis, is caused by a protozoan that's usually transmitted sexually.

Symptoms. The different infectious agents result in different types of vaginal discharge: for bacteria, thin and grey; for trichomoniasis, frothy and yellow-green; for yeast, thick and whitish, like cottage cheese. Yeast infection also produces intense itching or irritation. A doctor can easily identify the culprit under a microscope or by culture.

Prevention. The same daily washings and front-to-back wipings that head off cystitis can help prevent some vaginal infections. Other helpful measures include:
■ **Stay dry.** Avoid clothing that blocks ventilation of the genitals. Wear cotton underpants, and sleep with none.
■ **Be natural.** Don't use douches or feminine sprays, perfumed toilet paper, or deodorant tampons or sanitary pads.
■ **Eat yogurt.** A cup a day of yogurt that has live cultures of the bacteria *Lactobacillus acidophilus* may cut down on vaginal infections.

Treatment. Bacterial infections should be treated with a prescription vaginal cream containing the antibiotic clindamycin (*Cleocin*) or with metronidazole, either in vaginal gel (*MetroGel-Vaginal*) or oral form (*Flagyl, Protostat*). Trichomoniasis also calls for oral metronidazole. Neither of those infections will be cured by over-the-counter antifungal medications, which are intended for yeast infections. So unless you have had a yeast infection before and are absolutely certain about your symptoms, get a professional diagnosis before treating any vaginal infection yourself.

If you do have a yeast infection, you can choose from a variety of antifungal creams, suppositories, and tablets: butoconazole (*Femstat 3, Mycelex-3*), clotrimazole (*Gyne-Lotrimin, Mycelex-7*), and miconazole (*Monistat 3, Monistat 7*). A new entry, the ointment tioconazole (*Vagistat-1*), cuts treatment down from three or seven days to a single dose—though it can still take a few days for symptoms to clear up. Convenience costs a bit extra: about $17 versus roughly $9 for generic clotrimazole or miconazole.

If over-the-counter remedies fail, a doctor can prescribe terconazole vaginal creams or suppositories (*Terazol 3, Terazol 7*). A single oral dose of fluconazole (*Diflucan*) is more convenient, but somewhat more likely to cause side effects.

Steer clear of "homeopathically prepared" products, such as *Vaginex Yeast Care, Vagisil Yeast Itch Control*, and *Yeast Gard*, which have not been proved effective. And know that vinegar and yogurt douches are useless, too.

Substance Abuse: New Trends for Women

It is virtually impossible to pick up a newspaper or magazine or to listen to a newscast without hearing something about drugs or the "substance abuse problem." Today it almost appears trendy or alluring to have an addiction to something or someone. Hollywood stars wax poetic about their drugs of choice and their rehabilitation experiences while the high-fashion runway sports the gaunt, greasy, "heroin look."

Although the number of women who are addicted to alcohol and other drugs is almost as alarming as that of men, most experts agree that the treatment and recovery issues are markedly different. The demands of multiple roles: wife, mother, employee, daughter; the cultural expectation that "good" women, especially mothers, should not do drugs; the stigma attached when women do admit to having a problem—these are just a few of the many issues that make addiction in women a different entity.

The articles in this section were chosen for two major reasons. The first is that they present information on a wide variety of abusable substances. The second is that these selections do an excellent job of illustrating the differences between the sexes in terms of addiction. The opening article "What Does Being Female Have to Do with It?" sets the tone for the section. Here, Rokelle Lerner explicitly outlines how treatment programs need to be conducted in order to be of benefit to female clients. First, the program must deal with being female; the addiction is really secondary. The female addict as well as the society at large need to stop viewing the addicted woman as morally bankrupt and instead see her as an individual in need of help.

Since smoking has been identified as the single largest preventable cause of death and disease in this country, considerable emphasis in this chapter has been placed on tobacco use. "The Facts About . . . Women and Smoking" presents a broad overview of the health risks and the consequences of smoking. The next article examines the connection between tobacco use and self-image in women. In "Up in Smoke: Why Teen Girls Don't Quit," Mimi Frost examines the use of cigarettes by young girls as a way of not only coping with stress but of presenting a certain sophisticated, mature image to the world. This is another example of the tobacco industry's exploitation of women's fears and insecurities.

A phenomenon currently touted in the media is cigar smoking by women. "Cigars, Women, and Cancer" examines the serious health implications of this practice. Once again, concern for one's health takes a back seat to glamour. The risks are disguised behind the glossy cover of a trendy magazine.

By far the most provocative article dealing with tobacco is "A Smoker's Tale," which chronicles the hazards of secondhand smoke in a most unusual way. It presents the case of a woman who stands to lose custody of her asthmatic child because of her addiction to cigarettes. Time and again, she tries to quit and fails. She is not unwilling to quit; she is unable. Who is the real victim in this story?

Although a very common and certainly important issue, tobacco is not the only substance abused by women. "Alcohol and Health: Mixed Messages for Women" examines alcohol use by women. This article attempts to clear up some of the mixed messages women receive regarding risk versus benefit of alcohol consumption. An attempt is also made to clarify such terms as "moderate" and "excessive" use.

The final topic addressed here is illicit drug use. It would take an entire volume to begin to examine the various drugs on the street and their impact on women. This article was therefore chosen for its uniqueness. In "Way Out West and Under the Influence" Carey Goldberg discusses an illegal drug that is used more frequently by women than by men, which is not the norm. The drug is methamphetamine. Patterns of use are discussed as are

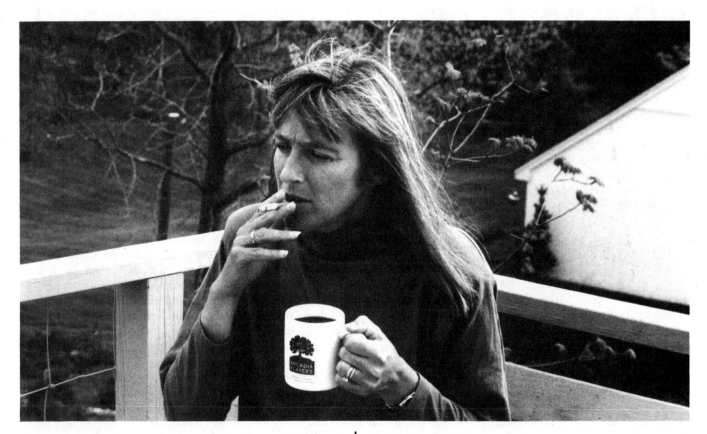

reasons why more women then men seem to fall victim to this drug.

Looking Ahead: Challenge Questions

Why are substance abuse treatment issues different for women than they are for men?

What are the specific health risks for women who smoke or use alcohol?

Why are young women such easy targets for the tobacco industry?

Why is smoking often used by women as a weight control device?

What attracts women to smoking cigars?

Should smoking be considered in terms of child custody?

Why are women, more than men, abusing methamphetamines?

What Does Being Female Have to Do With It?

ROKELLE LERNER

Rokelle Lerner is an international consultant, lecturer and author on addictions and family systems, and clinical advisor to Marworth Treatment Center and Sierra Tucson.

The developmental and psychological pathways that lead women to drug use are different than those followed by men. Female addicts and alcoholics exhibit more depression and more suicidal tendencies than males, and report a far greater incidence of physical or sexual abuse as well as a greater incidence of family substance abuse.

Women also tend to get to treatment at much later stages of the disease than men, due in part to our society's reluctance to acknowledge female alcoholics and addicts.

It starts early. One study revealed that the average age of a child when she or he learns of Dad's alcoholism is approximately 12.6 years. The average age of the child who recognizes that Mom is an alcoholic is 18.3 years. The fact that women hold many more menial positions in the workplace — or do their work in the confines of their home — helps them to more easily "hide."

We also have to acknowledge that culturally women have lower self-esteem than men. The shame of being a woman goes way back, as is evidenced by the quote of Thomas Aquinas: "A woman is a man gone wrong"; or the Orthodox Jewish prayer: "Dear God, thank you for not making me a woman."

Women who are addicted carry not only the cultural shame of being a woman, but also being a woman who is alcoholic or addicted. If a man drinks he may be considered to be funny, just acting foolish or simply having a good time. When a woman drinks she is called a lush, a "floozy," sometimes a whore.

Because of their sensitivity to relationships, women will often take care of others before they care for themselves. Recent studies on women's development reveal that this is not necessarily pathological. Men are trained to develop an ethic of "justice" while women are trained to develop an ethic of "care." Nevertheless, women are as often called codependent and, again, shamed because of their caring.

Many woman have medicated themselves with drugs or alcohol to avoid dealing with the pain of childhood sexual abuse. In fact, the *majority* of addicted women have a history of incest, sexual abuse and physical abuse. In these cases, women have used alcohol or drugs to self-induce a dissociative state. Once sober, these painful memories may recur.

Counselors who deal with women need to be aware of women's inherent shame and low self-esteem. Because of these feelings, it is possible that once a woman is sober, rather than feeling better many recovering women find that they need help for depression, obsessive compulsive disorders or eating disorders — all powerful triggers for relapse.

While delving into these issues may not be totally appropriate in early sobriety, women need to learn how to soothe themselves when flashbacks and anxiety occur. If a woman brings these issues forward in treatment, then it will be crucial for her to know she can get help.

Communication is the key to success. I suggest to women in recovery that if they find that during or after treatment they suffer from depression, anxiety, eating disorders or other problems, they should communicate this to their loved ones. It will not only help them to understand why the woman may be having a difficult time, but it will also provide the woman with the support she needs and deserves.

It is of utmost importance for women inpatients to talk about their relationships with their spouse and their children before returning home. One aspect of the homecoming that recovering women fear most is their ability to be intimate and sexual with their partners. Many women feel that they can only be romantic or sexual when they are using. We need to remind women to be gentle and patient with themselves while they discover their sober, recovering lives.

If a recovering woman is reluctant to return home, we cannot assume that her reluctance is simply a normal response to returning to family life; it may be violence or battering she fears.

If we ask a woman if she is being beaten at home, she will probably say no. However, if we ask specifically, "Have you been shoved, slapped, bruised or threatened?" we may get a very different response. If a woman is returning to a home where she is battered, then her sobriety and, quite possibly, her life are at risk. We must provide her with resources for help.

With most of the addictions research based on men, it is no surprise why many women have difficulty in the treatment and recovery process of addiction. Carol Gilligan, author of *In A Different Voice*, puts it eloquently: "It all goes back to Adam and Eve, a story which shows, of course, that if you make a woman out of a man, you're bound to get into trouble!"

Recovery means finding a way of living that works for us: spiritually, emotionally and physically. We need to attend to the special needs of women to help them find ways of making their lives more joyful, peaceful and loving.

The Facts About . . .
WOMEN AND SMOKING

Nancy Dreher

You're female, age 15. Just for a moment, picture yourself in the future. Not your future as in what you're doing this summer, but when you're about 30 years old. Would you like to see yourself in a good job? as a mom? traveling? living in a place of your own? as a drug addict with a killing habit?

A safe guess at your answers: Yes. Perhaps. Good idea. Yes. NO.

Of course you don't see drug dependence in your future. But when it comes to one of the most common and dangerous forms of drug addiction, many young women take the first step every day. They smoke their first cigarette.

A young woman's first cigarette may not lead to more, but it could. If young smokers continue to smoke, by age 20 they probably will be addicted to the habit. (In some cases, addiction occurs after only a few cigarettes.) And down the road, their habit could cost them

---

AN UGLY HABIT

Health concerns aren't the only convincing reasons not to take up smoking. The habit has other physical side effects. To name a few:

- bad breath
- smelly clothes
- stained teeth
- deep wrinkles around the eyes and lips caused by a reduction in blood circulation to the skin.

---

their good health—and ultimately their life, long before they reach old age.

The World Health Organization estimates that the number of women who die each year from smoking-related dis-

eases will double to more than 1 million over the next three decades. More troubling news:

- Recent research by British and Norwegian scientists indicates that women who smoke are more likely to develop lung cancer than are male smokers. In fact, scientists conducting the research say that preliminary evidence from the United States shows that women run about *twice* the risk that men do of getting lung cancer from smoking.
- Statistics produced by the Centers for Disease Control and Prevention (CDC) show that although increasing numbers of U.S. women are quitting the habit, this is not the case among female teens. More than 18 percent of female high school seniors smoked in 1993, about the same percentage as in 1988.

The Toll on Women

The toll that smoking takes on females is, however, hardly a new story. Fifteen

---

THE GENDER ISSUE

Is smoking a gender-neutral killer?

Among men, lung cancer death rates began to climb sharply in the 1930s, approximately 20 to 30 years after men began smoking in large numbers. Now, as fewer men smoke, lung cancer deaths for men are beginning to level off and are expected to decline.

Women experienced an increase in lung cancer deaths similar to men starting in the 1960s, approximately 20 to 30 years after greater numbers of women took up the habit. Lung cancer rates continue to increase among women. In 1987, lung cancer surpassed breast cancer as the leading cause of cancer deaths among women. This rising rate is expected to peak around the year 2010.

MORE QUITTERS, FEWER SMOKERS

When it comes to quitting smoking, women overall show greater willingness to take the step than men. That's another statistic revealed in a recent national survey by the CDC. Some other survey findings:

- Some 32 million Americans who smoke (70 percent of all adult smokers) report they want to quit. Women (73 percent) are more likely to want to quit smoking than men (67 percent).
- By 1993, half of all living U.S. adults who had ever smoked had quit.
- The higher a smoker's level of education, the greater the likelihood the person will quit the habit. By 1993, an estimated 38 percent of high school dropouts who had ever smoked had quit, compared to 45 percent of high school graduates and 65 percent of college graduates.

years ago, in 1980, the U.S. Surgeon General issued a report concentrating entirely on the effect that smoking has on a woman's health. The 359-page report cited hundreds of studies that reveal that women who smoke have increased risk of not only different types of cancer but of heart and respiratory diseases as well. There was more: Women who smoke face unique risks in pregnancy and are more likely than nonsmokers to give birth to babies who weigh less than normal.

Regardless of gender, smoking is an unhealthy venture. The tobacco in cigarettes contains at least 40 known carcinogens (cancer-causing chemicals). Lung cancer is not the only cancer caused by these chemicals but it is the most prevalent. Chemicals in tobacco smoke collect in the lungs and trigger the formation of cancerous growths.

In the lungs of a female, the recent British and Norwegian research found, tobacco smoke is especially damaging to the lung cells' DNA, the basic genetic

material. The team of scientists says their study indicates that smoke, specifically a group of carcinogens in smoke, does more damage to women's DNA than to that of males.

Were it not for tobacco, lung cancer would be far less common among both men and women. Approximately 90 percent of lung cancer cases in men and 79 percent in women are attributable to cigarette smoking. Sadly, nearly 90 percent of lung cancer patients die within five years of diagnosis. If lung cancer is detected early, survival chances improve somewhat, but few cases are detected early and there is no effective treatment for lung cancer.

Research has tied other cancers to smoking and its effects on women. Compared to nonsmokers, female smokers have three to four times more cervical cancer. Once a smoker has cervical cancer, radiation therapy is considered to be less effective. Other cancers associated with smoking include cancers of the larynx (voice box), esophagus, pancreas, and mouth.

Out of Breath

Cancer isn't the body's only payback for smoking. Smoking is a major cause of chronic obstructive pulmonary disease (COPD), the name given a series of diseases such as chronic bronchitis or emphysema, which occur more often in women who smoke than in those who don't.

COPD results in a permanent reduction of the amount of oxygen in the

blood. With less oxygen, a person with COPD is chronically short of breath and tires easily.

COPD is a major cause of smoking-related deaths in the United States today. Death rates for COPD have paralleled those for lung cancer and have been increasing over the past 25 years. Nearly 80,000 people die each year from this condition, according to the U.S. Public Health Service, and cigarette smoking accounts for 82 percent of these deaths.

But death rates alone don't tell the whole story about the toll COPD takes on those who suffer from it—and on their families. Death usually occurs only after a long period of disability, and in many cases COPD complicates other serious—and ultimately fatal—conditions.

Loss of a Unique Protection

And then there's the story of smoking and heart disease, the greatest overall killer of women as they grow older. Until she reaches menopause, a woman's female hormones give her unique protection against heart disease. This protection declines as the female body produces less of these hormones in later years. And even before menopause, a woman's coronary arteries can begin narrowing and hardening, a process that is speeded up when a person smokes.

Cancer, heart disease, a life of breathing difficulties: Women who smoke put themselves at a far greater risk for developing them than those who don't. Who wants these major problems in their future? Picture yours without them.

SECONDHAND SMOKE, FIRSTHAND RISK

A woman who smokes puts not only herself at risk, but others around her, too. Often the others are babies and children who have no choice but to inhale their mother's cigarette smoke.

In 1993, the U.S. Environmental Protection Agency (EPA) found that fumes given off from the tip of lighted cigarettes have higher concentrations of cancer-causing chemicals than the smoke that smokers inhale.

Numerous studies have linked secondhand smoke to health complications in nonsmokers, especially children. Because their bodies are still developing, exposure to the poisons in secondhand smoke puts children in danger of severe respiratory diseases and can hinder the growth of their lungs. On top of that, says the U.S. Public Health Service, the effects can last a lifetime.

Up in smoke

Why teen girls don't quit

We want them to butt out. They want us to butt out. How can we stop the women of tomorrow from smoking? By Mimi Frost with files from Susan Baxter

BEHIND THE MALL, ON THE BUTT-strewn steps that serve as the smoking lounge for the bargain outlets and busy food courts, four girls arrange themselves in a nearly closed circle. Jen, who has a model's figure and red ringlets that take at least 45 minutes out of her morning, sits in the centre, surrounded by friends who gather like ladies-in-waiting, laughing at her jokes, adding quips to her pronouncements. In unison, they reach for their cigarettes and commune in a cloud of nicotine.

For nearly a decade, scenes like this teen smoke-fest at Toronto's west-end Dufferin Mall had been on the decline. Cigarettes seemed be going the way of bell-bottoms. But in 1994, mysteriously, the percentage of girls who smoke rose to 29 percent, up from 21 percent just four years earlier. Now, teen girls represent the largest group of newly converted tobacco users—and the only group where female smokers outnumber males. This worries parents and public-health officials alike. Antismoking propaganda, smoke-apartheid bylaws and efforts to legislate tobacco out of teens' reach have not extinguished their cigarettes. More powerful forces entice kids to smoke: the pressures of adolescence, the confusion of growing up female, and potent messages from media and advertising. What's worse, girls are picking up the habit earlier. And the longer they smoke, the more likely they are to suffer from smoking-related illnesses.

It's a public-health nightmare waiting to happen. Already one Canadian woman dies every 35 minutes from smoking-related causes. Smoking puts women at higher risk for infertility, pelvic inflammatory disease, ectopic pregnancy and osteoporosis. For the first time, women's smoking deaths are increasing faster than men's. So why do these teens at the mall, along with a quarter of a million Canadian girls, continue to smoke?

"It's something to do," says Mandy.

"Everybody was doing it," blurts fast-talking Cathy.

Mandy makes a statement: "You're going to do things on your own and your parents can't do anything about it."

"It's better than biting your nails," says Jen, with a big laugh that's quickly joined by machine gun-like rounds of guffaws.

Jen would probably bite her nails if she really felt like it. Smoking for two years, the 15-year-old wears a short top, flaunting a landscape of skin and her boyfriend's key around her neck. Loaded with confidence, she probably started smoking to rebel. Her three friends may represent the other type of girl smokers, who puff to blend in. Unlike their willowy leader, they fear gaining weight if they quit, and say smoking instead of eating lunch saves money.

BOTH BOYS AND GIRLS LIKE THE buzz of nicotine, the promise of coolness, the soot of camaraderie. Still, girls have complicated reasons of their own for smoking, according to research published in the Journal of the American Medical Women's Association. Primarily, smoking helps girls control their weight, deal with negative emotions, develop an identity and create a mature self-image. "You have to look at the context of their whole lives to understand why girls smoke," says Dawn Hachey, head of Health Canada's tobacco reduction division. Pressures at school, trouble at home or low self-esteem can cause them to light up. And when girls do, they often smoke together—finding sociability in malls or doughnut shops brimming with nicotine and caffeine.

Sitting in a neighborhood doughnut shop, a flimsy aluminum ashtray before her, 14-year-old Terra has been smoking for three years. A basketball and soccer player, Terra wears a black T-shirt and leather jacket. Her brown hair has been lightened a few shades. In Grade 5, she and her friends used to light butts her parents left in ashtrays: "We all thought it was cool, and if we did it we were so much older and more mature . . . we would talk like we were grown-ups and have coffee." For many kids, cigarettes serve as a rite of passage, one deep drag into the grown-up world. Vancouver pediatrician Roger Tonkin, head of the division of adolescent health at the University of British Columbia's department of pediatrics, says, "In the absence of clear social customs, young people in Western society use alcohol and cigarettes as a sign of growing up." Just like Terra, girls typically take up smoking between the ages of 11 and 13. According to Dr. Michele Bloch of the American Medical Women's Association, they want to feel adult faster than boys. And the earlier they start, the more likely they are to get addicted.

Admitting she's addicted, Terra, like many women smokers—and unlike men—sometimes puffs to help deal with negative emotions. And bad moments strike often on the teen threshold. A couple of weeks ago, I felt fat and ugly. The friends I hang out with are skinny. I just felt bad about myself." So the 120-pound girl stopped eating, smoked constantly and didn't sleep. Worried that Terra might have bulimia or anorexia, friends told Terra's mother. (Although they probably didn't know it, eating disorders and smoking have been linked by a 1994 French study published in the International Journal of Eating Disorders.)

"Kids use cigarettes to cope with tough lives."

Besides experiencing bad feelings about her body, Terra is staring to notice a difference between how boys and girls

are treated. "People say things about you, for instance, a guy can start sleeping around at 13 and he's a stud, but a girl's a slut." Psychologist Carol Gilligan has written that girls Terra's age withdraw as they start to perceive women's still-unequal place in the world. This realization could be another factor in making girls more vulnerable to smoking, says Lorraine Greaves, a London, Ont., sociologist who studies women and smoking.

Images in the media make smoking look normal.

A top-drawer student, Terra feels stupid if she gets a B, yet at the same time, she's been suspended a few times for things such as telling off teachers and laughing at the principal. Terra's coach threatens to throw her off the basketball team if he catches her smoking. She even gets peer pressure from kids who are militant antismokers. On top of all that, today's teens must navigate a landscape mined with drugs; besides marijuana, which is commonly diluted with tobacco, high school kids are doing cocaine, ecstasy and acid. "These kids are using cigarettes to cope with difficult lives," says Phyllis Jensen, a Toronto addiction counselor and health researcher who has studied girl smokers and worked with girls in quitting programs. Pointing to family responsibilities and preferential treatment of boys, Jensen says, "Just because they're kids doesn't mean their lives are easy."

Terra's life certainly wasn't easy at the gifted school she left. When she started wearing jewelry and makeup, the other kids—the ones she called nerds—teased her. And along with this more grown-up person came cigarettes. It seemed like a perfectly reasonable thing to do, because as Richard Pollay, a professor of marketing at the University of British Columbia who specializes in advertising, points out, kids think smoking is more prevalent than it really is.

The media help make it seem next-door to normal. Cigarettes star in the Guns N' Roses video. Movies cast ciga-

rettes regularly: smoking was featured in *The Client, Who Framed Roger Rabbit* and *The Mask*—which wowed kids with its famous heart-shaped smoke rings. Women smokers on the big screen seem powerful: Sharon Stone in *Basic Instinct,* computer whiz Sandra Bullock in *The Net.* In the past, Hollywood awarded cigarettes plum roles because

Nipping it in the butt

If you're concerned about a teen's smoking, talk with her and really listen. Ask her about what's going on in her life. And when it comes to smoking, be honest about the facts—stress the dangers without getting hysterical.

● Acknowledge how addictive nicotine can be and how difficult quitting really is. Nearly three-quarters of drug and alcohol abusers participating in a study by the Addiction Research Foundation said that stopping smoking is at least as difficult as quitting their problem substance.

● Discuss the cost of smoking and calculate the cost of the teen's cigarettes for one year. If it amounts to the price of a new bike or stereo, offer such a reward if she'll quit.

● Arrange a chat with the doctor. In more than 50 studies with adults, when physicians ask patients about smoking and offer some help in quitting, six of 10 try and up to 6 percent succeed. An article in the Journal of the American Medical Women's Association devoted to female smokers suggests that doctors give teens these reasons to stop smoking: bad breath, ▷

tobacco companies paid for it. That practice, called product placement, gave cigarettes movie-star glamour.

"It never tasted so good, it's more the way I felt. I loved doing it, it was fun holding the cigarette in my hand—pretending I was all that." Terra would smoke in her room, taking in her reflection, watching her hand, thinking how she blew out the smoke made her look "sophisticated." She says, "I liked the way it looked. That was the main thing." The glamorous grown-up woman Terra saw in her mirror actually reflects back much recent advertising. Teen girls see plenty of U.S. women's magazines—where 7 percent of ads sell tobacco, according to a 1995 report. The Canadian study Women, Tobacco and the Media reported that ads fill women with images of sociability, relaxation and fashionability. Advertising expert Pollay says campaigns with funky Joe Camel and Marlboro machismo stress the independence kids crave.

Canadian teens are no longer immune to such images after the Supreme Court of Canada voted to allow cigarettes on billboards: in fact, last winter, an advertising company placed a billboard for cigarettes directly opposite a school in Hull, Que.—public outcry quickly brought it down. Plus, in Canada, tobacco companies spend $62 million on sponsorships that get their brands in the public eye. (Like many publications, Chatelaine accepts ads for tobacco-sponsored awards and events, believing the benefit outweighs the harm.) Kids are influenced by them. A 20-year study published in the Journal of Marketing found teens are three times as likely to respond to cigarette ads as adults.

AT THE DOUGHNUT SHOP, TERRA and her mom talk about their smoking. Neither of them lights up, trying to ignore an issue they mostly avoid. Terra's mother, Sandy Pellizzer, 39, started smoking back when cigarettes were everywhere. And like 61 percent of teen smokers, Terra comes from a smoking household. Like many smoking parents, Terra's mom is perturbed that her daughter follows her example: "I don't want your teeth to be yellow, I don't want to hear you cough. I'd like to give you money without thinking where you

spend it. I don't want to check up on you to see if you're eating."

Saying that her mother is cool and doesn't hound her, Terra understands her mom's fears. "I think she did all the same things I do. She knows what I'm up to without my telling her anything." In turn, Terra worries about her 12-year-old sister who occasionally gets a buzz from smoking to fit in. "I can't stop her, she sees me doing it all the time." Sandy, a mother of three, imagines that Terra, whose teachers say she could go to any school or get athletic scholarships, will be sucked into the teenage vacuum. Since she works as an assistant manager of a store, Sandy often checks on her daughter at school or at her lunch spot. When the kids see her coming, says Pellizzer, they drop their cigarettes out of respect.

But when Sandy suggests the two of them drop the habit together and make a quitting pact, Terra replies, "I can't imagine you without a cigarette. I don't care if you quit."

Messages from adults, whether from parents or commercials, fall on deaf ears.

Back at the mall, Jen's group of be-jeaned girls laugh at doom-and-gloom antismoking ads. Describing one where a woman morphs into a wrinkled monster, the redhead says, "You see all these pretty girls at 50 years old and they've still got glamorous faces. I know it kills your lungs, but I don't think it does anything to your features." These Lolitas in makeup don't buy the finger-wagging propaganda. The number of girl smokers has in fact risen since Health Canada's educational push began in 1993. Girls puff away—despite being aware of the risks. A 1995 survey on smoking shows that 97 percent of Canadians aged 15 and over realize smoking is addictive and 91 percent know it's unhealthy.

What's more, Health Canada's multi-million-dollar campaign on the dangers of secondhand smoke may have backfired and helped teens rationalize smoking. Many teens repeat the perverse logic Nicole offers: "Secondhand smoking is worse, so why not get it firsthand?" The mall smokers shout defiantly that planes kill. High cholesterol too. Plus, the girls get tired of being nagged by parents and school. "They're obsessed with drugs and smoking," says Jen. "Sure, you're going to have black lungs, but would you rather be walking around with a kid or having AIDS?"

stained teeth, cost, cough, sore throats and respiratory infections. Furthermore, cigarettes affect their ability to exercise.

● Find a nonjudgmental adult to mentor the teen: a guidance counselor, teacher or relative who respects her. Teens may not be able to talk about all the issues and pressures in their lives with a parent. Phyllis Jensen, an addiction counselor who developed the first women-only smoking-cessation program, says having individual counseling can help people quit.

● Help teens find ways of building confidence through sports, art, music or dance.

● Call Health Canada at 1/800/300-8449 for details on quitting programs across the country. Or call your local Lung Association branch or public-health unit for local programs.

● Suggest the teen visit CyberIsle, the teen-made Web site on prevention and cessation, at: *http://teennet1. med.utoronto.ca/welcome*

● Become political. Lobby to keep the price of cigarettes high. For help, write to your local branch of the Canadian Cancer Society or call 613/565-2522 ext. 303 to request a copy of their community action guide, Preventing Tobacco Sales to Young People, which costs $25, plus $8 for the accompanying video.

TERRA'S MOTHER WOULD PREFER not to choose. She hates to think of her daughter smoking and wants the law to help. Several times, Sandy Pellizzer has called police to report local stores that sell cigarettes to minors—but there's no action. It's common across Canada: 60 percent of retailers are willing to sell cigarettes to minors, according to a nationwide compliance check by the Canadian Cancer Society. If police don't enforce the law, it's back in the parents' hands, and Terra's parents don't let her smoke at home.

Trying to make her kick the habit, Sandy has cut off Terra's lunch money, to no avail. "Cigarettes are so cheap now," Sandy says. Her daughter actually brags that she can get cigarettes for $2.80 at the local milk store—less than what her mother pays.

In her mom's concern, Terra sees hypocrisy. "It's okay for grown-ups but not for kids. It shouldn't be that way. You should be stressing it for everybody. Then, maybe the kids would think, 'It's not good for them, it's not good for me.'"

That contradiction remains a part of the problem. "The policies don't back up our educational message," says Heather Selin, a policy analyst for the Non-Smokers' Rights Association, the antitobacco lobby group. Cigarettes sell for three bucks a pack, whereas nicotine patches cost about $75. In the same month Health Canada announced its $104 million tobacco-reduction plan, the government lowered cigarette taxes. "Regulation must accompany education," says Selin.

IF MOTHERS CAN'T PERSUADE their daughters not to smoke, what can? No single solution will do; smoking needs to be attacked on all fronts. "Looking at it as simply a health problem won't work," says sociologist Lorraine Greaves, author of *Smoke Screen: Women's Smoking and Social Control*. Greaves says we need to understand the issues behind girls' smoking—such as body image, inequality, social needs—and address them as well. As more and more girls smoke, Health Canada has finally responded by creating an initiative on women and tobacco. This year, it unveils three special programs developed especially for girls—which teach media literacy, promote sport and teach coping skills. Although new, they're a move in the right direction. So are antismoking policies with real teeth that bite.

If cigarette prices went up again, Jen from the mall circle says she would stock up on gum. "Without question, the evidence shows that pricing dictates consumption," says Les Hagen of Ac-

tion on Smoking & Health in Alberta. After the federal government lowered cigarette taxes in 1994, cigarette consumption jumped almost 10 percent, whereas the western provinces and Newfoundland, which did not follow suit, lacked such dramatic surges.

Raising cigarette prices curbs teen smoking, as does enforcing laws that prohibit sales to minors. With the country's toughest such bylaw, Edmonton has revoked the licenses of a half-dozen retailers. Smoking among the city's teens has decreased to 13 percent; in neighboring St. Albert, Alta., a full 23 percent of teens smoke. Inspired by Edmonton's success, St. Albert's citizens are proposing a similar bylaw.

RATHER THAN GETTING GIRLS into quitting programs, it's better to dissuade them before they start. Teaching girls how the media and advertising influence their decisions may help. That's the aim of Back Talk, a Health Canada program now being prepared. This media-literacy program will have girls rate magazine articles, analyze cigarette ads in U.S. magazines and tape TV shows. It has not been tested yet, but the similarly themed Thumbs Up! Thumbs Down! has been used in several B.C. schools. One graduate, 12-year-old Keri McKinney, turned into an antismoking activist who has preached to an assembly of hundreds at her school. Teens respond well, says health educator Joanne Lamoureux, who has also helped kids with critical viewing skills. "They can't believe they're being pulled in, they don't notice subliminal messages." Making girls aware might deflect their rebelliousness away from smoking and onto the media and tobacco companies.

Other antismoking policy makers suggest replacing cigarettes with sports. Sports can help with weight and stress, and provide camaraderie, says Marg McGregor of the Canadian Association for the Advancement of Women and Sports (CAAWS)—replacing three things that girls think smoking does for them. CAAWS has developed a program called Evening the Odds to encourage girls to get physical. So has the Canadian Intramural Recreation Association—with a peer-led program called HIP (Health in Perspective).

Getting active can bolster girls' self-image, says McGregor, who suggests that rock climbing or snowboarding can provide girls with a healthier way to rebel against societal pressure to assume a passive role. No hard evidence proves the approach works. However, a smoking-prevention program called Break-Free All Stars gets kids active. Aimed at kids aged 6 to 12, it uses rap songs and games to build self-esteem and improve body image. A pilot study shows 10 percent fewer kids in the program say they will smoke, compared with kids in control groups. But getting girls more active may not counteract the powerful enticements to smoke: two girls from the mall klatch have quit their teams; even Terra, a star player, says that given the choice between smoking and basketball, she would choose smoking. At least, for the present.

"I will quit one day," says one Vancouver girl, "when I'm around 20, when I'm on my own and can't afford it." Although 80 percent of teens say they want to quit eventually, getting them to butt out remains difficult because traditional quitting programs aren't really designed for youth. Cheryl Moyer of the national Women and Tobacco Working Group says, "We've told them to resist peer pressure, but that's when young people are longing to be part of society." Lamoureux says that many kids won't participate in quitting sessions if other kids know: for one seminar this year, only two out of 35 kids showed.

However, tailoring quitting programs to teens can make a difference. Close to 100,000 teens have ordered a quit-smoking kit advertised on MuchMusic and during popular TV shows. Quit 4 Life comes packaged like a CD and includes a wheel that shows kids how much money they could save—12 months of cigarettes adds up to one stereo. (Health Canada has not determined its future distribution.) Six months after receiving the kit, 85 percent of teens reported they'd tried to quit.

Like the outdated quitting programs, messages about health must be rehauled as well. Like most students, Jen has seen slides of blackened lungs but still has doubts. "They say it causes cancer," Jen says, "but there's a lot of old people who smoke—look at George Burns. He lived to 100, and he smoked cigars."

And appealing to girls not to harm their health doesn't move those who experience negative feelings about their bodies—remember Terra's week-long nicotine bender when she traded food for cigarettes. Now that researchers are finally starting to study the physiological differences of women smokers, their findings could play a part. Girls already know the long-term effects of smoking, says addiction counselor Phyllis Jensen, who has suggested girls might respond if they were shown how smoking affects their health now. The possibility of menstrual irregularities and discomfort might provide a more compelling argument than visions of polluted lungs in a faraway future.

GETTING GIRLS TO BUTT OUT ALSO requires quitting and prevention programs just for girls. Preliminary results from an ongoing University of Waterloo study suggest coed prevention programs don't affect high school girls' smoking rates. "Most of the programs have worked for boys but not for girls," says Moyer of the Women and Tobacco Working Group. "We have to do something different for girls—something extra."

Moyer explains that girls need help dealing with body image and negative emotion. Addressing that difference seems to work. Indeed, the country's first girl-directed smoking-cessation program, Project Vogue, proved very effective. Developed in eastern Ontario, where 38 percent of the women smoke, the Vogue program decreased the percentage of girls who smoke from 17 percent to 10 percent by dealing with such issues as self-esteem, body image and diet fallacies—and paired girls with buddies for support. It's no longer used in eastern Ontario because the boys felt left out! However, schools across Canada still use the kit, which has inspired a new prevention program. Aimed at Grades 6, 7 and 8, Improving the Odds devotes half the material to girls' issues and segregates the sexes. It has girls do innovative things such as interview women about smoking and mentor younger girls in danger of smoking. Rather than lecturing to deaf ears, this program asks girls to brainstorm their own solutions.

For Terra, smoking means she can't sing anymore. She may get kicked off the basketball team she loves. She gets lectures from teachers and scoldings from her father. But she continues to puff away. "Right now, I don't think anything can make me quit unless I want to quit." It seems that even locking up cigarettes, inoculating girls with self-esteem and teaching them sports may not put out their cigarettes, if those measures don't get to the root of the larger problem—which is the very difficult task of growing up. As Lorraine Greaves says, "We must recognize the deep meaning of smoking for girls and start from there."

a smoker's tale

Susan Tanner grew up with the ads that equated smoking with female independence. Sixteen years later, as a result of her unbroken habit, she's fighting for custody of her daughter. Tanner feels like a victim. Is she? **Steve Fishman** reports on the latest skirmish in the war on smoking

The squib in the newspaper was short, direct, and astounding: A Sacramento woman who smoked about a pack of cigarettes a day was in danger of losing custody of her asthmatic daughter. Susan Tanner, a divorced 30-year-old nurse, had long been eight-year-old Elysa's guardian. And now, at her ex-husband's request, a family court judge was considering taking Tanner's daughter away—because she smoked.

Smoking, as everyone knows, is self-defeating behavior. Cigarettes kill 430,000 people a year, half the population of, say, the city of Sacramento. Secondhand smoke—the fumes that nonsmokers breathe in—may kill another 53,000. And just last year the Environmental Protection Agency added a new dimension to the hazards of cigarette fumes: They are especially harmful to children like Elysa, who suffer symptoms of asthma. The explosive report prompted John Banzhaf III, executive director of Action on Smoking and Health, to declare that "smoking is the most pervasive form of child abuse," a charge that will no doubt be heard more and more. Already judges in at least eleven states have stopped parents from lighting up when their kids are around.

Where should smokers be permitted to smoke? That question—which in Tanner's case was raised in family court—is being decided by city councils and county boards across the country these days. Nonsmokers want smokers out of shopping malls, restaurants, even private offices. For the first time, a national smoking ban will be taken up in Congress this year. Cigarette-makers, naturally, are busy fighting the trend. Perhaps nowhere has the battle been more ferocious than in Tanner's hometown of Sacramento, where the tobacco industry inaugurated a little-publicized strategy of lavishly funding front groups that fought for "smokers' rights."

To some, Susan Tanner has become a symbol of the embattled smoker. Tanner hardly sees it that way. She isn't *for* smoking. "I'm a nurse," she says. "I, of all people, know what smoking does to you." If anything, Tanner is among a generation of women who feels taken in, "like a victim," she says sometimes.

This winter a landmark study in *The Journal of the American Medical Association* essentially agreed. Tanner was among the first women targeted by the cigarette industry. And as the *JAMA* article demonstrated, when the industry goes after women, teenage girls

start smoking in droves. The surgeon general reported in February that the person who takes up smoking is most often a woman under eighteen, just as Tanner was when she began.

These days Tanner's child obeys the voice of Judge Nancy Sweet, and that breaks her heart. Last October Sweet decided Elysa should live in a "neutral home" until final custody is decided. She gave Tanner and her ex-husband equal visitation rights. As school let out one January day, Elysa's father picked up the chubby-cheeked second grader and took her to his mother's house. "Elysa used to live *here*," says Tanner. "Now I get to see her every other weekend. How do you live with that? It's so painful."

And yet under the emotion, Tanner seems, like many smokers, more careworn than angry. "Why don't I just quit smoking?" she asks herself time and again. "I desperately want to. It's just so damned hard."

By the time she was fourteen, Tanner had shot up to nearly her full height of five feet eight inches. People commented on her clear blue eyes, her perfect nose. She had lovely shoulder-length brown hair with bangs. "I was really bright and I was beautiful. I could've gone anywhere. I had the world in the palm of my hand," she says. "I just didn't know it." That was in 1977, which was also the year she moved. She was from the city of Sacramento, California's capital, and didn't exactly fit into Arden Manor, an affluent suburb of Sacramento County. "The most important thing to me was my friends," she says, "and whether or not I had any." Teenage girls are probably more sensitive to fitting in than adolescent boys—their stock of self-esteem is often reported to be lower. Tanner's parents had divorced when she was two; maybe that made her feel like more of a loose thread. "To be accepted," she says, "was the most important thing."

Tanner's friends smoked. So she tried, too. Smoking, as one small study reported, is "a bonding agent." Her first cigarette was nauseating. "Why does anybody do that?" she still wonders. She persisted. (Up to half of those who even experiment with cigarettes will become regular smokers, says Michael Eriksen, who worked on the Surgeon General's 1994 Report on Youths and Tobacco Use.) Tanner's friends smoked Marlboros. Tanner, though, liked the ads for another Philip Morris brand, Virginia Slims—one of the first cigarettes to target women and still one of the five most-advertised brands in the country. Something about the ads was sexy, Tanner thought. Virginia Slims women looked independent and confident. YOU'VE COME A LONG WAY, BABY was the feminist-sounding slogan. Virginia Slims took off like a rocket.

Cigarette manufacturers insist that their ads only pitch brand loyalty. The adolescent Tanner was too young even to buy cigarettes legally. Yet the most recent studies show that at fourteen, Tanner was actually at the top end of the "age of smoking experimentation." Girls of eleven are starting now. "As a teenager, your body is betraying you. You're awkward. You feel you have to adopt more adult behaviors. And here are these thin, groomed, gorgeous, self-confident, popular women smoking cigarettes," says Regina Penna, a former smoker who now directs Women and Girls Against Tobacco in Berkeley, California, the most prominent group to organize women against smoking.

That Virginia Slims was suddenly offering Tanner role models who smoked was no coincidence. For decades, the typical smoker had been a man. But since the 1964 surgeon general's report linked cigarettes to cancer, men had been quitting at ever-increasing rates. Who was to step in? One manufacturer pointed out the obvious: The women's market is "probably the largest opportunity."

What now seems undeniable is that when the industry talks of the women's market, it means teenagers, too. "We can't speak for manufacturers' intentions, but we can speak for their actions," says John Pierce, lead author of the most comprehensive study ever to examine the smoking habits of women, released in February. "Their advertising differentially hits teens. The data are very clear." In fact, virtually no one in America begins to smoke after age 20 anymore. The economics of this shift are compelling: On average, Pierce says, the industry spends $3,000 to hook a teenager who over the lifetime of her habit will spend $20,000 on cigarettes.

Through the 1960s, the tobacco industry placed 90 percent of its

Cigarette manufacturers insist that their ads pitch only brand loyalty. Yet studies show that at fourteen, when Tanner started smoking, she was at the top end of the "age of smoking experimentation." Girls of eleven are starting now

magazine ads in publications aimed mainly at men. By the late 1970s, when an adolescent Tanner was looking for adult role models, the industry was placing half its ads in women's magazines (including *Vogue*). The strategy paid off. By the time Tanner graduated from high school in 1980, female high school seniors were smoking more than their male counterparts. Older smokers might have been quitting at record rates, but as Tanner took up the habit, Americans consumed more cigarettes than ever—12,854 cigarettes per smoker per year, one every waking half hour. "Young women have picked up the slack," says Nancy Kaufman, vice president of the Robert Wood Johnson Foundation, the largest health-care foundation in the country. These days, about 2,000 teenage women light up for the first time every day. The younger a smoker begins, the more likely she is to become a heavy smoker.

Within a dozen years female smokers will outnumber male smokers, and that trend will continue to rearrange the demographics of disease. Though lung cancer is rarely seen as a women's issue, it has recently passed breast cancer as the leading cancer killer of women. (Lung cancer is more deadly, with only 13 out of 100 people surviving more than 5 years with the disease.) "If a woman walks in here with lung cancer, what can I say?" says Pierce, the head of cancer prevention at the University of California at San Diego. " 'You should have thought about that 20 years ago. I can't help you now.' "

Tanner, who is now into her sixteenth year of Virginia Slims, never

thought she'd end up a smoker. In that she was also typical—92 percent of teenage women smokers say they don't expect to continue through the next year. The truth is that two-thirds of all smokers don't really want to smoke. "Who in their right mind would want to?" asks Tanner. Every year one third try to kick the habit; half of young women smokers make an attempt. The grim news is that less than 2 percent of teenage women actually succeed in quitting. "Cigarettes enslave young women," Kaufman wrote in *JAMA* last February.

Is she overstating the case? Not really. To judge by relapse rates, stopping smoking is tougher than giving up heroin. "I've taken care of heroin addicts, and they quit more easily than smokers," says John Robbins, M.D., chief of general medicine at the University of California Davis Medical Center. He runs quit-smoking groups in Sacramento, where the success rate is about 30 percent. "If there's enough motivation," says Robbins, "people quit."

Motivation, though, is tough to come by. Often it arrives only by degrees. Eighty percent of women who smoke don't give up the habit when pregnant—Tanner couldn't—even though most know smoking reduces birthweight and increases miscarriages and infant mortality. Eriksen, director of the Centers for Disease Control's office of smoking and health, tried to quit for five years. "I felt like I didn't have control of my right hand," he said. Then his uncle died of cancer. He never smoked again.

Tanner had already tried to quit three, maybe four times before the custody hearing. She sometimes talks as if she is just waiting to quit. Once she went two entire years without a cigarette. She was young and interested in someone who didn't smoke. "What got me back on? One cigarette. Just one drag. That's it. That's all it took," she says.

On average, people who succeed at quitting try four or six or eight times, each time rearranging their lives, dropping the rituals that involve cigarettes, like what they drink in the morning and where they go at night, and developing new responses to stress. In surveys women say one of the two reasons they smoke is stress reduction. (The other is weight control; cigarettes are an appetite suppressant.) In 1993 Tanner enrolled in a stop-smoking course. She paid $180 to be hypnotized over a period of a month. She had exercises to follow at home. Then the custody turmoil began. "Maybe it's a cop-out," she says, "but with all the stress, I didn't think I'd succeed." She dropped the course.

Tanner had once entertained the idea of becoming a physician. Her mother is a nurse. Medical school, though, soon seemed like a luxury. By the age of 20, she was supporting a young son from a short-lived relationship. She didn't have much money. And she had other worries: like, who would be interested in a young woman with a baby? Then along came an attractive, charismatic guy who was willing. Steven Masone was eleven years older. She knew he wasn't perfect. "I was 21," she says. "I thought I could change the world." They married in 1985. Their daughter, Elysa, was born the next year. "She's really cute, very energetic, outgoing, *very* precocious, very bright," says Tanner. Baby pictures of Elysa look just like Tanner's own. Even Tanner's mother can't tell the difference. The marriage ended in 1986; Tanner kept the two children. The divorce is the one thing the couple agrees on. "We never should have been married," says Masone.

"I'm a survivor," says Tanner. "You either make it or you curl up in a little ball and go away." After the separation, she attended nursing classes at American River Junior College in Sacramento. Her grandmother fixed her meals; her grandfather fixed her car. She got loans to buy books, grants to raise her family. (Masone, whose child support bill was $75 a month, often didn't pay that.) For the past three years, Tanner has been an emergency-room nurse at Kaiser Permanente North. "You're doing something that's going to make a difference and you're doing it right and you make a reasonable wage," she says. "I love it."

While Tanner waited to quit smoking, she figured she'd limit the effect on others. The hospital already required smokers to take their cigarettes outside. At home, she'd open doors or windows, go into another room, take care to stay downwind of Elysa. But smoking became one of the things she and her ex-husband fought about. Masone, who had supervised visiting rights every other week, said their daughter was asthmatic. While Tanner disputed the severity of her asthma, Elysa did wheeze and cough at least a few times a year. In 1988 Masone took the dispute to court. The judge ordered Tanner not to smoke in front of Elysa. "I can go outside and smoke," she says. "I have a little bench I sit on out there." This, more than the confident woman at the cocktail parties, may be the realistic image of the contemporary smoker: chased to a bench in the brisk night air.

Certainly there is reason to worry about cigarette fumes. Over the past decade, a dozen studies have examined the effect of secondhand smoke on wives of smokers. The women turned out to have a one-third greater chance of developing lung cancer than women who lived with nonsmokers. In 1990 the Environmental Protection Agency concluded that cigarette fumes cause 3,000 lung cancer deaths a year in people who *don't* smoke. More recently, Stanton Glantz, a heart researcher at the University of California at San Francisco, fingered secondhand smoke as the cause of 37,000 fatal cases of heart disease a year, which would make it the third leading cause of preventable death from the disease. (Smoking is first, alcohol second.)

The health threat of secondhand smoke has, as a by-product, created perhaps the largest special-interest group ever: nonsmokers. After all, 75 percent of the adult population doesn't smoke. In Tanner's home county in 1990, nonsmoking citizens proposed a complete ban on smoking in restaurants and offices. "We wanted our law to be a model for the nation," says Paul Knepprath, spokesman for the Sacramento chapter of the American Lung Association. "Even a company president's office has got to be smoke-free." The Sacramento County Board of Supervisors passed a rigorous smoking ban by a vote of three to two.

The tobacco industry often battles communities that want to restrict smoking. If they lose, they almost always move on. But in Sacramento, the fight to overturn the ordinance became one of the costliest ever.

What was at stake in Sacramento (as with any such ban) was more than where smokers could have a cigarette. Restrict where people can smoke and they smoke less. A study last year in the *Archives of Internal Medicine* reported that if all California workplaces became smoke-free, employees would smoke 41 percent less—a $406 million annual loss in sales in one state.

Three days after the vote on the ban, Sacramentans for Fair Business Policy was launched. It claimed to be mostly local restaurant owners afraid business would be hurt by a smoking ban (a widespread but false fear, studies now show). Its aim was to force a general vote on the ban: By California law, if 30,433 signatures were presented to the county within 30 days, then the ordinance had to be suspended and either rescinded, changed, or put a general vote.

But the Fair Sacramentans—as investigators from the University of California at San Francisco learned and reported in *JAMA* last year—were funded almost exclusively by tobacco interests. (Philip Morris, manufacturer of Tanner's Virginia Slims, would contribute $124,963.) Why use a cover? As cigarette lobbyist Ron Saldana once remarked, "I've learned from experience that as soon as I'm identified as a representative of the Tobacco Institute, I lose all credibility."

The money bought the services of professional petition gatherers, who swooped into town and earned between $3 and $5 a signature. Petitions with 60,000 names were presented to the county clerk within the 30-day limit. A referendum was scheduled for June 1992.

The tobacco industry is very good at reaching the public. Its annual $4 billion ad and promotion budget has resulted in six-year-olds knowing Joe Camel as well as Mickey Mouse, according to one study. (R. J. Reynolds recently introduced Josephine Camel.) To promote its cause in Sacramento County, the industry poured in $2 million—twice the annual budget of the county's tobacco education program.

A group of doctors, hospitals, and health groups retaliated with Citizens for a Healthier Sacramento. They raised $65,000. An early poll showed 72 percent of the people supported the county ordinance. But that was before the industry really got going.

Industry front groups—sometimes organized by public-relations firms—placed 472 30-second local TV spots. "Tobacco is something my friends and neighbors choose to enjoy" is how Thomas Lauria of the industry's Tobacco Institute sometimes explained the industry's stance. "It's their business." The campaign emphasized that government would be getting into people's business. It featured a Cigarette Patrol, which ads suggested, would hunt out and ticket smokers, attacking a person's privacy rights.

Citizens for a Healthier Sacramento responded that smoking wasn't private; it was pollution. "Smoking is a public-health issue," says Knepprath. "We kept the public informed that the tobacco industry's bottom line was to make profits off addicted smokers."

Tanner looked on from the sidelines. She wasn't about to go fight *for* the right to smoke. A well-regarded emergency-room nurse, she was witness to a daily shuffle of emphysema cases: two-pack-a-day types who at 55 were circling the drain. Every case brought her up short. She liked to smoke; that was the problem. (The psychoactive drug nicotine suppresses the anxiety of nicotine withdrawal: that translates into "pleasure" for smokers.) But she was ashamed of smoking. She sometimes said she'd give anything to *want* to quit. She thought of herself as individualistic, headstrong, confident. She couldn't make smoking fit, though, couldn't make it seem part of the planned outrageousness of, say, the very, very short hair—the Sinéad look—she'd strolled into work with one day. "Smokers are outcasts," she says.

The Sacramento ordinance restricting smoking won, 56 percent to 44 percent—a landslide, though not, perhaps, compared with the head start it had enjoyed. In the end, the tobacco industry spent $17 for each "no" vote. The citizens group spent 37 cents per "yes" vote.

Sacramento County is one of the country's largest communities—population 1.2 million—to go smoke-free, joining a list of cities and counties more than 100 names long. This year smoking bans are expected to show up on state agendas. Vermont, Maryland, and Utah have already passed statewide restrictions. In Pennsylvania, a bill has been introduced to prohibit smoking in a car with anyone sixteen or younger. Violators would risk a $50 fine.

The battle, however, is as constant and contested as ever. The tobacco industry contributes to political campaigns at every level. And a study in California headed by Michael Begay, now at the University of Massachusetts, shows that contributions to politicians tend to result in votes for industry positions. Other tactics are more unconventional. In California, under cover of the Freedom of Information Act, industry representatives have wheeled copy machines into county health department offices and demanded loads of documents. "They're basically harassing," says Alyonik Hrushow, director of the Tobacco Free Project in San Francisco. In February, Philip Morris moved into the open, suing San Francisco over its new no-smoking ordinance. "The forces of darkness and evil are pulling out all the stops," charges UCSF's Glantz.

Lauria, the nonsmoking tobacco spokesman, protests that the enthusiasms of the antismokers are misguided. Perhaps some studies of spouses show the nonsmoker has a higher risk of lung cancer. But, he says, what does that have to do with customers who spend a short time in a restaurant? There's no "safe" exposure level to any carcinogen, but even Pierce says, "it's yet to be proved that one hour exposure is going to lead to major disease." Last summer, though, Michael Siegel of the Centers for Disease Control found that nonsmokers who work in bars and restaurants had a 50 percent greater chance of developing lung cancer. News like this means that secondhand smoke may pose a risk to the financial well-being of employers. "Employers are clearly negligent for permitting employees to be exposed to a carcinogen," says Richard Daynard, chairman of the Tobacco Products Liability Project. "It's like not taking steps to protect them from asbestos." Daynard's forecast has already come true in at least one case. A nonsmoking waiter who worked in a smoky bar for five years recently won a $95,000 settlement after getting sick with heart disease.

It's difficult to deny that the data on spouses have bearing on a situation like Tanner's. Children live with smokers the same way spouses do. And, being little, kids are hit with a bigger wallop from the same dose of smoke. Lung cancer is not the issue. But last year the federal government told parents: Smoke, and your children suffer. The fumes of others contribute to as many as 300,000 respiratory infections in babies. They also trigger up to 26,000 new cases of asthma a year and worsen symptoms in up to a million children. Mark Witten, Ph.D., of the University of Arizona exposed rabbits to burning cigarettes fifteen minutes a day for 20 days—about the amount breathed in by kids of smoking parents. Cells in the rabbits' airways degenerated. It resembled an asthmatic reaction, the kind that Elysa sometimes had. Even scarier, scientists this winter demonstrated for the first time that nicotine from secondhand smoke is measurable in a fetus.

"Secondhand smoke is killing children, and I think it's time for the courts of this country to help these children," said a Florida circuit court judge who then ordered a seven-year-old asthmatic boy taken from the home of his mother, whose new husband smoked. Already, courts have ordered parents not to smoke in front of kids in New Jersey and Michigan. In Texas a smoking mother and a nonsmoking father fought for custody, until the father testified that the child's pediatrician couldn't find any other reason for the little girl to have so many upper respiratory diseases, except smoke. The father won sole

custody. In Tennessee a woman lost her asthmatic daughter to the father, in part because she smoked. She quit smoking but still couldn't get her child back. If she'd really been a good mother, the court seemed to say, she would have stopped earlier.

More than anyone else, Joseph Lamacchia of Watertown, Massachusetts, may be responsible for pushing nonsmoking parents into the courts. Lamacchia asked his ex-wife not to smoke around their son, who lived with her. (Dawn O'Brien, Lamacchia's ex-wife, says, "If that's what's best for my son, then I want to do it.") Then Lamacchia formed Parents Against Second-hand Smoke—PASS—which he runs out of his home. For $8, he'll send a photocopied booklet with a step-by-step strategy for "building your case." Last year he mailed off 1,300 of them. One page is titled, "Nicotine Test: Get This Done for Your Child."

Tanner's ex-husband, Steven Masone, was one of those who got in touch with Lamacchia. He wasn't convinced that Tanner was doing all of her smoking outside. Early this year, he took a sample of Elysa's urine for a nicotine test and took the results back to family court. The test was flawed but still showed enough nicotine—exposure to half a pack a day, Masone says—to alarm Judge Sweet. Tanner protested that she didn't smoke near Elysa. "I'm going to keep her with her paternal grandmother as long as I can," says David Miller, the attorney appointed by the court to represent Elysa. "She's in a smoke-free environment. That's a strong issue in this case."

It may be true that when family courts factor smoking into custody battles, women are at a disadvantage. Says Frances Olsen, a law professor at University of California at Los Angeles, "Women smokers are judged more harshly." It may be unconscious, but judges hold women up to an ideal of motherhood, and that mother doesn't smoke, says Olsen.

It also may be true that the court will eventually return Elysa to the environment she grew up in—including her brother and dog and friends—as long as Susan Tanner sticks to her cigarette bench outside the house. Tanner is, after all, competing against an ex-husband on probation for resisting arrest. (The charge stems from a complaint that was later dropped of cruelty to a child.) And he lost in a previous attempt to get custody. "That was on some psychological evaluation that was not thorough," he says.

Yet custody fights involving secondhand smoke—like any fight over who can smoke where—start with another issue, and that is addiction. Amid her willfulness and her poise, Tanner returns these days to the fact that she has spent more than half her life asking herself the same question: "How can you *be* in this world not smoking?" She doesn't know. In February she called the American Lung Association, the group that spearheaded the Sacramento smoking ban, to inquire about quit-smoking classes. Perhaps in the past her motivation had been imperfect. Now they've taken Elysa. "The courts are chopping my daughter up into little pieces," she says.

Perhaps that is motivation enough.

Cigars, women, and glamour CANCER

"It's a woman thing" is the latest slogan for Virginia Slims cigarettes, and now cigars, too, are becoming a woman thing. Demi Moore, Julie Andrews, Diane Keaton, Goldie Hawn, Whoopi Goldberg, and Bette Midler, as well as other glamorous screen personalities, singers, and models, have appeared on posters, in films, and in a string of advertisements with stogies in their mouths or held at rakish angles. This is not as new as it seems. Marlene Dietrich used to smoke cigars, and so did George Sand, the very symbol of female rebellion in nineteenth-century France. Amy Lowell, the poet, puffed away on this side of the Atlantic.

The marketing push to sell cigars to women is also not new. According to Dr. Stanton Glantz, a tobacco expert at the University of California at San Francisco, cigar makers are simply using the tactics long employed by cigarette companies. These include getting famous people to endorse the product, thus persuading women that putting a poisonous wad of tobacco in their mouths will bring them success in the boardroom and private club—male strongholds until recently—and associating cigars with images of luxury and power.

According to an article in *Advertising Age* last August, premium cigar sales are booming, after languishing for more than a decade. Nobody knows, or is telling, how many women contributed to the sales spike. *Cigar Aficionado*, a slick magazine that exists to promote cigars, has found a growing audience among women, according to an article in *Marketing News*. These women tend to be young and well-educated. They may smoke cigars to make business contacts. And no doubt they enjoy breaking taboos, much as Madame Sand did.

Cigars, of course, do seem less harmful than cigarettes. Most cigar smokers, it's thought, and particularly women, are only occasional smokers. And cigar smokers usually don't inhale, but simply hold the smoke in their mouths, or don't inhale deeply. Scientific studies have shown, however, that former cigarette smokers who switch to cigars do inhale, and in many European countries cigar smokers inhale.

Behind the glamorous images, a big cancer risk
Cigar smokers who don't inhale are at lower risk for lung cancer than cigarette smokers. But cigars do increase the risk substantially: women who regularly smoke cigars triple their chances of getting lung cancer. In addition, cigar smoking boosts the risk of heart disease and cancers of the mouth and lips: it increases the risk of oral cancer anywhere from four- to tenfold.

Another problem with cigars: they are much more polluting than cigarettes. For instance, cigar smoke is higher in carbon monoxide—one cigar, on average, produces more of the gas than three cigarettes. This "sidestream" smoke is worse not only for others who happen to be in the room, but for the smoker herself, who also breathes it.

We don't know of any famous women who've actually died from smoking cigars, but plenty of famous men have, including Ulysses S. Grant, Sigmund Freud, and Babe Ruth. When Virginia Slims tells us that smoking is a "woman thing," they neglect to add that dying of lung cancer has now become a woman thing, too. Once rare among women, lung cancer (thanks to the upsurge in cigarette smoking among women after World War II) kills more American women every year than breast cancer.

An opportunity women should pass up. *Oral cancers occur most frequently in men over 40; twice as many men as women get the diseases. Now, alas, women have a chance to catch up.*

Reprinted with permission from the *University of California at Berkeley Wellness Letter*, January 1997, p. 2. © 1997 by Health Letter Associates.

As far as women's hearts are concerned, the road to health may run through a vineyard or two. But nothing is ever simple: Drinking carries considerable risks—breast cancer among them—and moderation is key.

Alcohol and Health: Mixed Messages for Women

Temperance leader Carrie Nation would be appalled: Thanks to findings about alcohol's heart-healthy benefits, U.S. dietary guidelines now endorse moderate alcohol consumption.

Though early evidence of alcoholic cardiac benefits came from studies on men, several recent studies suggest that the benefits apply to women as well—at least to those women at risk of developing heart disease.

However, this rosy picture is not without thorns. Though the cardiac benefits appear to be real, many physicians are reluctant to endorse a practice that can have such devastat-ing physical, emotional, and social consequences when carried too far.

Says New York cardiologist Marianne Legato, "The incidence of alcoholism is increasing among women. It's a much-underestimated addiction in this country. Alcohol is the last thing I would recommend for coronary artery disease."

And even when alcoholism is exclud-ed, any assessment of alcohol's bene-fits for women must be balanced against the potential risks. Heavier drinking is associated with an increased risk of breast cancer and with a host of other serious health problems (see "Good Reasons to Cork It"). Moreover, a woman's body is especially vulnerable to alcohol abuse, sustaining damage at lower levels of consumption than a man's.

Good in Small Doses

The sticking point for most critics is the concept of moderation—and how well or poorly it may be applied in the real world (see "How Much is Too Much?").

During the last two years, several studies have found lower death rates among light to moderate drinkers (generally defined as one to two drinks per day). The findings point to a "U-shaped curve"—that is, risk is lowest for moderate drinkers, who fall in the middle, and highest for teetotalers and heavy drinkers.

A recent report from the massive Nurses' Health Study supports these findings. In that study, published in the May 11, 1995 *New England Journal of Medicine*, light drinkers (one to three drinks per week) had a 17% lower risk of death than non-drinkers. The risk was 12% lower for moderate drinkers (four drinks per week to about two drinks per day). Heavy drinkers had a 19% higher risk of dying.

The survival advantage of modest drinking was primarily attributable to fewer deaths from heart attacks. However, it applied only to women at risk of heart disease—those who were over 50 or who had other coro-nary risk factors, such as smoking,

---

How Much Is Too Much?

Alcohol researchers define moderate alcohol consumption as one to two drinks per day. That's easy enough. But many of us kid ourselves about how much we drink, especially when it comes to sipping wine from tall goblets or to free-pouring an evening cocktail. Here's what "moderate" alcohol con-sumption really means on a daily basis:

Beer	Wine	Spirits
one to two 12-ounce cans	one to two five-ounce glasses	one to two 1.5-ounce shots

If your favorite wine glass holds eight ounces of wine, for example, and you drink two glasses a day, you're pushing beyond moderate consumption. By some definitions, you would be considered a heavy drinker.

---

high cholesterol, high blood pressure, obesity, or a family history of heart disease. (Much of the increased risk of death among heavy drinkers was due to breast cancer.)

How alcohol protects the heart isn't entirely clear. Several studies have suggested that alcohol discourages clot formation. A key factor, however, appears to be its favorable effects on cholesterol levels.

Specifically, alcohol consumption increases high-density lipoprotein (HDL, the so-called good cholesterol). Before menopause, women have higher HDL levels than men do—a fact that's believed to explain premenopausal women's relative protection from heart disease. When estrogen production declines at menopause, however, HDL levels begin to fall and heart attack rates begin to climb. By the time women reach age 65, we're as likely as men to die of heart attacks.

Estrogen appears to be a key link in the alcohol-HDL connection. Women who drink have higher circulating levels of estrogen than do non-drinkers—a factor that presumably boosts their HDL and reduces the risk of heart disease. But that estrogen upswing might also contribute to the increased incidence of breast cancer seen in heavy drinkers.

Further complicating the picture is the fact that even modest amounts of alcohol raise triglycerides. High triglycerides are a particularly ominous coronary risk factor in women. For a woman whose triglyceride level is on the high side (a level consistently over 200 mg/dl), moderate drinking might do more harm than good.

The Gender Gap

In the women and alcohol debate, one thing is clear: Women pay a heavy price for heavy drinking. And in research circles, "heavy drinking" means as few as three drinks a night.

Because of gender differences in

Good Reasons to Cork It

Heavy drinking takes a toll on women's health. Liver disease, weakened hearts, damage to unborn children, and accidents are the better-known risks. But heavy alcohol consumption also is believed to aggravate or contribute to the following conditions:

- stroke
- cancers of the liver, head and neck, pancreas, and breast
- osteoporosis
- high blood pressure
- depression
- anxiety

- insomnia
- premenstrual syndrome
- infertility
- nutritional deficiencies

A final—and important—consideration is alcohol's long-term effects on the brain. "The cognitive effects of heavy drinking are greatly underestimated," says New York cardiologist Marianne Legato. "People stop being able to think clearly, they lose their memory, and they have little blackout spells. Though they seem to be 'functional,' they're not if you measure them very carefully in terms of what they once were."

body composition and metabolism, women suffer alcohol-related physical problems at lower levels of consumption than men. And these medical problems may remain hidden longer for several reasons.

For one, many women are closet drinkers. And some doctors may still be reluctant to broach the "indelicate" subject of alcohol abuse with a woman—or when they do, her reported amount of drinking may not raise a red flag.

In reality, however, it takes less alcohol to damage a woman's liver and heart. "There's no question that alcohol has a bigger impact on women than men in terms of cirrhosis," says Dr. Legato, an associate professor of clinical medicine at Columbia Presbyterian College of Physicians and Surgeons.

Moreover, a serious heart condition called alcoholic cardiomyopathy is a problem for both men and women who drink heavily. In this condition, chronic alcohol consumption weakens heart muscles, compromising heart function and leading to heart

failure in many patients. According to a report in the July 12, 1995 *Journal of the American Medical Association*, it takes much less alcohol to cause this damage in women than it does in men.

Gender differences in metabolism appear to be to blame for alcohol's exaggerated effects in women. Women have less of an enzyme called alcohol dehydrogenase, which breaks down alcohol first in the stomach and then in the liver. As a result, less alcohol is processed at these sites, and more passes to the liver, brain, and other parts of the body.

And the lower fluid content of a woman's body also contributes to their inability to handle alcohol, according to a recent report. Less fluid means less opportunity for the alcohol to dissolve and more opportunity for alcohol molecules to reach the brain. In practical terms, a woman may have fewer drinks than a man but end up with a blood alcohol level as high or higher than his.

Weighing the Risks

So what are women to do? Given the

public's proclivity to grab a headline and run with it, many cardiologists are decidedly uncomfortable with stories on alcohol's heart benefits.

For Dr. Legato, the entire issue is at best overblown and at worst potentially dangerous. "Alcohol is such a problem in our society," she emphasizes. Attempts to legitimize alcohol as a medical intervention for heart disease are "like using morphine to treat a migraine."

If you don't drink at all, don't start in hopes of reducing your heart disease risk. Other lifestyle modifications are far more important—stopping smoking, getting regular exercise, losing weight if you're overweight, keeping high blood pressure and diabetes in control, and watching dietary fat intake.

If you do drink, you're best off leaning toward the "light" side of moderation—one drink a day or less.

That level of consumption shouldn't elevate your breast cancer risk, says breast cancer surgeon Laura Esserman, M.D., M.B.A. "Everything has to be put in perspective," says Dr. Esserman, an assistant professor of surgery and co-director of the Breast Cancer Center at Mt. Zion Hospital and the University of California, San Francisco. "Modest amounts of alcohol are associated with improvements in cardiac risk factors, and cardiac problems are a much more significant health risk for women than breast cancer."

However, "heavy drinking—three to four drinks a day—clearly is associated with breast cancer," she continues. "In fact, moderate to heavy alcohol use increases a woman's breast cancer risk as much as family history. But someone who drinks three to five glasses of wine a week should be fine."

Way Out West and Under the Influence

CAREY GOLDBERG

SPOKANE, Wash.

It was like the buzz of 1,000 cups of coffee, Joy said. It kept her up for days at a time, and set her to cleaning the house like the old white tornado commercials for Ajax. It whisked away her postpartum depression and made staying slim a breeze.

The only problem, said Joy, who asked that her last name not be used, was that it wrecked her life, costing her custody of her 3-year old son Conor (she is now fighting to get him back) and it proved so hard to kick that she went through four in-patient programs to get to the point where she is now, with six drug-free months behind her.

"I was a garbage pit," she said.

The illegal drug that seduced and almost destroyed Joy is methamphetamine—also known as crank, speed or meth.

Its growing popularity, almost entirely in the West and Midwest, has brought warnings from Federal officials that it could become the 1990's version of crack cocaine. It is easy to make, cheap, powerfully addictive and so long-lasting that $25 can buy a four-day high.

From Crack to Crank

The biggest difference between crack and crank, experts say, is the constituency: Crank users are mainly white and come from rural or suburban areas.

And crank appears to be popular among women in unheard-of proportions.

At a recent regional conference on methamphetamine held in San Francisco, researchers from the National Institute of Justice, a Federal research center, reported that crank users in their 20's were likelier to be women than men. In eight Western cities, they said, methamphetamine was found more often in bloodstreams of women than in men who had been arrested, and women were likelier to use it than any other drug.

The statistics are still preliminary, researchers say, and it's not yet established why women are especially drawn to it. Popularized by bikers and truckers as long ago as the 1950's and nicknamed crank because it was often hidden in their crankcases, it was also once known as "blue-collar cocaine." Later it became popular among gay men.

But now, said Gen. Barry McCaffrey, director of drug policy for the Clinton Administration, "women are testing positive at a higher rate than men, and that's the first time we've seen that on any drug.

"There may be a piece of it related to weight loss," he said, and "a piece of it related to enabling prostitution—it's a drug that allows you to deal with your feelings of remorse."

The spread of methamphetamines also fits into a broader picture of rising drug use among women, he said. Last summer the National Center on Addiction and Substance Abuse at Columbia University issued a report showing that 3.1 million American women regularly used illegal drugs, that 40 percent of crack addicts were women and that among teen-agers, girls and boys were equally likely to have used drugs.

Mr. McCaffrey said he found the spread of methamphetamines among women especially scary because crank users, like crack users, are prone to violence and child abuse. It is, he said, one of the few things "powerful enough to shatter a mother's love for her child."

Speaking at the San Francisco conference, Senator Dianne Feinstein of California noted that in one Sacramento hospital, there are now more babies addicted to methamphetamines than to crack.

Spokane, a regional center of 400,000 on the sparsely settled eastern edge of Washington state, typifies the kind of territory where methamphetamine use is increasing rapidly. Barb Richey, an outreach worker who helps mainly pregnant women on drugs, said that many women have gotten hooked on crank—which can be smoked, injected or snorted—as a weight-loss drug. Of the 335 pregnant women she has helped get into drug treatment since November of 1995, she said, about 40 percent of them were on crank.

"Eight years ago I thought injectable cocaine was the worst drug in the world," said Lynn Everson, who staffs a needle exchange program in Spokane. "Six years ago I thought crack was the worst and now I think it's crank."

Joy said the drug is readily available at bars or through small groups of casual friends. Users don't often have to deal with violent gangs to get it, because small-time manufacturers and distributors abound.

That is part of its appeal to women and other users, said Thomas Constantine, head of the Federal Drug Enforcement Agency, in an interview at the San Francisco conference. "It can be bought in rural and suburban areas, without venturing into a high-crime area," he said.

The prevalence of women on crank also seems to hark back to old patterns. Women, who suffer disproportionately from anxiety and depression, have long been prone to abusing prescription tranquilizers, anti-depressants and weight loss pills, researchers say. The only difference is that crank, which delivers a much more potent and long-lasting high, is illegal.

Mother's Little Helper

Crank "is kind of a drug of the times in that it's a drug for people who don't have enough time," said Michael Gorman, a University of Washington researcher running a study of methamphetamine use in Seattle. "You have the sense that it's moms trying to juggle jobs and three kids and day care, and women working as waitresses on their feet for 12 hours a day. And it's truck drivers, carpet layers, people who work long hours doing tedious, repetitive tasks."

Dr. Gorman's research has focused mainly on crank's prevalence among gay men who sometimes use it to enhance sex. But he said it was clear that among women, the weight-loss component of crank was also very strong. In Hawaii, where "ice"— a smokeable form of methamphetamine—has been in wide use since the late 1980's, doctors and the police have become much more familiar than their mainland colleagues with its effects on users, and have noticed a peculiar difference between the sexes.

Dr. Tom Leland, a psychiatrist at Queens Hospital in Honolulu, said one can often tell where ice is being smoked, because the woman in the house will be a compulsive cleaner, and the place will be spick-and-span. The man, meanwhile, will have become what police officers call a "tweaker," overcome with a manic urge to take things apart, and so car and machine parts will often be scattered on an immaculate lawn.

That urge to clean is what Joy, a 36-year-old janitorial supervisor, experienced in her Spokane home, where she tended her tiny garden and cleaned compulsively.

"Things got done," she said. "It's not like cocaine where you use it and automatically you're out looking for more."

For days at a time, she said, she would be gloriously numb, able to forget all her troubles. But whenever she would stop using it, she would be forced to face "the wreckage of the last 15 or 17 days."

Joy, who weighed 130 pounds on crank, is now at 200 pounds and struggling toward recovery, thankful she was never arrested and trying to win custody of her son from her mother.

But she knows she is fighting the odds: "They say that with crank, there's such a high rate of recidivism they just about write you off," she said.

Violence in Women's Lives

Violence in women's lives can take many forms. It can be images of violence in the media; it can be the fear of being out late at night; or it can be fear at home because of a violent partner. Violence can also take the form of culturally accepted rituals that involve violence. Whatever the form, most women report some experience with violence and take as a necessary part of life the need to deal with it.

In this section we have tried to highlight some of the most pressing issues facing women today. It is important to recognize that there are other forms of violence that we have not been able to touch on, particularly the issue of violence in relationships between teenagers.

As the world is made smaller, through travel and technology, we become aware of cultural practices that are violent and yet are clung to. One of these is female genital mutilation or clitoridectomy. In "Female Genital Mutilation," Layli Bashir discusses how health care providers should respond when encountering patients who have been mutilated or who practice mutilation. How are tolerance and respect for cultural differences balanced with our concept of the ethical practice of medicine? Can a violent practice ever be justified by cultural norms?

Violence within a relationship does not begin overnight. Violence can be seen at all stages of a relationship and can take many forms. In "Dangerous Men," Gavin De Becker examines the warning signs of men who may be potential stalkers. Although focused on the dating relationship, many of the behaviors he describes are also those of a partner who will batter. Yet many women accept these controlling behaviors because of a conditioning "not to make waves."

Rosemary Black notes that somewhere in the world a woman is battered every 9 seconds. Recent research has found that a woman who is killed in New York is more likely to be killed by her partner than by a stranger. Often the woman is trying to leave the relationship at the time of her death. The articles, "Domestic Violence: Why It's Every Woman's Issue" and "A Woman's Killer Is Likely to Be Her Partner," both touch on the fact that women are more at risk from a family member or partner than from a stranger. Yet as Black notes, many women find it hard to get help due to the fact that domestic violence has been hidden "behind closed doors." She encourages us to bring the discussion into the open.

Trying to leave a battering relationship can be dangerous. Pam Belluck reports that in the New York City data examined, many of the women who were killed by a partner were in the process of ending the abusive relationship at the time of their death. One of the significant findings of this study was the aggressive nature of the killings wherein the killers expressed a high level of anger.

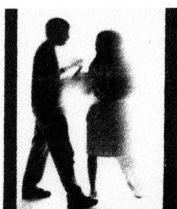 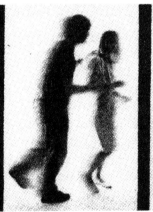

While many abusers say they love their victim, the extreme nature of these killings speaks to the need for power and control that overwhelms the relationship.

The article "I Was Raped," by Lori Robinson, also addresses the role of power and aggression in relationships. In her examination of a rape that divided two colleges and revived her own memories of rape, the author touches upon all the issues of acquaintance rape. According to the Centers for Disease Control, 15–25 percent of male college students admit to involvement in some form of sexual aggression, and 80 percent of rapes on college campuses are committed by someone known to the victim. By addressing the issues of responsibility, alcohol use, racism, and institutional attitudes, the author raises as many issues as she resolves.

Looking Ahead: Challenge Questions

Female genital mutilation is justified by its practitioners as a cultural tradition. How do tradition and health collide when people emigrate to a new country?

What can be done to make the issue of violence against women more easily discussed?

Victims of rape are often told that they brought it upon themselves through their dress or behavior. Do you think this is ever true? Why or why not?

Many cultural images show violence against women. Do you think that these images promote or cause actual violence?

A groups' history often helps to form its views on issues such as violence. How does the history of African Americans in the United States help to shape their view on aggression against African American women?

What is the role of health care providers in responding to and preventing violence against women?

Lex et Feminae

Female Genital Mutilation: Balancing Intolerance of the Practice with Tolerance of Culture

LAYLI MILLER BASHIR, J.D., M.A.*

Female genital mutilation (FGM)** is a cultural rite of passage performed in many African and some Asian countries[1] on an estimated 114 million girls and women. Typically performed under unclean ritual circumstances and without anesthetic, FGM often causes serious medical complications, pain, and sometimes death.

Recently, the influx of immigrants from countries where FGM is performed has caused the practice to gain increased attention in the United States. This is reflected in the recent media spotlight given to women requesting asylum in the United States in order to avoid the ritual and women requesting that FGM be performed on their daughters at American hospitals.[2] The World Health Organization (WHO) declared in 1994 that, because of recent immigration patterns, FGM has become a public health issue in the United States.[3] In addition, the Centers for Disease Control and Prevention estimated that in 1996 more than 150,000 women and girls in the United States were at risk of genital mutilation.[4]

The growing presence of FGM has placed the medical community—particularly women's health practitioners—in the middle of this cultural, ethical, and now, legal dilemma. Last fall, Congress passed a law making FGM a felony,[5] following similar action in several states. In addition, medical associations recently have spoken out against the practice. Practitioners should be aware of their legal liabilities and ethical responsibilities in this area, as well as the cultural circumstances that surround this practice.

WHAT IS FGM?

FGM has several forms, which may vary in severity but always result in permanent damage to the clitoris. Nahid Toubia, M.D., a Sudanese physician at the Columbia University School of Public Health, advanced a system of classification that groups the most common forms of FGM into two broad categories: clitoridectomies and infibulations.[6] Type I clitoridectomy (Sunna circumcision) is the least severe form of FGM and involves the partial or complete removal of the clitoris. Type II clitoridectomy (excision) involves the excision of

---

*Ms. Bashir received her Juris Doctor from the Washington College of Law at American University and her Masters degree in International Relations from American University in 1996. She currently works at the United States Department of Justice, Board of Immigration Appeals. The opinions expressed in this column are solely those of the author and are not intended to represent those of her employer.

**There is a controversy over the terms used to refer to this practice. Some feel that the description of the ritual as mutilation is offensive and insulting, while others argue that the use of the term "female circumcision" evokes improper comparison to male circumcision. I follow the usage of the Inter-African Committee, which voted that "female circumcision" did not accurately reflect the ritual practice and decided that it should be referred to as "female genital mutilation" (Marilyn Milos, NOCIRC Newsletter, Fall 1993 at 2). I must note, however, that I feel that no suitable term for this ritual practice has been identified.

the clitoris and part of the labia minora. In a type III infibulation (modified infibulation), the clitoris, labia minora, and parts of the labia majora are removed, and the anterior two-thirds of the labia majora are sutured together, leaving a posterior opening. Type IV infibulation (total infibulation), the most severe form of FGM, involves the same amount of cutting as a type III, but the labia majora are sutured together to cover the urethra and the vagina, leaving a very small opening for the passage of urine and menstrual blood.

FGM frequently causes serious and prolonged physical complications. In a 1993 Kenyan study, more than 80% of women reported at least one medical complication after undergoing FGM.[7] Other reports estimate that between 15% and 30% of all girls and women who endure FGM die from bleeding or infection.[8] Serious early adverse effects include severe pain and vaginal hemorrhage, which sometimes may lead to shock and death. Other effects include wound infections, abscesses, ulcers, septicemia, tetanus, and gangrene. A serious long-term consequence of FGM is hematocolpos, which may lead to chronic pelvic infections, back pain, dysmenorrhea, infertility, and urinary tract infections. The most common long-term complication is the formation of painful dermoid cysts and keloid scarring. Childbirth creates additional risks, particularly among immigrants in the United States, as most American obstetricians have not been trained to deal with infibulated women.[9] If an infibulated woman is not properly cared for during childbirth, complications, including perineal tears, vesicovaginal fistula, and even fetal death, may result.

The rationale behind FGM is a matrix of superstitions, perceptions of gender roles, beliefs regarding health, and religious customs. The most frequently cited reason for the continuation of FGM, however, is that it is perceived to preserve virginity, prevent promiscuity, and, consequently, preserve family honor. Parents who insist on this ritual for their daughters frequently state that if the ritual was not performed, their daughters would be perceived as immoral, would be unable to find a husband, and would be ostracized by the community.

LEGAL AND ETHICAL OBLIGATIONS

In September 1996, Congress passed a law that makes FGM a felony punishable by up to 5 years in prison.[5] The bill authorizes the prosecution of anyone who "circumcises, excises, or infibulates the whole or any part of the labia majora or labia minora or clitoris of another person who has not attained the age of 18." The law punishes both the parents who arrange for their daughters to be cut and those who perform the procedure.

Th[e] new federal law also seeks to prevent FGM through a process of education and cultural sensitivity. It requires the Secretary of the Department of Health and Human Services to identify ethnic communities in the United States that practice FGM and to engage in outreach activities to educate these communities on the physical and psychologic effects of FGM. These activities must be "designed and implemented in collaboration with representatives of the ethnic groups practicing such mutilation." The law also requires the Secretary to develop recommendations for the education of medical students regarding FGM. The federal law will go into effect on March 30, 1997.

In the past 2 years, numerous states have passed laws that criminalize FGM. Such states include California, Minnesota, Tennessee, Rhode Island, and North Dakota. South Carolina and Colorado are currently considering similar laws.

In addition to criminal penalties for performing FGM, medical practitioners also must be cognizant of ethical statements on the practice, recently developed by national and international medical organizations. The WHO has declared it unethical for a physician to perform FGM.[9] In 1994, the International Federation of Gynecology and Obstetrics passed a resolution that calls on all doctors to refuse to perform FGM.[10] In addition, the American Medical Association (AMA), in Policy 525.987(A-91), pronounced that it "opposes all forms of medically unnecessary surgical modification of female genitalia."[11] The AMA recommends that "[p]hy-sicians who are requested to perform female genital mutilation on a patient provide culturally sensitive counseling to educate the patient and her family members about the negative health consequences of the procedure, trying to discourage them from proceeding. If possible, physicians should refer the patient to social support groups that can help them cope with changing societal mores."

THE REAL SOLUTION

Criminalization of FGM is one step toward its eradication and may assist in fostering an environment in the United States that is clearly intolerant to FGM. The example of other Western nations that have criminalized FGM, however, demonstrates the inadequacy of merely making it illegal.[12] In Britain, for example, FGM has been a crime for more than 11 years, and despite this, there have been no convictions, and the rate of the mutilation of immigrant girls is reportedly on the rise.

While criminalization will assist in deterring the practice, the medical community can play a prominent role in protecting young girls and women from FGM by educating its members about the anatomic and psychological effects of FGM. The psychological and emotional side effects of FGM are particularly important to understand. A failure to appreciate the loss of dignity an FGM victim often feels when going to the doctor, let alone undergoing a pelvic examination, may contribute to poor patient attendance at prenatal care obstetrics services, or for routine physical exams.

When faced with a request to perform FGM, the practitioner must balance the legal and ethical obligation to emphatically refuse to perform the ritual with a sensitivity for the family's perspective. A reaction of anger or disgust will likely embarrass or alienate the patient and her family, and jeopardize the physician/patient relationship. The health care professional, in this situation, should explain to the patient and her family the serious dangers to the life, health, and well-being of a victim of FGM. Also, the practitioner should inform the patient and family that the practice is a crime in the United States.

Health care professionals should understand that many immigrants are surprised by what they perceive to be the flagrant sexual behavior of American youth and an apparent moral decay of our society. They are genuinely and seriously concerned that having moved into a culture where their values of virginity and chastity are in the minority, their children may fall victim to American immorality. To some families, FGM may be seen as even more important once in the United States in order to safeguard their family honor and culture against the contrasting tendencies of American society.

Although the criminalization of FGM may intimidate those who want to have the ritual performed on their daughters, health care professionals can have the greatest impact by understanding the root causes of FGM and, through culturally sensitive education and counseling, communicating its dangers to patients and their families. Health care professionals can help convey to a family requesting that their daughter undergo the ritual that, although the family's values are legitimate and their concerns are understandable, a girl or a woman has the ability to make rational decisions regarding sexuality and, if she shares her family's values, will be able to remain chaste and uphold her family's honor with her clitoris intact.

ACKNOWLEDGMENT

I am grateful for the invaluable assistance of R. Martin Bashir, M.D., in the preparation of this column.

REFERENCES

1. According to the World Health Organization, over 30 African countries and Muslim populations in Indonesia, Malaysia, India, Pakistan, Oman, South Yemen, and the United Arab Emirates practice FGM.
2. See, e.g., Ostrom CM. Doctors at Seattle hospitals consider circumcising Muslim girls. Seattle Times, September 29, 1996 (describing the dilemma of Seattle doctors at Harborview Medical Center faced with requests to perform FGM on Somali girls); Dugger C. Women's plea for asylum puts tribal ritual on trial, New York Times, April 15, 1996 (discussing the case of Fauziya Kasinga who fled from Togo to escape FGM and requested asylum in the United States).

3. UN calls for end to female genital mutilation. Chicago Tribune, May 5, 1994.
4. Dugger CV. Tug of taboos: African genital rite vs. American law. New York Times, December 28, 1996.
5. Federal prohibition of female genital mutilation act of 1996, Pub. L. 104-140, 110 Stat 1327 (1996).
6. Toubia N. Female circumcision as a public health issue. N Engl J Med 1994;331:712.
7. Okie S. Female circumcision persists: Tribal rite worries Kenyan health officials. Washington Post, April 13, 1993.
8. H. Lightfoot-Klein H. Pharaonic circumcision of females in the Sudan. Med Law 1983;2:353. (estimating that one-third of all Sudanese FGM victims die); Mann J. Torturing girls is not a cultural right. Washington Post, February 23, 1994 (quoting Rosemary Mburu, a Kenyan gynecologist, who estimates that 15% of all circumcised females die of bleeding or infections).
9. Female circumcision: state of World Health Organization position and activities. Submitted to the UN sub-commission on the prevention of discrimination and protection of minorities (Press Release WHO/10, June 1982).
10. Adolph C. Doctors must become advocates for women, conference is told. The Gazette (Montreal), October 1, 1994.
11. Report of the Council on Scientific Affairs. CSA Report 5-I-94, 1994.
12. For a broader discussion of European legislation against FGM and its effectiveness, see Bashir LM. Female genital mutilation in the United States: an examination of criminal and asylum law. Am UJ Gender L. 1996;4:415, 433.

Address correspondence to:
Lynn Sargent Berner, J.D., M.P.H.
Editor of Lex et Feminae
The Cleveland Clinic Foundation
9500 Euclid Avenue-KK53
Cleveland, OH 44195

Domestic Violence: Why It's Every Woman's Issue . . . and What *You* Can Do

ROSEMARY BLACK

When Lisa Luciano was killed by her estranged husband, Marco, in front of their two children last year, her family was devastated, but not surprised. It wasn't the

first time Marco had acted violently toward Lisa, a 27-year-old computer programming student.

For several years, Marco, 33, had stalked his wife and abused her in front of their children. He was arrested twice for violating orders of protection and attacking her. Each time he pleaded guilty to harassment, a violation that carried a maximum 15-day jail term. He sidestepped a serious prison sentence, only to attack her again.

On March 13, 1996, Marco went to the Woodside, NY, apartment house where Lisa lived with Melissa, 5, and Marco, Jr., 9. When she returned from class at about 4 p.m. and saw Marco outside, Lisa called her brother Willie and asked him to come over. After Willie arrived, though, Marco managed to get into the apartment. According to police, he turned on Willie, slashing him in the legs, then stabbed Lisa repeatedly with a kitchen knife when she came to her brother's defense. Marco was arraigned on a murder charge, and at press time he was awaiting trial.

Each year more than 1,400 American women die at the hands of an abusive partner, according to the U.S. Department of Justice. On average a woman is battered every nine seconds. But even if we aren't among the victims, it's likely that we are silent witnesses. In a 1995 poll conducted for the San Francisco–based Family Violence Prevention Fund, more than one-third of those surveyed said they know someone who is a victim of domestic violence. And many more of us may suspect a friend, neighbor or coworker is in such a situation.

Thanks to the Violence Against Women Act signed by President Clinton in 1994, more funds than ever before are available to help victims escape batterers and rebuild

DOMESTIC VIOLENCE AND THE DOCTOR'S OFFICE

An American Medical Association poll found that a woman would rather discuss domestic violence with her doctor than with the police, a pastor or rabbi, or a lawyer. Yet health professionals are often ill equipped to diagnose and treat domestic violence. The next time you visit your doctor, ask if she's aware of the AMA's guidelines for treating domestic violence. "Our goal is to have every physician ask every patient at every visit a question such as 'Are you in a safe relationship?'" says John C. Nelson, M.D., an AMA trustee in Salt Lake City. Suggest your doctor do this. Also urge her to do the following:

◆ Put a domestic violence awareness poster in the waiting room.
◆ Include questions about abuse on all medical history questionnaires.
◆ Develop a list of specialists who provide low-cost care for abuse victims (for example, a plastic surgeon who treats facial wounds).
◆ Call the Health Resource Center on Domestic Violence (888-RX-ABUSE), an information line for physicians run by the Family Violence Prevention Fund in San Francisco.

shattered lives. But money alone can't buy safety. All of us must fight to end domestic violence. Getting involved not only saves lives today, but can also prevent our sons from growing up to be batterers and our daughters from becoming victims. Here's how you can help stop the violence.

In Your Own Backyard **Know the warning signs.** Domestic violence knows no racial, ethnic or socioeconomic boundaries. Someone you know may be a victim if she has frequent unexplained physical injuries; if she or her child is often withdrawn or upset; or if she often cancels plans at the last minute without saying why, or seems afraid of making her partner angry, according to Joan Sculli, director of education and community services at the Nassau County Coalition against Domestic Violence in New York.

Help a friend open up. If you suspect that someone you know is facing violence, question her gently and in private. Sculli suggests opening the conversation like this: "I'm concerned because you don't look like yourself and I noticed a bruise on your face. I've been hearing a lot about domestic violence and wondered if you might be a victim." At first she may be afraid to talk, so ask again a few days later.

If she tells you she is being abused, listen without judging. A battered woman often believes her abuser's negative comments about her, says Marissa Ghez, associate director of the Family Violence Prevention Fund. She may fear that you too will judge her. Let her know that you know the abuse isn't her fault. Tell her that she can choose whether to leave the relationship. Emphasize that domestic violence tends to become more frequent and severe over time. Provide her with the number of a local domestic violence hot line. (For information on groups to contact, see "Keeping Women Safe and Sound.")

Give her shelter. Encourage your friend to find a safe place to stay (your home, perhaps) for future use. She should have her own key to her safe place and should store money, copies of important documents, prescription medication and a change of clothes there in case she and her children must flee.

Encourage an abuser to talk. If you suspect a man of abusing his partner, don't confront him directly—doing so could be dangerous, says Sculli. Instead ask him how the relationship is going and whether he and his wife are having problems. This might lead to a conversation about violence. If he admits to using controlling tactics, let him know that what he's doing is wrong and make sure he knows that hitting his wife or girlfriend is a crime that could land him in jail. Ask a local shelter about programs in your community that work with batterers, and tell him that help is available.

Take it to the streets. If you see or hear an assault in progress, call the police. If you witness an attack while in your car, Ghez suggests that you stop and honk your horn repeatedly until a crowd forms and police arrive.

In Your Own Home **Teach your children well.** Model the behavior you want your children to learn, advises Diana Barnett, director of the Coalition on Child Abuse and Neglect in Hempstead, NY. "Tell them that problems aren't solved with their fists." Adds Sculli, "Avoid the use of physical discipline, because if you are bigger and stronger, it's okay to hit." Tell your son that it's never okay to hit a girl and that it's a crime for a man to strike his partner.

In Your Community **Volunteer.** Hospitals, courts and shelters all need your help. Volunteers at battered women's shelters give clients emotional support, help them find housing or legal services, even provide child care. Hospital or court advocates act as liaisons between battered women and law enforcement officers or medical personnel. These programs generally require hours of training, but the work is tremendously rewarding, notes Sculli.

Raise money. Call local groups to find out where fund-raising services are needed. You could sell tickets for a banquet, make telephone calls to solicit contributions or help run an event to benefit a local shelter.

Raise consciousness. Invite community leaders to speak against domestic abuse in schools. Ask your PTA to sponsor speakers who will discuss safe dating. Re-

---

Keeping Women Safe and Sound

- **Family Violence Prevention Fund,** 383 Rhode Island St., Suite 304, San Francisco, CA, 94103-5133; 800-END-ABUSE. Call or write for a free kit detailing ways to help stop domestic violence.

- **National Domestic Violence hot line,** 800-799-SAFE. Staffers can put you in touch with domestic violence programs in your area.

- **Silent Witness National Initiative,** 1319 Riverside Dr. N., Hudson, WI 54016. Contact director Jane Zeller to learn about the exhibit and march on Washington.

- **National Organization for Victim Assistance,** in Washington, 202-232-6682, provides referrals to crime victim assistance programs nationwide.

- **Childhelp/IOF,** 800-4-A-CHILD, provides 24-hour child abuse crisis counseling for kids and adults.

quest that your pastor or rabbi make domestic violence the subject of a sermon. Make sure that places in your community where women spend time—gyms, libraries—have information posted about domestic violence. Post literature in rest rooms so women can read it in private.

Assess community support systems. Call your local police department to find out if officers have been trained to respond appropriately to domestic violence calls. At work, ask your benefits manager if your company's employee assistance program includes domestic violence services; also inquire into whether security guards have been trained to shield women who may be stalked on the job. Request that your employer donate money and allow employees time off to volunteer.

On Capitol Hill
Be a newshound. Watch the news for information on the Battered Women's Employment Protection Act. This law would extend family and medical leave protection to women affected by domestic violence. It would also provide unemployment benefits to women who are fired or must quit their jobs because of domestic violence.

Write letters. Be on the lookout for portrayals of violence against women in music, television, movies and video games. Contact manufacturers of offensive products to urge them to develop a policy on violence against women. Ask filmmakers to put an NC-17 rating on movies that show a woman being beaten or killed. Also send a letter to every insurance company you deal with, urging policymakers to avoid discrimination against battered women. Some women are denied coverage; others are charged higher premiums for insurance when medical records indicate a history of abuse. (To their credit, some insurers have responded to public criticism and are working to improve policies.)

March on Washington. The silent Witness is a traveling exhibit begun as a memorial to women murdered in Minnesota in 1990 in acts of domestic violence; it has since expanded to 41 other states. (For information, see "Keeping Women Safe and Sound.") A national march in Washington is planned for October [1997]. Be there to show your support.

Rosemary Black is an editor at the New York Daily News.

A Woman's Killer Is Likely to Be Her Partner, a New Study in New York Finds

PAM BELLUCK

More women in New York City are killed by their husbands or boyfriends than in robberies, disputes, sexual assaults, drug violence, random attacks or any other crime in cases where the relationship between the murderer and victim is known.

That conclusion, long suspected by family violence and criminal justice experts, has been confirmed by a study of every woman killed in New York City over five years, one of the first studies of its kind in the country.

To piece together a portrait of these women, researchers from the New York City Department of Health spent nine months teasing clues out of the documents that are the residue of murder: autopsy findings, crime scene reports, witness statements, toxicological and sexual assault tests, ballistics reports, and descriptions of stab wounds and strangulation marks.

For a study that has yet to be released, researchers looked at files on each of the 1,156 women age 16 and over killed in New York City from 1990 through 1994. In only 484 murders could investigators determine the killer's relationship to the victim—friend, stranger, acquaintance or relative. From that narrower pool, researchers learned that nearly half of the women were killed by current or former husbands or boyfriends, a much higher proportion than expected. Nationally, the figure is 40 percent, compared with 6 percent of men who were killed by wives or girlfriends.

The portrait derived from the homicide files is telling in its details of how the women lived and graphic in the specifics of how they died.

More than half the women killed in the city during those years died in private homes, usually their own. In the majority of the cases in which the killer was identified, the murderers were people they knew.

When they were killed by their husbands, one-third of the time the women appeared to be trying to end the relationships. In one-quarter of the cases where husbands or boyfriends were the killers, children were also killed or injured, or they watched the murders or found their mothers' bodies.

And, unlike men, who are killed most often by guns, women "are very likely to be punched and hit and burned and thrown out of windows," said the leader of the study, Dr. Susan A. Wilt, the director of epidemiology and surveillance for the Health Department's injury and prevention program. "We were surprised by the degree to which some of these murders just spoke of enormous rage. Some women were stabbed and also strangled," she said.

"What's very clear is that female homicides are so different from male homicides," Dr. Wilt added, noting that her research staff attended monthly support group sessions and deliberately avoided looking at gruesome autopsy photographs.

Understanding the women's deaths, city health officials say, will help map a plan for hospitals, law enforcement officials, clinics and community organizations to identify and protect women at risk.

The study also provides concrete information at a time when domestic violence policy is a heated issue, with victims' advocates pressuring city and state officials for more help for battered women and more serious penalties for their batterers.

Dr. Margaret A. Hamburg, the New York City Health Commissioner, said the study showed a need for different strategies to protect women. "On-the-street police strength is not effective when the majority of women are killed in an individual's home," Dr. Hamburg said. "Health care providers should be trying to identify women who are at risk for domestic violence because often women do have early contact with the medical system. And we need to reexamine laws that apply to domestic violence."

Two-thirds of the domestic violence killings were in the poorest boroughs, the Bronx and Brooklyn, and three-quarters of the women killed by husbands and boyfriends were black or Hispanic. These findings run counter to the public impression that "domestic violence knows no class and color boundaries," said Dr. Jeff Fagan, director of the Center for Violence, Research and Prevention at Columbia University's School of Public Health.

"The myth of classlessness of domestic violence is one that has persisted since the 1960's," Dr. Fagan said. "The truth is, it is a problem of poverty, associated with other characteristics like low marriage rates, high unemployment and social problems. Whatever we've done to prevent domestic violence has been more effective for white women and we have to figure out how to make it apply to poor women in poor areas."

Also surprising was that in nearly one-third of the cases where husbands and boyfriends killed women, the men also tried to kill themselves.

"Now, when a man comes into a psych clinic and acts like he's suicidal, we should know to screen him to see if he has a family and what kind of relationship it is," Dr. Wilt said. "And women who come into an emergency room because they get hurt by their intimate partners should be aware of the risk to children in the house."

The fact that one-third of the women killed by their husbands were not living with them suggested to Dr. Wilt that these women were trying to leave the relationships.

Overall, many fewer women are killed than men—during the five years in the study, the proportion was nearly seven to one. As total crime decreased in those years, murders of women decreased also, but not as sharply as those of men. At the same time, the number of domestic violence murders increased slightly.

Public health officials worry that the incidence of domestic violence has not dropped as precipitously as the overall crime rate in the past few years. And they are finding that domestic violence rates are not responding to the most common types of crime fighting techniques.

Vivid stories sprang out of the files and forms and documents used in the study.

A 35-year-old woman in Brooklyn was stabbed 12 times with a hunting knife and bludgeoned with a baseball bat by her boyfriend in a case described as "very typical" by Dr. Wilt, who said confidentiality concerns kept her from proving names or identifying details of the victims. The Brooklyn woman's boyfriend killed her on a night he had come home drinking and accused her of having an affair. He also stabbed the woman's sister, who survived.

In another typical domestic violence case, Dr. Wilt said, a 28-year-old woman in the Bronx was killed by her live-in boyfriend after they argued about her leaving him. Neighbors said the boyfriend had abused the woman before and that there was a protection order barring him from seeing her. The boyfriend hit the woman in the face, shot her with a .38 caliber handgun and then shot himself in the head. When the police arrived,

they found two children, 5 and 7, in the home with the bodies.

The researchers also looked, of course, at the highly publicized murder cases of those five years, but said that many of them were not typical. Those included the deaths of 87 clubgoers (31 women, 56 men) in the Happy Land Social Club in the Bronx in 1990, which was set on fire by the ex-boyfriend of an employee. And the 1993 murder of Danielle Almonor, a Federal probation officer shot in the back of her head by her estranged husband at the Brooklyn Family Courthouse while she was waiting for their case to be called.

Other unusual cases were the deaths of a woman whose doctor was accused of malpractice and a 16-year-old girl who died of AIDS after being infected through childhood sexual abuse.

Of the 1,156 women killed in New York over the five-year period, more than half were black, even though only one-quarter of the city's female population is black. Sixteen percent of the victims were white, although they make up nearly half the city's female population. And 29 percent of the victims were Hispanic, about the same as their proportion of all women in the city.

Black women were likely to be younger, in their 20's or 30's, and to live in poorer neighborhoods. White women were likely to be older (nearly half were over 50).

Almost one-third of all the murders of women were in the Bronx, even though only 16 percent of the city's women live in there.

Sixty-eight women were killed by their children, grandchildren or other family members who were not husbands or boyfriends. Those murders tended to be more brutal than "intimate partner" murders and other killings because women were more likely to be stabbed—and stabbed more than 10 times.

Domestic violence victims were much less likely to be using cocaine, marijuana or other illegal drugs than other women who were killed. But they were just as likely to be drinking. Dr. Gelles said if a woman in a troubled relationship used alcohol to help her cope, she would be "less able to perceive a threat, more vulnerable to a lethal assault."

Still to be studied, Dr. Wilt said, was whether these victims had sought help from hospitals, the police or other places.

THE TALLY

A Demographic Portrait

Of 8,932 victims of homicide in New York City from 1990 to 1994, 1,156, or 13 percent, were female. Some predominant characteristics:

Most female victims were black ...

Black	52%
Hispanic	29
White	16
Other	3

... and 21 to 40 years old.

21–40	58%
Other	42

Nearly half were killed by an "intimate partner"* ...

An intimate partner was almost always a current or former husband or boyfriend.

Intimate partner	49%
Stranger	17
Acquaintance	15
Relative	14
Other	6

*For the 484 homicides for which the relationship between the victim and the assailant could be identified.

... and in their homes.

Home	50%
Public place	37
Other home	10
Unknown	3

Percentages may not add up to 100 because of rounding.

Source: City Department of Health

"We're very interested to know," she said, "if women didn't avail themselves of the system, or if the system doesn't work, or if the system can't save them at all."

"I Was Raped"

A survivor explores an accusation that has divided the Spelman and Morehouse family

LORI S. ROBINSON

A BRISK NOVEMBER WIND GREETED ME when I returned to Spelman College last year. Fall in Atlanta was cooler than what I remembered as a freshman at the historically Black, all-women's school. But that was a decade ago, and much more than the weather had changed. A three-story parking deck sat on what was an asphalt lot in my day. The tiny Guest House near the entrance of the small, fenced campus was gone, replaced by the year-old Camille Olivia Hanks Cosby Academic Center, an elegant five-story building with a museum and auditorium. Even Johnnetta Cole, affectionately known as Sister President, had announced her resignation after 10 years.

Still, as I strolled past the new guard booth, I easily slipped back into the campus' comforting energy. College anywhere is a special time. I was blessed that my time was spent at Spelman, where people didn't assume they were smarter or better than me because of the color of my skin. All around me that November day, young women raced in and out of red brick buildings and cut across lush green grass with confident strides. Spelman strides. I was home again.

And my heart was crumbling because of what had brought me back. I was home to write about rape.

For nearly a month, Spelman and its brother school, Morehouse College, had been in an uproar over a freshman student's accusation that four Morehouse men had sexually assaulted her in a Morehouse dorm late one Friday night. The two schools are educational meccas for the Black middle class and share a special relationship. They are next to each other, and Morehouse men and Spelman women often marry. But in the weeks before my return, the schools had been rocked as rape allegations garnered newspaper headlines and were reported on local television newscasts, packed courtrooms and seriously strained their bond.

There was irony in my returning for the case. In May of 1995, I was supposed to attend my five-year reunion at Spelman. I didn't make it. That was the week that I was raped. In my Washington, D.C., apartment. On my bed. By two men with a gun who accosted me on my doorstep. I was 26 and forever changed.

More than a year later, when I suggested during an *Emerge* staff meeting that we write about rape, I had no idea that in a matter of weeks I would be back in Atlanta. I had mentioned the Spelman–Morehouse case as another example of how serious and complicated the issue is for African–American communities. When senior editors called me back for a private meeting to ask if I would return to Spelman to write the story, I hesitated. They knew about my rape, but there were many issues to consider. Could I write fairly? Could I handle it emotionally? Would it be safe for me? After all, my attackers had never been caught, and *Emerge*'s offices are not far from my old apartment. My editors assured me they would respect whatever I decided.

I thought about those issues during the next few days, but what I thought about most was whether I wanted people to know. My family, my close friends and a few of my colleagues knew I had been attacked, but that was all. Was I ready to give them — and countless strangers — the whole story? Was I ready to write it down in black and white for them the way it had been written in memory for me?

SPELMAN and its brother school, Morehouse College, had been in an uproar over a freshman student's accusation that four Morehouse men had sexually assaulted her.

. I was at my desk when the phone rang. Pamela Crockett, an Alexandria, Va., lawyer and rape activist I had been trying to reach for weeks, was on the other end. Shortly after my attack, I had thrown myself head on into healing. Part of the medicine is keeping in contact with women who work on this issue. She and

From *Emerge: Black America's Newsmagazine*, May 1997, pp. 42-53. © 1997 by Emerge Communications, Inc. Reprinted by permission.

I had met when we both spoke to high school girls about careers. In her opening comments, Pamela had mentioned sexual assault as an important issue, and we both noticed how the girls had responded with a keen interest.

I told Pamela what I was considering. In the past we had talked about the silences and the shame in our communities. How Black women are raped at the same rate as White women but are less likely to report it. How we debate the issue when "heroes" such as Mike Tyson are the accused, but never seem able to find our voices when the victim is our mother, or our daughter, or our sister, our niece, or ourselves. I am still amazed at how many women have a story to tell, either about themselves or someone they know.

I went over my concerns with her about doing a story — not only about Spelman and Morehouse, but about me. Finally, Pamela said simply, "I would do it if I were you."

MAY 19, 1995

I T WAS EXHILARATING being on my own. It hadn't been easy living with my parents for two years, saving up money for an apartment. But I had stuck it out and wound up with a comfortable, one-bedroom apartment in Northeast Washington near Catholic University of America. It was a quiet neighborhood and considered relatively safe.

It was my four-month anniversary of independent living, and I was looking forward to attending my college reunion later that week. After visiting friends that Monday night, I drove home a little before 11:30. As I drove, I prayed for inner peace, hoping to quell the ordinary anxieties that left me feeling down from time to time. I believe now that prayer enabled me to get through what was about to become the worst hour of my life.

"Great, a space across the street from my apartment building," I thought as I drove up. Usually, street parking filled up by 8 or 9 p.m., and I would have to park behind the small, two-story apartment building where I lived. It was always too dark and spooky back there for my taste. Pleased at my good fortune, I parked and walked toward my building, thinking about the exercise video I was going to play and the dishes that needed washing.

I jumped slightly when I saw two brothers. "Funny, I didn't notice anybody walking when I parked," I thought once I had crossed the street. Then I reminded myself that I didn't have any reason to be afraid of two men just because they were Black. I didn't give them a second thought. But as I reached my doorstep, one of them jumped up behind me and said something I didn't understand. I turned around to the barrel of a gun pointing at my head. It took me a second to focus. My eyes bulged as I started to look at who was on the other end of the gun.

"You better not look at me," he spat out.

My heart was pounding hard and fast. I felt weak, as if all the wind had left my body. It struck me then that this is what it felt like to have your life threatened. I handed over my purse.

"You can have anything you want," I squeezed out of my burning, deflated lungs.

They ordered me to open the door, but I couldn't get the key to work. That lock always jammed. My hands were shaking. I was talking out loud. "I know it's this key next to the silver one." After several of my futile tries, one of the men said, "It better open this time."

I stopped struggling with the lock and surrendered to God. This time the key turned. They rushed me up the stairs to my apartment. Once inside, they told me to lie on the floor, then they walked around spouting questions.

"Anybody else live here? Anybody else have a key? You supposed to call anybody when you got home?"

They led me to my bedroom, sat me on my bed and continued asking questions about my belongings, reminding me not to talk so loud. "You better not be lying," one said.

Then I was ordered to lie face down on my full-size bed. They tied my feet to the bottom corners of the bed, and my right arm to the upper right corner. When one asked me for something else to use to tie my left hand, I told him where my belts were. Then they wrapped thick duct tape around my head, covering my eyes and mouth.

"Are they doing this so they can shoot me? Maybe they just want to make sure they have plenty of get-away time." My thoughts raced. What was about to happen hadn't occurred to me. Then, with a knife from my kitchen, one of them spliced up the back of the right leg of my black stretch pants. Then it became clear.

"I'm about to be raped."

I never felt so powerless as at that moment. My underwear was snipped at the side and pulled out from under me. Then I heard the sound of a zipper.

One of the rapists climbed on top of me and barked another order.

"Open it up."

He penetrated vaginally for a few seconds, then anally.

The first guy didn't take as long as the second one. He climbed on top of me and started vaginally, too. Then he jammed his penis into my anus. He also talked a lot.

"We're not crazy or nothing.... Does your boyfriend do this to you?"

The time they pounded at me was probably a matter of minutes, but for me, those minutes seemed like hours. Every second I thought I couldn't take any more of the pain.

"Can I come inside you?" he asked several times. Then, as if he had heard me answer through the duct tape across my mouth, he said simply — and pathetically — "Okay, I'll pull out."

The semen poured over my behind.

I remember wondering what it would feel like if they shot me. Maybe a single bullet in the back of my head. I thought about how terrible it would be if I just didn't show up for work for a few days and people came looking for me. They would find me dead, tied to my bed with no underwear. Then I tried not to think about being shot. I tried not to feel any more of the pain and terror that were consuming me. At some point, I simply let go. I realized that I was powerless and helpless. Who I was, the Lori I had known all my life, receded at that moment. All I wanted was for them to leave. All I wanted was to live.

I waited until the apartment was quiet and I was sure they were gone. Ordinarily a hopeless crier, I wasn't crying at all as I worked to untie myself from the bed. I looked at the clock and noticed only an hour had passed since I had parked my car.

All the electronics from my apartment were gone. So was my car. They took the phone cord, so I summoned up the courage and humility to walk down the stairs and knock on my neighbor's door. When I had to face people, that's when I started to cry.

After calling the police, I called my sister and began the long road to healing.

SPELMAN AND MOREHOUSE

ON NOV. 12, I was on USAir Flight 1161 headed south to a place where Black girls are molded into women and sent out to make their mark in the world. I do not know how ready for the world the 17–year–old I met last fall will be when — and if — she graduates from Spelman. If what she says is true, that four Morehouse men raped her and three of them sodomized her, the road to self–realization will be difficult. Thinking about the case reminds me that, in a perverse way, I'm one of the lucky ones. My attackers were armed strangers who forced their way into my home and into my body. No one doubted my story or suggested that the assault was my fault. Statistics show, however, that 60 to 80 percent of rape victims know their attacker. For them, the story is very different.

Except for a brief delay caused by the chaos of the 1996 Summer Olympics, the school year had started off like the others. There was a "freshman week" of activities for all the students in the Atlanta University Center, the six–member college association that includes Spelman and Morehouse. There were special bonding events, such as the annual brother–sister tea for Spelman and Morehouse. Shortly after the semester began, President Cole announced her plans to resign after the academic year. When she took the job in 1987, she promised to stay for 10 years.

She was going out with an incredible record, having exceeded the $81 million capital fund-raising goal by almost $33 million. That, with an endowment of about $143 million, gave Spelman, one of two Black all-women's colleges in the country, one of the richest endowments for a Black college. Who would've guessed that Cole would leave another special mark[?] How many college presidents testify at bond hearings for alleged rape defendants?

When the school year began, the Spelman teenager, who spoke to *Emerge* on condition that her identity not be disclosed, settled into her freshman dorm room with the normal anxieties and excitement of new college students. That summer she had worried about whether she and her roommate would get along, but they hit it off immediately. She was excited about the opportunities college would offer—the new experiences, the new friends. Plus, that September she had celebrated her 17th birthday. She was away from home, away from her sheltered family life and ready to take full advantage of her new independence.

Then late one Friday night, she says, it all changed.

At a hearing on Oct. 30, she told her side of the story. She spoke so softly, court records show, that officials had to repeatedly ask her to speak up. This is her courtroom account:

Somewhere between 9 and 9:30 p.m. on Friday, Sept. 27, the freshman, her roommate and several other friends boarded a shuttle bus to go party at The Casino, a nightclub on Auburn Avenue N.E. Spelman freshmen who live on campus are not allowed to have cars, so piling onto a party–destined bus is virtually a weekend ritual. At The Casino, the young woman said she shared two or three drinks with friends. After a few hours, a male acquaintance — whose name she told the court she does not remember — drove the group to the International House of Pancakes for a late–night meal. That same guy dropped her off at Morehouse's Frank Forbes Hall, where she visited a friend,

"I'M ONE of the lucky ones. My attackers were armed strangers who forced their way into my home and into my body. No one doubted my story...."

Lorenzo McFadden, also a freshman. His roommate and another young woman, whom she didn't know, were also there. The four of them played cards in McFadden's third–floor dorm room, then she and the other woman played "Bust–A–Move," a video game. After McFadden fell asleep, the Spelman freshman left, deciding to walk the short distance to her dorm alone.

At the bottom of Forbes' stairwell, she told the court, she bumped into Herman Lamar Banks, a senior and member of Morehouse's basketball team. They had met briefly before at the Robert W. Woodruff Library, which is shared by the six colleges of the Atlanta University Center. At Forbes, Banks was standing with Darren Peter Marshall and Dadon Kimontte Dodd, both sophomore basketball players. She'd never met either of them, she testified. Banks offered to walk her back to Spelman but asked her to wait in his room for a few minutes because he had to get something from another room. It was about 15 minutes before Morehouse's 2 a.m. curfew for Friday and Saturday nights, which requires all visitors to leave the dorms.

Banks never walked her home.

While waiting in his first-floor room in the same hallway where the resident director resides, the young woman testified that she heard a loud banging at the window. Then it shattered. Banks, the Morehouse basketball team's starting point guard, had broken it from the outside, she said. Why he broke it has never been explained.

She was about to leave when the few guys now gathered in the room urged her to wait in another room while they cleaned up the glass. Then she would be walked home. She decided to visit another friend in Forbes Hall, but he was not in. She left him a note before going to wait in Dodd's room.

The room was empty for five to 10 minutes before Dodd came in, she said. His name, he had told her, was Suave. When he sat on the bed, she stood up. She looked through his CDs, selected one and he put it on his disc player. He noticed her looking at his bottle of rum. He offered her some. She told him she couldn't drink it straight. Then they began to hunt for change to buy Cokes. She went to the vending machines in the lobby to get the sodas. She saw Banks and Marshall near the machines.

THE INCIDENT

WHEN SHE BROUGHT THE DRINKS to Dodd's room, he left to find some glasses. He came back with one and told her they'd have to do shots. The young woman said she didn't do shots. She poured the rum and Coke into the glass and took two sips; Dodd drank the rest. In court testimony, she also would say that she had had a couple of hits off a friend's bottle of Boones Farm wine before arriving at Morehouse.

Victims of Rape/Sexual Assault
Based on surveys of state prisoners

By Sex

Rape victims are...

5.5% Male

94.5% Female

Sexual assault victims are...

15.2% Male

84.8% Female

SOURCE: U.S. DEPARTMENT OF JUSTICE

Relationship to offender	Victims of rape	Sexual assault victims
Family	20.3%	37.7%
Spouse	1.2%	0.6%
Child/stepchild	14.0%	25.9%
Other relative	5.1%	11.2%
Intimate	9.1%	6.2%
Boyfriend/girlfriend	8.8%	5.4%
Ex–spouse	0.3%	0.8%
Acquaintance	40.8%	41.2%
Stranger	29.8%	14.9%

By Age	Victims of rape	Sexual assault victims
12 or younger	15.2%	44.7%
13–17	21.8%	33.0%
18–24	25.1%	9.4%
25–34	25.4%	7.7%
35–54	10.2%	4.3%
55 or older	2.3%	0.9%

CHART: ROD LITTLE FOR EMERGE

Dodd sat down on the bed again and they began to browse through a photo album, she said. They talked casually about majors. Dodd asked her to sit on the bed. When she did, he asked why she sat so far away. She told him she was leaving soon. By that time, curfew had passed.

Morehouse's curfews are routinely broken. The rules for male visitors on Spelman's campus are strict. Men must be off the grounds by midnight. Guards keep track of male visitors by signing them in and out and by collecting identification. Morehouse is on an honor system, and guards don't track women visitors, a policy officials now say they are re–evaluating.

Dodd slid close to her and began touching her pants, she told the court. He asked what type of material it was. She said she didn't know. He said he thought it was silk. She said she didn't think so. He put his hand in her lap and began to touch her vagina through her pants, she testified. She said she didn't think they should be doing this because they'd just met. He said sometimes people click. She said she didn't feel like they had clicked.

In hearing the testimony, a lawyer asked the Spelman student why, at that point, she didn't leave. She said she still felt safe, that if she asked him to stop he would. Then she added, "Now that I think about things, I look back and say there's so much I could have done but I didn't."

Dodd, she said, reached above his head and turned off the light and began pulling down her pants. She tried to pull them back up, but the 6'6" basketball player eventually got them off, she testified. He stood over her and stuck his penis in her vagina against her will, she testified. She objected and told him that she wanted to go home.

Banks and Marshall entered the room at that point and spoke to each other in whispers, she testified. Then Marshall, also 6'6", stood next to the bed. His pants were off. "This is all for you," she said he told her as he pushed her head toward his penis and stuck it in her mouth. Marshall raped her as Banks put his penis in her mouth, she said.

Morehouse junior Tony Carnell Clark came into the room, the Spelman student said. He stood in the doorway for a moment before telling Banks that his brother was on the phone.

The Spelmanite doesn't recall Banks responding. Marshall got off her and Clark then stuck his penis in her vagina, she testified. While Banks was on top of her, Clark stuck his penis in her mouth. Clark also sodomized her, she testified.

She repeatedly said, "I do not want to do this. I want to go home," she told the court. But the young men ignored her.

When they did back off, she was in tears. She grabbed her clothes and ran to the door. Clark stopped her there. "Haven't I seen you before?" he asked her. Disgusted, she shook her head, but he continued. "I remember meeting you at the library, that was the last time I saw you." Marshall wouldn't look at her, she said. Dodd focused on a closet. She did not account for Banks.

She ran outside Forbes Hall, but there was a crowd of people there and she couldn't bear to walk past them, so she ran back upstairs to her friend McFadden's room, she testified. She banged on the door, but there was no answer. She called from the pay phone down the hall, but there was still no answer. She banged on the door again. This time his roommate answered. Still crying, she woke McFadden and told him she needed him to walk her home.

"He kept on asking me what was wrong...and I couldn't tell him. I said I just need for you to walk me home," she said. He told her he wasn't going to walk her home until he knew why she was crying. She finally told him.

She also told her roommate, Jackie Holland, daughter of Spelman board chairman Bob Holland, former CEO of ice cream–maker Ben & Jerry's Homemade Inc. It was Holland who called a cab and took her to Grady Memorial Hospital's rape crisis center, where she underwent a rape examination.

The examinations can be physically and emotionally painful. Far worse than any gynecological exam, doctors must scrape inside the body for "evidence." What I remember most about my exam is that it felt like another rape.

Early that Saturday morning, the young woman reported the incident to Spelman's security force. Five days later, on Oct. 2, she filed a report with Atlanta's police department. Banks, Clark, Dodd and Marshall were arrested the next day.

FACE TO FACE

FINDING HER IS EASIER than I thought it would be. I ask around and am eventually directed to her dorm door. I introduce myself to a young woman standing in the door. I tell her who I am looking for and she shakes her head. "I'm just a friend," she says and points to another young woman who is sitting on a bed, talking on the phone. She is a petite, attractive woman. I introduce myself, explain that I am a journalist. I tell her that I am a rape victim, too, but spare her details, saying only that I was attacked at gunpoint in my home. I mention, too, that I am a Spelmanite.

Our situations are so different. She is 17, in her first semester of college. I am already a woman, out of college, working. My story has never been questioned. For her, others' doubts are a given, and their accusatory questions are a fact of life. What was she wearing? What was she doing in the dorm so late? And why was she alone?

Even I must reserve judgment. The four accused men are innocent until proven guilty in a court of law.

Her soft, quiet voice does not fill the tiny room where we sit. The floor is cluttered with magazines, shoes and other items you'd expect to find in a college dorm room. There are lots of pictures of her family and friends on the wall above her bed. She and her mother. Her sister, who is older, out of college and working, like me. Family and friends have been with her in court, and her sister testified at one hearing.

During our brief time together, friends drop in to check on her. She tells me that she rarely goes to class and sees a private therapist. She slowly shakes her head at how much of a spectacle this whole thing has become.

I am not sure if I could have stayed on campus. I never returned to the apartment where I was assaulted. My sister, my boyfriend and other friends moved my things. Police found my car, which the attackers used to get away. I drove it once, from the police station to my parents' home. A short time later, it was traded.

I think, too, about the 15–year–old high school student at New York's Manhattan Center for Math and Science who was forced to perform oral sex on the school's basketball star, Richie Parker, and one of Parker's friends, in January 1994. She was harassed so much that eventually she was forced to transfer. The Spelman freshman has received an anonymous letter implying that she was ruining the lives of four promising Black men.

So why does she stay? "They've already taken so much from me," she says.

The four young men tell a different story. Three say they engaged in consensual sex with the Spelman freshman. The fourth, Marshall, says he had no sexual contact with her at all. They have all pleaded not guilty. Though I have had several conversations with their lawyers, I have not had access to the young men. But within hours of being on campus, I learn that they are well–liked.

On Thursday, Oct. 3, Atlanta police arrested the four on Morehouse's campus, and took them to the Atlanta City Detention Center before eventually moving them to the Fulton County Jail. They would spend nearly a month and a half in jail, their names and faces flashed across television screens, their alleged crimes recounted in print.

The first time I see them it is at a bond hearing. It is Nov. 14, the day before they will be released from jail. They are marched into a crowded courtroom, each wearing a blue prison jumpsuit with "Fulton County Jail" emblazoned in white.

Banks, the shortest of the four at 5'7", is Morehouse's starting point guard. His youthful, light–brown face belies his age. He turned 21 the day before he was freed on bail. Banks grew up in Cambridge, Mass., where his father is a retired police officer. His mother works in the registrar's office of Roxbury Community College. And his sister, Chandra Banks, a 1991 Spelman graduate, is president of the Boston chapter of the National Alumnae Association of Spelman College.

Clark is a Morehouse junior who also grew up in Cambridge, and like Banks, spent his 21st birthday behind bars. He is on academic scholarship and the only defendant not on the basketball team. His father is deceased and his mother teaches preschool.

Dodd, a 20–year–old sophomore, is the youngest and one of the tallest at 6'6". His parents are divorced. His mother, an administrative assistant, now lives in Stone Mountain, Ga., near Atlanta. His father is vice president of a steel company in Detroit. His basketball skills were good enough to win him a scholarship to Morehouse.

Darren Marshall is also a sophomore, but is the oldest of the four at 26. Even with his long, brown face and mustache, he appears younger. A native of Trinidad, he was required to surrender his passport as a condition of his release on bail. A younger brother is also a Morehouse student, and their parents live in New York, but unlike the parents of the other young men, they cannot make the trip to Atlanta.

They are Morehouse men, with family and friends who love them. And, according to a young African–American woman, they are the four men who raped her. For young Black men to successfully navigate the pitfalls and dangers that ensnare so many others, it is particularly painful for their family and friends to believe that their lives may be destroyed. If convicted, they face a minimum sentence of 10 years with no probation or parole, up to life in prison, the maximum for rape in Georgia. At an Oct. 30 court hearing, the sodomy charges, which also carry a minimum 10 years to life, were dropped because the judge believed it would be impos-

"THAT was one of the most emotional courtrooms I've sat in in a long time." People "would run out of the room."

sible for the accuser to say which of the students committed it.

In this drama, their lives and futures have been pitted against the life and future of their accuser.

I have squeezed into a seat in the back of the courtroom. As it was for a hearing nearly a month earlier, on Oct. 16, the room is packed. By all accounts, that October hearing was an emotional, tense and dramatic scene. The Spelman freshman's parents and three of the four defendants' mothers were there. President Cole's testimony that day played a pivotal role in the initial denial of bail.

Spelman senior Cara Grayer, a friend of Clark's, was there.

"That was one of the most emotional courtrooms I've sat in in a long time," says Grayer, whose father is a lawyer. "I was sitting next to Dadon Dodd's mother. . . . They would say 25 years to life. Dadon Dodd's mother would run out of the room. . . . The mother of the girl—[when] they would say [the charge of] 'sodomy', she would . . . run out of the room."

A month later, emotions would be just as high, but there had been a development in the days before that had bolstered the young men's supporters. There had been reports that a security guard had found their accuser in her friend McFadden's dorm room days before the November hearing. She was hiding in a closet, supposedly, with her pants down around her knees.

When I hear this, I, like many, begin to have doubts. I ask her about the accusation when we meet. She does not deny being in McFadden's room. They have grown closer—platonically, she stresses—since the attack. He has become one of the people she talks to and that is what they were doing when she was found in his room. And her pants being down? "He's lying," she says of the security guard's accusation.

At the bond hearing, defense attorneys bring one character witness after another to testify for their clients. Among them were Banks' sister, Dodd's former boss and a Morehouse assistant basketball coach. The young men also take the stand to answer questions about their character. No details of that night are discussed. The most dramatic moment comes when an attorney asks all those present in support of the defendants to stand.

The display of support stuns me. I try to count the people still in their seats, but can't see in front of me because there are so many people standing. I would learn later that the Spelmanite also had been in the courtroom.

The hearing was enough to persuade Judge Gail S. Tusan, a Black woman, to set bail at $30,000 for each of the accused.

In an interview later, Ted Lackland, Tony Clark's lawyer, tells me this case reminds him of the Scottsboro Boys, nine young Black men who in 1931 were falsely accused of raping two White girls. Eight received death sentences and one received life in prison. Their case inspired a successful international campaign for their freedom. "The presumption is that it must have been a rape because that kind of thing is beneath her," he says of this case.

His point leaves me wondering about questions I do not ask. What if the young men accused had been White fraternity boys? What would he have said then? But Black women have always been put in the position of choosing between racial and sexual oppression.

Grayer, like many students on Spelman's campus, is torn. "It's very, very difficult and that's where a lot of students are being put in that position," she says. "They're being asked to choose. ...you either have to stand behind the women or you have to stand behind the men, there's no middle ground. I stand firmly against rape. At the same time, I stand firmly that I hold one of the young men in my heart. And that's what's most disturbing about this case.

"That's what makes it high–profile, when you see the mothers and they're in tears, all of them.... That is a mother's worst nightmare...to send your daughter away to college, and then at the same time to have your young man that you've raised...to know that they've assaulted another woman. I think that that has to be the hardest thing on earth."

Grayer says she has chosen to support her friend, Clark. The circumstances, she says, are questionable anyway, and she does not want to see his future lost.

Hers is a view not foreign to African–American women. I am a Black woman, too, and I understand. I, too, cringe at the thought of one more Black man being turned over to a flawed criminal justice system. I have a brother and a father and other Black men in my life whom I love and respect. My brother was falsely accused and arrested once for mugging an elderly White

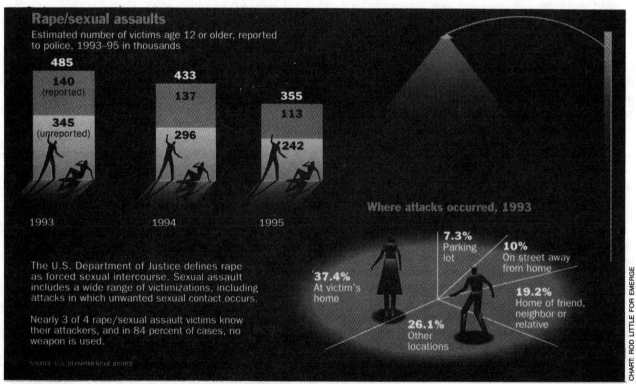

Rape/sexual assaults

Estimated number of victims age 12 or older, reported to police, 1993–95 in thousands

485
140 (reported)
345 (unreported)
1993

433
137
296
1994

355
113
242
1995

Where attacks occurred, 1993

37.4% At victim's home

7.3% Parking lot

10% On street away from home

19.2% Home of friend, neighbor or relative

26.1% Other locations

The U.S. Department of Justice defines rape as forced sexual intercourse. Sexual assault includes a wide range of victimizations, including attacks in which unwanted sexual contact occurs.

Nearly 3 of 4 rape/sexual assault victims know their attackers, and in 84 percent of cases, no weapon is used.

SOURCE: U.S. DEPARTMENT OF JUSTICE

CHART: ROD LITTLE FOR EMERGE

woman when he was in college in Tacoma, Wash. If my father had not had the money to fly across the country and hire a lawyer, who knows how long my brother would have been in jail. The thought of any of my loved ones behind bars — or the thousands of men wrongly jailed — ties me in knots of sadness and anger. But I also know this: One of my greatest fantasies is to castrate the men who raped me.

Evelyn C. White, author of *Chain Chain Change: For Black Women in Abusive Relationships*, says there is a "great sense of racial loyalty that exists among Black women. Black women, because of racism, are very, very aware and understanding and empathetic toward the African–American men who sexually assault us."

Still, questions remain. What if the Spelmanite is lying? It has happened, though I don't understand why someone would put themselves through the emotional or physical horrors of doing such a thing. No matter what, her college years have been ruined. College will not be the wonderful experience it should be. But I am forced to concede that anything is possible.

But what if she is telling the truth? This type of hell I already know the answer to. Rape is a violation that forever changes you. To confront it on a campus or in a courtroom, takes tremendous fortitude. I could not imagine being in a courtroom where a sea of people stand up against me.

A final question comes to me: What if she's telling the truth, and so are the defendants — at least that they believe they are innocent? What if they think that what happened is okay? Nathan McCall writes, in *Makes Me Wanna Holler*, about "running trains" on women — women who may not have fought or resisted, but who were certainly tricked or coerced into a situation that devalued and demeaned them. I listen to students such as Grayer and conclude that that would be the worst of all.

THE CAMPUS

THE SISTER–BROTHER bonds between Spelman and Morehouse have been strained. The case has forced a tight–knit community to examine its attitudes about sexual violence. Some Morehouse students have said they felt betrayed by President Cole's strong support of the Spelman student. They are disappointed, too, in what they consider their own administration's lack of support for their four schoolmates.

"Everybody becomes consumed by it, students, faculty, staff, it's almost like a struggle to try to understand, and people hold on to beliefs," says Vice Provost Eddie Gaffney, a Morehouse graduate who worked at the University of South Carolina for 17 years. "At the University of South Carolina, they'd see [this] as an individual problem. Here, it's a family problem."

For a while it seemed the family was divided into two camps.

Cole set the tone at Spelman. She took the freshman into her home for a few days immediately after the incident. At a town hall meeting, she urged students to support their schoolmate. And when she testified at the hearing where bail for the four accused men was denied, she got the best of a defense lawyer who tried to spar with her. Spelman students followed her lead, attending public meetings and holding discussions on sexual violence. They decorated a board of supportive wishes in the Manley College Student Center. The young woman's friends rallied around her, supporting her decision to remain on campus, get-

SHE recalls Spelmanites complaining about an offensive image on a flier advertising a club. But by the next week, they were back partying at the same spot.

ting her assignments from professors, turning them in for her, as she rarely left her dorm.

There were about 80 women and fewer than a dozen men at a speak–out against sexual violence sponsored by the Women's Research and Resource Center when I was on campus. SGA president Ardenia Johnson talked a lot about personal accountability. She recalled Spelmanites complaining about an offensive image on a flier advertising a club. She said students were ready to burn bras, Snoop Doggy Dogg tapes and anything they could get their hands on that denigrated women. But by the next week, she says, they were back partying at the same spot.

Morehouse's administration wasn't far behind Cole. The school began its own investigation into the matter on Sept. 30. Administrators immediately suspended the four students for the academic year for violation of college rules. It said the suspensions were not related to the criminal charges but the violation of the campus rules regarding conduct.

"For generations, Morehouse has set very high standards of ethics and morality for its students, staff and faculty, standards that must be upheld at all times," said the school's Oct. 7 statement. "The College determined through its investigation that the behavior of the students in this case was not consistent with behavior expected and demanded of Morehouse students.

"The College is deeply concerned and saddened that anyone, especially a student at our sister institution, Spelman College, may have been the victim of violence or abuse. Inappropriate sexual conduct has never been acceptable on the Morehouse campus and will not be tolerated now."

At a school assembly that same day, John H. Hopps, provost of Morehouse College, made similar remarks. Faculty members answered questions about the incident at a forum that night in King Chapel. At least 1,500 students attended the town hall meeting and what faculty and staff heard that night took some by surprise, says Gaffney. "That's when we really found out that a lot of young men had no idea about the sexual politics of present times," he says.

If statistics from the U.S. Centers for Disease Control and Prevention are any indication, such educational efforts are desperately needed on all college campuses, not just African–American ones. From 15 percent to 25 percent of male college students admit to involvement in some level of sexual aggression. Additionally, more than 80 percent of rapes on college campuses are committed by someone the victim knows.

At Morehouse, while there was tough talk about the abuse of women, there was also another side to the discussion. In handouts distributed on college stationery, the administration said it was considering a defense fund for the four accused students. Five lawyers volunteered to teach students about their legal rights.

7. VIOLENCE IN WOMEN'S LIVES

Beverly Guy-Sheftall, founding director of Spelman's Women's Research and Resource Center, wants to know who will teach young African-American men at Morehouse and around the country about respecting Black women?

"There is an assumption that Black men are being targeted, or that there's actually some conspiracy to destroy Black men," she says. "I think that's the scenario around which these cases get framed and that it's very difficult to separate those notions."

Lawrence Edward Carter, dean of the Morehouse chapel, didn't help the campus friction much. During regular worship services, a day before the Oct. 7 assembly, Carter suggested that women bring abuse upon themselves because of their attitudes and their dress. Some Spelman students walked out. Later, nine Spelmanites responded in a pointed letter that was printed Oct. 14 in Morehouse's newspaper, *The Maroon Tiger*:

"We found your understanding of the true issues involved in the violent crime of rape to be faulty. As evidence of this, we point to the particularly offensive description of the woman wearing 'a strip of tape,' the woman whose skirt was 'sprayed on,' and that she was 'an accident waiting to happen.' ...You victimized the victim in your remarks, and this was unfair, inappropriate and un-Christian.

"...You suggested that a heinous crime of violence perpetrated against a Spelman woman by Morehouse men should be excused or even justified because the sisters are 'loose,' and the brothers are weak and must be expected to succumb to 'temptation.' Rape is not about lust or attire; it is about power and control."

They demanded an apology. Carter was suspended for an unspecified period. He issued a five-paragraph response/apology, which *The Maroon Tiger* printed the same day, and agreed to attend a joint worship service at Spelman's Sisters Chapel but he did not show up.

Says Hopps: "Let me be very clear. Morehouse College absolutely rejects any such notion. No individual, no man or woman, ever deserves to be abused by virtue of the clothing they choose. We abhor any suggestion to the contrary."

Says Antonio Johnson, Morehouse's student government association president, whose mother was raped when he was a child, "Dean Carter, in my opinion, should be fired. Those statements, I think, were extremely insensitive to women. He knew of the sensitivity of the moment, and that's why I'm so outraged about it."

Some students were disappointed in the Morehouse administration for other reasons.

"I didn't like the positions the college took," says Baimba Norman, a junior from Liberia, who believes Morehouse turned its back on the young men. "I don't think they should have suspended them.... Other people break curfew rules. If it was based on that, on breaking curfew rules, hundreds of people would be suspended because that happens daily."

Another junior, Darnik McAlpin, expressed a common attitude toward the Spelman freshman. "Why was she over here at that time by herself?" asks the Augusta, Ga., native. "Maybe [she] got mad afterwards.... There's no justification for doing that, don't get me wrong.... But I think she was there, and she had sex with all those guys, and afterwards, maybe she was feeling guilty.

" ... Like Mike Tyson and Desiree [Washington] ... one of those things where after they finished with her, instead of letting her stay over or whatever, they're like, 'You better go ahead and get out....' She got mad.

"The law is messed up for the simple fact that a girl can lie. I can have sex with her one night, and then the next day we get in an argument and then she accuses you of rape the night before.... My word against hers. I'm already in jail. It's already on my record."

Craig Boyd, who works for Morehouse's sports medicine department and knows all four defendants, says, "Someone

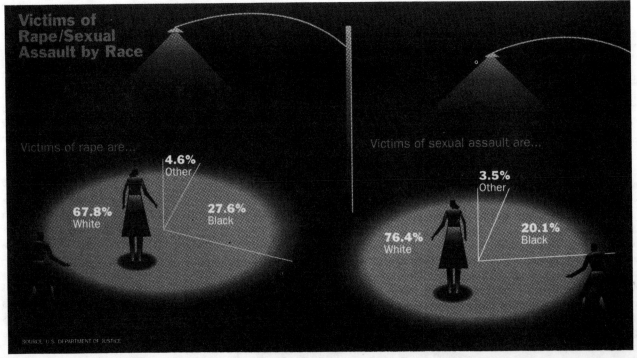

Victims of Rape/Sexual Assault by Race

Victims of rape are...

67.8% White   4.6% Other   27.6% Black

Victims of sexual assault are...

76.4% White   3.5% Other   20.1% Black

SOURCE: U.S. DEPARTMENT OF JUSTICE

CHART: ROD LITTLE FOR EMERGE

"I DON'T like the positions the college took. I don't think they should have suspended them."

should have said this is wrong," but he does not believe a crime was committed that night.

Kevin Ladaris, a senior and a leader of the campus group Men for the Eradication of Sexism, says he believes so many male students doubt that a rape occurred because they see themselves in similar situations. That is parallel to women blaming the victim, he says, because if the men didn't do anything wrong, then any woman is vulnerable to rape.

Says Rev. Aubra Love, director of the Black Church and Domestic Violence Task Force at the Center for the Prevention of Sexual and Domestic Violence in Seattle, "We have a rape culture which does not accept rape as violence and treats rape as if it has something to do with sex, when in fact, if we could talk plainly, it's like mugging with a body, assault with a penis."

For Kevin Ladaris, of Morehouse, the campus incident has

irony. It occurred the same weekend that his organization hosted its forum on violence against women.

At press time, the four men had not been indicted and no court date had been set. "The investigation is still on–going," says Terri Lawson–Adams, a spokesperson for the Fulton County district attorney's office. Atlanta police also are still investigating the charges.

Morehouse officials, meanwhile, have readmitted the four to classes and extracurricular activities. Their original one–year suspensions — for violating college rules and standards of conduct — were appealed and later reduced to one semester.

RECOVERING

THE DAY I LEAVE CAMPUS I am exhausted. I have spent my last hours trying to arrange to speak with the four men. It never works out. I also try to call the accuser, but there is no answer. I walk across the campus and remember that this is where I first learned what it meant to believe in myself and my dreams. For me, like it is for so

---

Haunted by History

IN ADDITION to the guilt and shame that can accompany sexual assault, Black women often face the additional burdens of race and history, which can encourage them to minimize their own pain and excuse or protect their attacker, say some who have studied the issue. Whether it is the case of Celia, a teenage slave girl who was hanged in Missouri for killing her White rapist, or the film, *Birth of a Nation*, conceived to perpetuate the myth of the Black rapist, African-American women have learned to be silent about sexual assault.

"One of the reasons that historically rape has been more complicated for Black people [is] there is the history . . . of Black men being falsely accused of rape, even though most of that memory is [of being] falsely accused by White women," says Beverly Guy-Sheftall, founding director of Spelman's Women's Research and Resource Center. "So I think that the whole issue of rape is already a contested terrain within the Black community."

Stereotypes of hypersexual African-Americans grew out of the slavery-era ethos. For the first centuries of this nation's existence, it was accepted, even expected for White men to sexually assault Black women slaves, a way for owners to produce more "property" and constantly demonstrate their total ownership of Africans.

One of the most egregious and documented cases was that of Celia, who in 1850, at the age of 14, was bought by Robert Newsom, a 70-year-old farmer. After years of repeated rapes by Newsom, Celia killed him. The court rejected the notion that she had the right to resist. She was charged with first-degree murder and hanged.

Once slavery ended, myths about Black sexuality festered, and the protection of White women's virtue became another rationalization for brutalizing African-American men and women.

In the 1890s, journalist Ida B. Wells reported that about one-fourth of lynching victims were accused of attempted rape or rape. Recorded lynchings from 1882 to 1962 number nearly 5,000, and many more unrecorded murders by White mobs cut short Black lives. Whites also lynched Black men who had attempted to avenge their loved ones who had been raped.

D. W. Griffith's 1915 work, *Birth of a Nation*, went a long way toward immortalizing such ideas. That movie dramatized Civil War and Reconstruction history from a White southerner's perspective, and fictionalized the origin of the Ku Klux Klan. In the film, a lecherous Black man attempts to harm White women. The film concludes with Klan members gallantly riding to the rescue.

Griffith said he wanted "to create a feeling of abhorrence in White people, especially White women, against Colored men."

Considered the technically sophisticated forerunner of today's feature films, the blockbuster grossed more than $18 million and was the first movie screened at the White House. More than anything, however, it reinforced a violent, racist and sexist culture that African-Americans continue to navigate today.

Conversely, Guy-Sheftall says, "Historically, we know that the rape of Black women has been paid absolutely no attention to by the larger society."

That legacy is never far behind, Guy-Sheftall says, arguing that it plays itself out between African-American men and women, both in high-profile media cases and those cases where the rape is never reported.

Says Guy-Sheftall, "In an ironic kind of way, when Black men get accused of rape, the Black woman almost gets put in the same category as White women who accuse Black men of rape, and she becomes the enemy, too."

—Lori S. Robinson

many women, it was an academic and social haven. I try to calm my stomach by telling myself if there is a place where lessons will be learned about confronting sexual violence in our communities, it will be here. If we do not, it will continue to eat away at us. The government reports a recent drop in rapes, but the crime remains a serious problem. As it has been true here, as it is true in my own life and the lives of others, rape — or even the allegation of rape — touches more than the accuser and accused. It devastates families, friends, communities.

I do not know how the Spelman student — or even the four from Morehouse — will fare. My own recovery continues and I believe it is a lifelong struggle.

Although I was blessed to never have nightmares, the fears of my waking hours — the fear of disease, of my family being tracked down and hurt by the rapists, of unknowingly bumping into them — left me drained of energy and happiness for months. After all, I never got a good look at the gunman's face, and never saw the other rapist's face. The police told me that the assailants were believed to have raped at least three other women. To my knowledge, they have not been caught.

My biggest obstacles in healing became lingering fears of being harmed again, by the rapists or other men. And I was furious over the disruption in my life, the loss of my treasured independence. I had to change my car, my home, and alter my psyche. My life was turned upside down.

The day after the attack, after I had told my family, I began telling the other people close to me. A girlfriend shocked me with her response, a shrill shriek and then uncontrollable sobbing. It confirmed my concern that even though the rape was not my fault, I now had no choice but to cause pain for those close to me.

When I told my mom, she looked as if she might pass out for a second, then she immediately began to talk about what needed to be done. My boyfriend repeated it back to me. "Did you just say you were robbed and raped?" he said, as if he was hoping he heard wrong. I remember begging for his friendship and support, fully expecting him not to want to deal with a basket case. "This will only bring us closer together," he told me. Nothing could have been more comforting. My family and friends, and the love and tender care of my boyfriend, have helped me survive and to grow stronger in spirit and resolve.

I guess more than anything, what I carry with me as I walk out of this valley in my life is a commitment to help end the silence. A close male member of my family could not bring himself to speak to me about my rape for an entire year. The last time we were both at Spelman was on my graduation day.

I have learned that he cried when told about my rape. I wonder what it would have been like if we had cried — and healed — together.

Where to Find Help

THE RAPE, ABUSE & INCEST NATIONAL NETWORK (RAINN)
24–hour national hot line for instant referrals to local organizations
1–800–656–HOPE

**NORTHEAST / NEW YORK
RAPE INTERVENTION PROGRAM**
Mount Sinai Medical Center
(212) 241–5461

VICTIM SERVICES
Hot line: (212) 577–7777

**NEW JERSEY
SEXUAL ASSAULT AND RAPE ANALYSTS**
Newark
(201) 733–7273

**MID–ATLANTIC / PENNSYLVANIA
WOMEN ORGANIZED AGAINST RAPE**
Philadelphia
Hot line: (215) 985–3333

**MARYLAND
SEXUAL ASSAULT & DOMESTIC VIOLENCE CENTER**
Baltimore
Hot line: (410) 828–6390

**WASHINGTON, D.C.
D.C. RAPE CRISIS CENTER**
Hot line: (202) 333–7273

**VIRGINIA
SEXUAL ASSAULT OUTREACH PROGRAM**
Richmond
Hot line: (804) 643–0888

**MIDWEST / OHIO
RAPE CRISIS CENTER**
Cleveland
Hot line: (216) 391–3912

**ILLINOIS
YWCA WOMEN'S SERVICES**
Chicago
(312) 372–4105

**MINNESOTA
SEXUAL VIOLENCE CENTER**
Minneapolis
(612) 871–5111

**WISCONSIN
SEXUAL ASSAULT TREATMENT CENTER**
Milwaukee
Hotline: (414) 937–5555

**MICHIGAN
DETROIT POLICE RAPE COUNSELING CENTER**
(313) 833–1660

**MISSOURI
METROPOLITAN ORGANIZATION TO COUNTER SEXUAL ASSAULT**
Kansas City
(816) 531–0233

**SOUTH / GEORGIA
GRADY RAPE CRISIS CENTER**
Atlanta
(404) 616–4861

**NORTH CAROLINA
RAPE CRISIS CENTER**

Charlotte
Hot line: (704) 375–9900

**FLORIDA
SEXUAL ASSAULT CRISIS CENTER (RESPONSE)**
Orlando
Hot line: (407) 740–5408

CRISIS CENTER OF HILLSBORO COUNTY, INC.
Tampa
(813) 238–8821

**LOUISIANA
YWCA RAPE CRISIS PROGRAM**
New Orleans
Hot line: (504) 483–8888

**TEXAS
HOUSTON–AREA WOMEN'S CENTER RAPE CRISIS CENTER**
Hot line: (713) 528–7273

**TENNESSEE
SEXUAL ASSAULT RESOURCE CENTER**
Memphis
(901) 272–2020

**WEST / CALIFORNIA
LOS ANGELES COMMISSION ON ASSAULTS AGAINST WOMEN**
(310) 392–8381

**COLORADO
RAPE ASSISTANCE & AWARENESS PROGRAM**
Denver
Hot line: (303) 322–7273

SOURCE: D. C. RAPE CRISIS CENTER

Dangerous Men: The Warning Signals You May Miss

The right way to respond and protect yourself from the kind of man who just won't let go. An excerpt from THE GIFT OF FEAR, a new book by one of the nation's leading experts on stalking behavior.

BY GAVIN DE BECKER

I WAS JUST TRYING TO let him down easy." With these words begins a story my firm hears several times each month. Before meeting me, this young woman, whose name is Katherine,* may have told it to her friends and her therapist, then a private detective, a lawyer, a police officer, maybe even a judge, but the problem persisted. It is the story of a dating situation that once seemed innocent, or at least manageable, but is now frightening. It is the story of a former boyfriend or acquaintance who seemed normal but was revealed to be something else.

Stalking is the way some men raise the stakes when a woman doesn't play along with their needs. It is a crime of power, control and intimidation very similar to date rape. Indeed, it could be described as an extended rape: It takes away a woman's freedom and disregards her wishes, honoring instead the wishes of the man. Whether he is an estranged husband, an ex-boyfriend, a former date, or an unwanted suitor, a stalker enforces society's cruel double standard: that a woman can say no to a man, but she can't make it stick.

It doesn't have to be that way. A woman can not only spot a potential stalker but can get away from him, if she follows her intuition right from the start.

Katherine's story illustrates some of the warning signs—listed here in brackets—of this type of stalker, the man who just won't let go:

* Names and details changed to disguise identities.

"I met Bryan* at a party given by a friend, and he must have asked somebody there for my number [researching the victim] because before I even got home, he'd left me three messages [overly invested]. I told him I didn't want to go out with him, but he was so enthusiastic that I really didn't have any choice [men who cannot let go choose women who cannot say no].

"In the beginning, he spent a lot of time listening and always seemed to know what I wanted. He remembered everything I ever said [hyperattentive]. It was flattering at first, but it also made me uncomfortable [victim intuitively feels smothered]. For example, I once mentioned needing more space for my books, and he just showed up one day with shelves and tools and all the stuff he needed, and just put them up [offering unsolicited help]. I couldn't say no [woman who can't say no]. He always read so much into whatever I said [projecting emotions]. Once he asked me to go to a basketball game, and I said maybe. Later, when I decided to stay home, he insisted that I'd 'promised' [enforcing casual or nonexistent commitments].

"We'd only gone out on a few dates when he began talking about serious things—living together and marriage and children [whirlwind pace, placing issues on the agenda prematurely]. He worried constantly about my safety and suggested that I get a car phone. I wasn't sure I wanted one, but he borrowed my car and just had the phone installed. It was a gift, so what could I say? And of course, he

called me whenever I was in the car [monitoring activity and whereabouts]. He was adamant that I never speak to my ex-boyfriend on that car phone. Later, he'd get angry if I spoke to my ex at all [jealousy]. There were also a couple of my friends he didn't like me to see [isolating his mark], and he stopped spending time with any of his own friends [making her responsible for his whole social world]. Finally, when I told him I didn't want to be his girlfriend, he refused to hear it [refusing to hear no]."

Katherine felt uncomfortable with this man right from the start, but like most victims ignored the warning signals. Instead of rejecting Bryan, she tried to let him down easy, at which point Bryan just tightened his hold. In doing so, he strangled the relationship, ensuring that it could never be what he said (and maybe even believed) he wanted. Still, his persistence paid off: Katherine remained involved with him longer than she ever intended. Nearly every victim I've met stayed in contact with her pursuer long after she wanted out.

While giving talks around the country, I sometimes ask the men in the audience, "How many of you have ever found out where a woman lived or worked by means other than asking her? How many have driven by a woman's house to see what cars were there, or called just to see who answered the phone and then hung up?"

The overwhelming show of hands tells me that the social acceptability of these behaviors—all of them techniques used by stalkers—is a matter of degree. An invisible line separates courting behavior that's charming from behavior that goes too far, and men and women don't always agree on where to place the line.

Many men believe that the best romantic strategy is persistence. Much of popular culture teaches men that if you just stay with it—even if she says she wants nothing to do with you—you'll eventually get the girl. If stalking cases teach us anything, though, it's that persistence only proves persistence—it does not prove love. The fact that a man is relentless in his pursuit doesn't mean you are special; more likely it means he is troubled.

In dating situations, women often say less than they mean or feel, while men often hear less than what is said. I've successfully lobbied and testified for stalking laws in several states, but I would trade them all for a school curriculum that would teach young men how to hear "no" and young women how to reject. If more women felt comfortable explicitly rejecting, stalking cases would decline dramatically.

One rule applies to all types of unwanted pursuit: Do not negotiate. Once you make the decision that you don't want a relationship with a particular man, tell him so, explicitly. But only tell him once. After that rejection, almost any further contact will be seen as negotiation.

If a woman tells a man over and over again that she doesn't want to talk to him, she should realize that she is talking to him, and every time she does it, she betrays her own resolve. If a woman ignores 30 messages from a pursuer and then finally gives in and returns his last call, no matter what she says to him in that conversation, what he has learned is that the cost of reaching her is leaving 30 messages. For this type of man, any contact will be seen as progress.

Of course, a victim may be worried that she'll provoke him by failing to respond and may try softening her rejection. Often the result is that he believes she is conflicted, uncertain, really likes him but just doesn't know it yet. When a woman says, "It's just that I don't want to be in a relationship right now," a potential stalker hears only the words "right now." To him, this means she will want to be in a relationship later. A more truthful, and effective, rejection would be, "I don't want to be in a relationship with *you.*" Unless it's that clear, and sometimes even when it is, he won't hear it.

If she says, "You're a great guy and you have a lot to offer, but I'm not the one for you; my head's just not in the right place these days," this man thinks: She really likes me, it's just that she's confused; I've got to prove to her that she's the one for me. He will challenge each reason she offers.

A woman should never explain *why* she doesn't want a relationship but should simply make clear that she has thought it over, that this is her final decision and that she expects him to respect it. Why should a woman have to explain intimate aspects of her life, plans and romantic choices to someone with whom she doesn't want a relationship? A rejection based on any condition—say, that she wants to move to another city—just gives him something to challenge. Conditional rejections are not rejections. They are discussions.

Let's imagine a woman has let pass several opportunities to pursue a relationship with a suitor. Every hint, response, action and inaction has communicated that she is not interested. If the man still pursues at this point, it is time for an unconditional and explicit rejection. Because few men have heard it and few women have spoken it, here is what an unconditional and explicit rejection sounds like: "No matter what you may have assumed until now, and no matter for what reason you assumed it, I have no romantic interest in you whatsoever. I am certain I never will. I expect that, now that you know this, you'll put your attention elsewhere, which I understand, because that's what I intend to do."

There is only one appropriate response to this: acceptance. However the man communicates this, the basic concept would ideally be: "I hear you, I understand, and while I am disappointed, I will certainly respect your decision."

I said there's only one appropriate reaction. Unfortunately, there are hundreds of inappropriate reactions, and while they take many forms, their basic message is: "I do not accept your decision." If a man debates, doubts, negotiates or attempts to change her mind, a woman should recognize that her decision to stop seeing this man was the right one. Instead of being challenged by his relentless pursuit, her resolve should be strengthened. No woman should be in a relationship with someone who does not hear what she says and who does not recognize her feelings. Moreover, if he has failed to understand a message this clear and explicit, his reaction to any ambiguous statements, the kind that are made when a man's being let down easy, can only be imagined.

What if a woman has explicitly said no and the man escalates his pursuit with persistent phone calls and messages; showing up uninvited at work, school or home; following her or even trying to enlist her friends or family in his campaign? Assuming she has communicated one explicit rejection, it is very important that no further response be given.

I repeat: When a woman chooses to communicate with someone she has explicitly rejected, her actions don't match her words. Her pursuer can then decide for himself which actions or words actually represent her feelings. Not surprisingly, he'll choose the ones that serve him. Often, such a man will leave phone messages that ostensibly offer closure, but that are actually crudely concealed efforts to get a response—and remember, he views any response as progress.

When the stalker is someone a woman has dated, she may have to listen to friends make unhelpful comments like, "You must have encouraged the guy in some way" or "You must enjoy being pursued." If the stalking continues, someone will inevitably advise her to change her phone number. Our office does *not* recommend this strategy, because as any victim will tell you, the stalker always manages to get the new number.

A better plan is to get a second phone line, give the new number to the people she wants to hear from and keep her old number hooked to an answering machine or voice mail so that the stalker is not even aware she has another number. She can check her messages, and when she receives calls from people she wants to speak with, she can call them back and give them her new number. Eventually, the only person leaving messages on the old number is the unwanted pursuer. In this way, his calls are documented. She should keep the message tapes in case she decides later to file a formal complaint with the police. More important, each time he leaves a message, he gets a message: that she can avoid the temptation to respond to his manipulations.

We also suggest that the outgoing message be recorded by a female friend, because he may be calling just to hear his object's voice. While people believe that an outgoing message with a male voice will lead the pursuer to believe his victim is in a new relationship, more commonly it leads him to investigate further.

When a pursuer has actually dated or

had a relationship with his victim, he may be so desperate to hold on that he'll settle for any kind of contact. Though he'd rather be her boyfriend, he'll accept being just a friend. Eventually, though he'd rather be a friend, he'll accept being an enemy if that's the only position available. As a stalking ex-boyfriend wrote to a young client of ours: "You'll be thinking of me. You may not be thinking good thoughts, but you'll be thinking of me."

Another rule: The only way to stop contact is to stop contact. As noted above, I suggest one explicit rejection, and after that, absolutely no contact. If you call the pursuer back, or agree to meet, or send him a note or have somebody warn him off, you buy another six weeks of his unwanted pursuit. Some victims think it will help to have a male friend, new boyfriend or male family member tell the stalker to stop. Most who try this learn that the stalker takes it as evidence that his love object must be conflicted. Otherwise she would have told him herself.

Sending the police to warn off a pursuer may seem the obvious thing to do, but it rarely has the desired effect, in my experience. Though pursuers may behave alarmingly, most have not broken the law, so the police have few options. When police visit and say, in effect, "Cut this out or you'll get into trouble," the pursuer intuitively knows that if they could have arrested him, they would have. So what's the message of the visit? That the greatest possible weapon in his victim's arsenal—sending the police after him—came and went without a problem. The cops stopped by, they talked to him and they left. Who got stronger, the victim or the pursuer?

Of course, the police should be involved if the stalker has committed an actionable crime that, if prosecuted, would result in improving the victim's safety or putting a high cost on the stalker's behavior. But the first time a stalker should see police is when they show up to arrest him, not when they stop by to chat.

Victims of stalking are often advised to get a restraining order. I would argue that, as with battered wives, it is important to evaluate which cases are likely to be improved by court intervention and which might be worsened. Much depends upon how far the case has escalated and how much the stalker has emotionally invested. If a man has been actively pursuing the same victim for years and has already ignored warnings and interventions, then a restraining order isn't likely to help. Antistalking laws differ from state to state but generally speaking, restraining orders obtained soon after a pursuer has ignored a single explicit rejection will be more effective and create less risk for the woman than those obtained after many months or years of stalking in which the pursuer has made a significant emotional investment.

Court orders frequently work with a naive pursuer, someone who simply does not realize the inappropriateness of his behavior. Being a bit thick and unsophisticated, he may think, I am in love with this person, I am only acting the way people in love act. The naive pursuer is usually distinguishable from other stalkers by his lack of machismo. He rarely displays anger at being rejected. He just seems to go along, happily believing he is courting someone. He stays with it until someone makes it completely clear to him that his approach is inappropriate, unacceptable and counterproductive.

Dating involves several risks: the risk of disappointment, the risk of boredom, the risk of rejection and the risk of letting some troubled, scary man into your life. I am not proposing a checklist of blunt questions, but I do suggest that all the information a woman needs is there on a first date, to be mined through artful conversation.

For example, during the date, a woman might turn the conversation to the man's most recent breakup and notice how he describes it. Does he accept responsibility for his part? Is he still invested? Was he slow to let go, slow to hear or accept what the woman communicated? Has he let go yet? Who broke up with whom? (This last question is an important one because stalkers rarely initiate breakups.) Has he had several love-at-first-sight relationships? Falling for people in a big way based on just a little exposure to them, particularly if this is a pattern, is a valuable sign. She should also observe how often the man tries to change her mind, even on little things.

Stalkers are by definition people who do not give up easily. But most do let go, if their victims avoid engaging them. Usually they have to attach a tentacle to someone else before totally detaching from their current object. Until that happens, the best approach is abstinence—no contact with him, no implied contact with him through intermediaries or letters. To put things in perspective, very few date-stalking cases end in violence. Romantic pursuers do not usually jump from harassment to homicide without apparent and detectable escalations along the way.

A woman can avoid these situations by saying what she means from the start, even if it means letting him down hard. Your intuition is now loaded, so listen.

Gavin de Becker, an expert in risk assessment, was a consultant to the prosecution in the O.J. Simpson trial. He is also the cochair of the Domestic Violence Council Advisory Board.

Special Issues for Older Women

In 1900 there were approximately 3 million Americans over the age of 65. Today that number has grown to 31 million and is expected to reach 66 million by 2030. The population is beginning to gray, and each of us will be left to deal with the problems and the potentials of growing older. Today, the average life expectancy is almost 80 for women and 73 for men. The difference in these numbers begins to illustrate why the aging process should be of particular concern to women. In general, the longer we live, the more prone to illness we become. The old adage, "if I had known I was going to live this long, I would have taken better care of myself," should strike a chord in most women. If women are likely to outlive their male partner by at least 7 years, who will care for them when they are ill or disabled? How can an older, frail woman care for an ailing spouse? What about the burden on family, particularly aging children?

If we are unable to avoid the inevitable decline associated with aging, perhaps we can at least slow it down. The goal should not simply be to live longer but to live better, to improve the quality of one's life and extend the independent years. What can a young woman do now to help ensure a healthier old age later? Is it ever too late for a woman to begin taking care of herself? These and other cogent questions are addressed in this final unit.

We begin with a broad perspective on the health of older women. In "Our Mothers, Ourselves: Older Women's Health Care," the author discusses the huge gap in research and knowledge about older women's health issues. Since the medical community has lagged behind in addressing this issue for younger women, it comes as no surprise that older women have also been neglected.

In "Who Age Better, Men or Women?" author Andrea Atkins says without hesitation, women. This article compares the aging process of men and women in terms of physical, cognitive, and emotional parameters. Also included in this piece is a description of what can be done now to help successfully navigate the changes that will occur later.

The remaining articles here address specific health problems commonly experienced by women as they age. "Hormone Therapy: When and for How Long?" examines menopause in terms of estrogen replacement. This article has a scientific point of view, presenting the often-conflicting arguments present in the literature.

Then, "Silent Sabotage" looks at another prevalent concern for aging women, osteoporosis. Although this article presents the usual risks and treatments, what separates it from the pack is the advice tailored to younger women. Judith Newman makes the point that women in their thirties and fourties should be actively engaged in preventing the disease. Now it is a matter of choice; later it will be one of necessity.

The next article looks at the mammography controversy: when and for whom? Few issues in modern medicine have presented as many conflicting points of view as this. This article explores some of the more pertinent reasons for the lack of agreement within the medical community.

Looking Ahead: Challenge Questions

Why can it be said that women age better than men?
Why do you think women live longer than men?
What do you think are the most serious health problems facing today's young woman as she ages?
What are the pros and cons of using "alternative" means of managing the effects of menopause?

UNIT 8

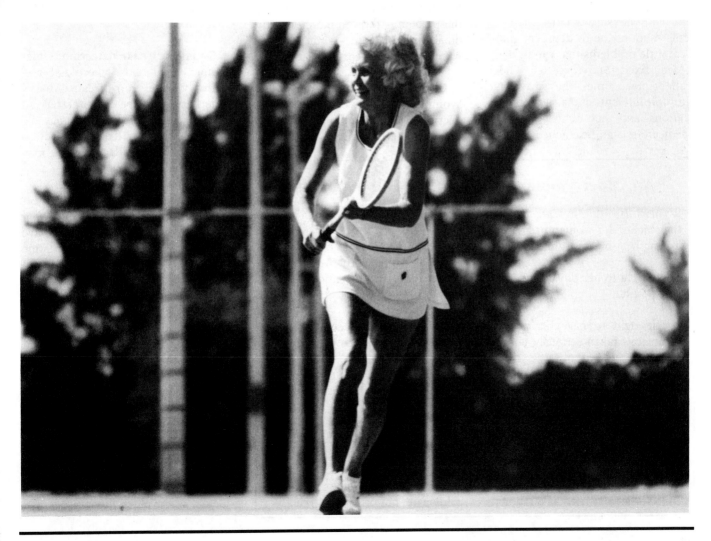

*Older women are the largest consumers of medical care, but they're often overlooked
by the health care system. It's time to close the gaps.*

Our Mothers, Ourselves:
Older Women's Health Care

She has been called the "invisible woman"—the compliant and complacent older woman who gets shuffled from one doctor to the next, without anyone ever really listening to her.

She wants what all women want from their health care providers: to be heard, to have her complaints taken seriously, to be respected as an individual, and to be offered a full range of choices for her health care.

But many physicians view her problems as mundane or depressing, not neat little problems that can be diagnosed, fixed, and forgotten. Older patients take time—they may have multiple ailments and a slew of medications, and they often come with Medicare-related headaches.

Critical Gaps

It's no wonder that older women often feel written off, discounted, and dismissed as patients. And this lack of respect and recognition can lead to serious deficiencies in their health care. These include:

• **Gaps in research.** Little is known about normal aging in women. For instance, when medicine finally woke up to the fact that research on aging was virtually nonexistent, one of the first major studies designed to rectify the problem—the Baltimore Longitudinal Study on Aging—didn't include women until 20 years after it began.

• **Gaps in physician knowledge.** Women's health advocates have long decried the lack of attention given to women's health problems in medical schools. The health problems of the elderly don't fare much better.

Despite an exploding population of people over 65, young physicians' interest in geriatrics languishes.

Moreover, a survey of practicing physicians found that fewer than 10% could cite accurate life expectancy figures for women. Most significantly underestimated life expectancy at various ages—miscalculations that could have serious ramifications for treatment decisions.

• **Gaps in disease detection.** Older women need both gynecologic and primary care. But because many elderly women see only one type of practitioner—and neither may be well-versed in geriatric care—potentially serious health problems may go undetected.

"Many women think of their gynecologist as their primary care physician, particularly if they don't have any other problems," notes Christine Cassel, M.D., professor and chairman of the department of geriatrics and adult development at Mount Sinai Medical Center in New York. "But as a woman gets older, she may need someone who can care for her blood pressure problems, heart disease, or osteoporosis, and gynecologists really aren't equipped to do that."

Switching to the average primary care physician won't necessarily solve this dilemma. "Most primary care physicians who do gynecology really aren't taught about the complexity of the older woman's gyneco-

---

An Older Woman's Health Care Bill of Rights

Women's Health Advocate believes that each older woman has the following health care rights:

• The right to her physician's interest and time.

• The right to have her physical complaints taken seriously, not dismissed as "just part of getting older."

• The right to receive comprehensive health care, including regular screening and prompt referral for diagnostic tests.

• The right to have any physical limitations understood and acknowledged—but not used as a rationale for less than optimal care.

• The right to be acknowledged as a sexual being, with the need for information and attention to this area of her life.

• The right to receive full and detailed explanations of all procedures and treatments.

• The right to be treated for a cure, if that is her desire.

• The right to refuse treatment and face death with dignity.

• Above all, the right to receive compassionate, not patronizing, care.

---

logic needs. So you have this odd situation where the gynecologists aren't interested and the primary care physicians aren't interested," says Dr. Cassel, who's also a member of *WHA*'s editorial board.

A gynecologist, for example, typically would not screen for diabetes, high cholesterol, or colon cancer. An elderly woman who sees only an internist, however, is less likely to receive a pelvic exam or a Pap test. And physicians in general are less likely to refer an older woman for mammography.

These are serious omissions in light of the still-substantial incidence of cervical cancer and the high incidence of breast cancer in older women. Older women account for 25% of new cases of cervical cancer and for 41% of cervical cancer deaths, presumably because of late detection.

Concerning breast cancer, Dr. Cassel says, "The incidence of breast cancer rises linearly with age, but the use of mammography goes down. Physicians probably aren't pushing it. Either they don't think about it or they think that women don't want it or it's awkward. Some don't understand the life expectancy figures for women and believe that someone 85 years old doesn't have many years left. But an 85-year-old could easily live another 15 years."

• **Gaps in treatment.** When a serious disease is diagnosed, older women aren't always offered the best treatment. Physician apprehension about drug side effects, concerns about anesthesia, or, again, misunderstandings about life expectancy may be to blame.

An elderly woman with breast cancer, for instance, is less likely to undergo lymph node dissection (considered crucial to accurate staging and treatment) and is more likely to undergo a mastectomy. Older women who do have lumpectomies are less likely to

Seeking Solutions

Increasing interest in women's health issues, an aging population of activist baby boomers, and ambitious studies already under way are expected to improve health care for future generations of older women.

Development of a women's health specialty, in which physicians would be trained in the special needs of women across the life span, might help, as might genuine multidisciplinary "women's health centers." In the meantime, however, women must advocate for themselves by taking the following steps:

1 Women of all ages need to safeguard their health and physical independence and prepare for the future, reminds Christine Cassel, M.D., professor and chairman of the department of geriatrics and adult development at Mount Sinai Medical Center in New York.

Proper diet and regular exercise—with particular attention to strength training and flexibility exercises—can significantly reduce the risk of frailty and disability in old age. These and other strategies also will help prevent heart disease, the biggest killer of older women, and osteoporosis, a major contributor to loss of mobility and independence.

2 In the absence of more geriatricians, many older women will have to ask for what they need. That may mean insisting that a doctor perform a pelvic exam, breast exam, or Pap test, or bringing up the subject of incontinence or sexual problems.

Advocating for yourself also means seeking out the best health care providers. Although board-certified geriatricians can be hard to find outside major cities, Dr. Cassel recommends contacting the nearest medical school for the names of its geriatricians. Those doctors may know someone in your community who, even though not certified in geriatrics, received additional training in the specialty.

3 "A lot of women in their 80s seem to have this kind of perverse loyalty to their doctors. They don't want to hurt their feelings. And they'll stay with someone even though they aren't getting good care and have their doubts," Dr. Cassel says.

"The message to give these women—and their adult daughters, who are often the people helping them—is that you always have the right to seek another opinion. If you have any doubts, especially if someone tells you 'it's just old age,' then you definitely should try another doctor."

4 As women's health care advocates, we can't afford to drop our guard on funding for breast cancer research. But we also can't afford to focus on only one issue. More research dollars need to be directed to the conditions that affect older women disproportionately.

As Dr. Cassel notes, although women survive longer, we also tend to have more chronic illness and disability, so we have a tougher time of it. "Research needs to be done in very simple things—things that don't kill people but that can cause enormous disability," she says, citing osteoarthritis, vision problems, and hearing loss as prime candidates.

Advocacy groups such as the Older Women's League (see Resources) offer one place to start.

receive radiation therapy, which is considered standard adjuvant treatment for younger women.

Treatment for cardiovascular diseases may be less than optimal as well. When compared to men, elderly women are less likely to be given clot-dissolving drugs during a heart attack; they're referred less often for carotid endarterectomy to prevent stroke; and they're less likely to be prescribed drugs to control hypertension.

Overall, however, prescription drug use is higher in older women than in older men, creating more problems with drug interactions. Because drug studies traditionally have been based on men—and women metabolize some drugs differently—women run the risk of being overmedicated on standard dosages of certain medica-

tions. Overmedication, in turn, can lead to falls and hip fractures.

• **Gaps in understanding.** Older women are often told that "it's just old age" or asked "what do you expect at your age?" But "old" does not necessarily mean "sick," and a woman shouldn't have her aches and pains dismissed just because she's no longer 35.

As the ranks of older patients increase, it's increasingly clear that "biological age" doesn't always correlate with chronological age. Says Dr. Cassel, "There's an expression: If you've seen one 90-year-old, you've seen *one* 90-year-old. A 90-year-old can be hitting 18 holes of golf or be at death's door in a nursing home—and everything in between."

No matter where she sits on this health care continuum, each older woman deserves to be treated with a personalized approach. Above all, she deserves to be treated with dignity.

Resources:

Older Women's League. OWL was the first national organization to focus solely on the concerns of mid-life and older women. For information on publications and programs, write OWL at 666 11th Street N.W., Suite 700, Washington, D.C. 20001.

Ourselves, Growing Older: Women Aging with Knowledge and Power by Paula Brown Doress and Diana Laskin Siegal (New York: Touchstone, 1994). Covers health care and includes a substantial resource section. ♀

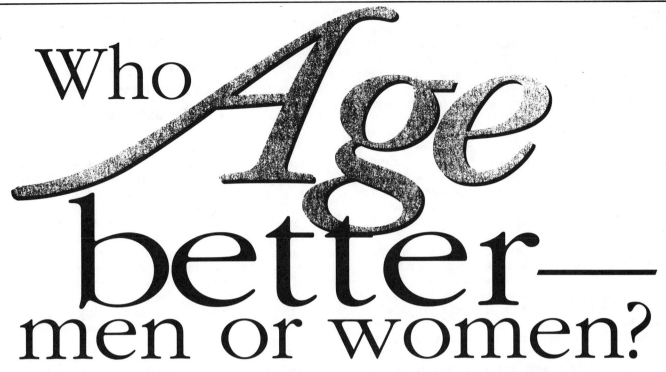

Who Age better— men or women?

Experts rate the sexes on their ability to hold off physical and mental changes—and report on the latest in anti-aging research

You know the typical images from movies and TV: The older man is distinguished, wise and virile. The older woman is bent, cranky and usually a victim. Then again, on average, men die six and a half years sooner than women. So who age better—women or men?

British researcher and Oxford University professor Richard Doll, M.D., gives the prize to women. In fact, says Doll, women consistently have a better shot at living at least one more year than men—until age 105. Only then, he says, is the mortality rate for men and women equal.

Since most of us won't get that old, here's a look at some things that happen as we age, how men and women fare and what, if anything, we can do about it.

PHYSICAL CHANGES
SKIN

Aging skin loses elasticity, collagen, fat and oil glands. The skin itself becomes thinner and often feels and appears dryer. On top of that, according to Marianne Berwick, Ph.D., of Memorial Sloan-Kettering Cancer Center in New York City, skin cancer is a major concern for older people. In fact, more than half of all new cases of squamous cell and basal cell skin cancer are diagnosed in people over 65 each year.

Men versus women: According to some surveys, men spend more time in the sun than women and are less likely to use sunscreen. By age 80, men have twice as many melanomas, a potentially fatal form of skin cancer, as women. Women also tend to see a doctor when skin lesions are smaller, which may explain why women's survival rate for this form of skin cancer is better.

Yet men have better-looking skin than women as they age—owing to one unlikely-to-change difference between the sexes: shaving. As men take whiskers from their face each day, they also slough away dead cells, which can make skin look old and dull.

What you can do: Most melanomas, experts agree, are caused by an intermittent pattern of exposure to the sun, but the way it works is baffling. At this point, the best advice remains to use caution. Whether or not sunscreens can prevent skin cancer in adults is a subject of hot debate among researchers, but it certainly won't hurt to use a sunscreen. Of course, stay out of the sun between 11 A.M. and 2 P.M., and wear hats, long sleeves and long pants. In addition, on every birthday, have your birthday suit checked for moles or new growths.

As for day-to-day wear and tear on your skin, use gentle skin-care products and avoid overscrubbing. And, in lieu of shaving, women can use a skin-care product formulated with alpha hydroxy acids to freshen the look of their skin.

B Y   A N D R E A   A T K I N S

MUSCLES

After age 30, muscles begin to atrophy. The change, subtle at first, becomes noticeable over time in both men and women. "Even Arnold Schwarzenegger is not as strong today as he was a few years ago," says James Fozard, Ph.D., of the National Institute on Aging.

"Strength and endurance fall off after age 30," agrees John A. Faulkner, Ph.D., of the University of Michigan.

Muscle cells and tissue—unlike skin—says Fozard, do not reproduce. Once they're gone, others won't take their place. That's significant because, as muscle cells weaken and atrophy, you become less able to do everyday chores such as walking up stairs or lifting luggage into the overhead compartment of an airplane. Worse than that, says Faulkner, "weak muscles are much more likely to be injured."

Men versus women: Men develop bigger muscles, so the decline of strength takes longer, according to Faulkner. Hence, a woman in her 70s may find it difficult to walk to the grocery store, but her husband may be able to take over the shopping for an additional 10 years.

What you can do: "You can't do anything about the change in muscle," says Faulkner, "but you can ameliorate it with conditioning. And I would give the same advice to both men and women." Stressing the muscle is the only way to strengthen it, so if you're not involved in some form of strength training, either at home or at a gym or health club, you're not doing anything to stop muscle loss, notes Faulkner.

BONES

With age, bones become more brittle and lose their density. The result: increased chance of fracture. An estimated 250,000 Americans suffer hip fractures each year, most often due to falls.

Men versus women: As with muscle mass, men start out with greater bone density. "Men start getting fractures about a decade later than women," says University of Chicago's Murray Favus, M.D. "Since men live shorter lives, they may not reach that stage."

"After menopause, women lose bone more quickly. Estrogen replacement therapy slows bone loss, which is why so many doctors recommend it," says Fozard.

What you can do: Exercise, exercise—and more exercise. "Studies have shown that a week of bed rest equals two years of aging on the skeleton," says William Evans, Ph.D., of Pennsylvania State University. The good news is that it doesn't take much exercise to have a positive effect. "Three to four days a week of walking for 40 to 45 minutes per day slows down the rate of bone loss—primarily from the spine," Evans says.

Do men or women exercise more consistently? No studies have answered that question, but Evans notes that when his center sets up exercise programs in the community, women enrollees far outnumber men.

HORMONES

Hormones, those chemical substances that travel around your body causing all kinds of reactions in everything from sex organs to memory to physique, decrease as you age. Scientists are unsure whether the

The good news: It doesn't take much exercise to slow bone and muscle loss

body suffers without them or simply has no use for them any longer. But hordes of researchers are trying to figure that out. A 1990 study by Daniel Rudman, M.D., found that men over the age of 60 given human growth hormone (hGH) for six months had improved energy, less body fat and more muscle mass. Unfortunately, a study released this year stripped hGH of some of its Fountain of Youth pizzazz. Although most of the men in this study who received the hormone showed the same physical gains, none gained strength, endurance or muscle ability, according to Dennis Black, Ph.D., of the University of California at San Francisco.

But the hormone hunt is far from over. "The potential is great," enthuses Owen Wolkowitz, M.D., also of the University of California at San Francisco. For example, Wolkowitz recently administered another hormone, DHEA, to a small group of depressed men and women between the ages of 50 and 75. The hormone not only lifted depression but improved memory as well, Wolkowitz says. Some researchers also believe that DHEA blocks the decline of the immune system.

Melatonin, a hormone on the research hot list, has been shown in some studies to improve sleep and even sexual function. You can buy it in health food stores, but its real benefits—like those of most hormones—remain unknown.

Men versus women: In the 1940s, doctors discovered the dramatic loss of estrogen suffered by women at the time of menopause. Researchers are just beginning to understand the loss of hormones in men. Reduced levels of testosterone, for instance, have been associated with decreased libido and, possibly, stroke.

What you can do: If you're a woman, you've probably made your choice about estrogen replacement therapy. But beyond that, for the moment, you can do very little about hormone replacement on your own. If you're a man, keep posted for news about testosterone studies.

One benefit credited to melatonin, however, is that it acts as an antioxidant, and both men and women can up their intake of antioxidants. Antioxidants seek out the body's free radicals, the result of normal metabolic changes, believed to damage the body. You can eat your antioxidants in foods, such as whole-grain cereals and breads, green leafy vegetables and citrus fruits, (which contain high concentrations of beta carotene and vitamins C and E), as well as take them in pill form. What's more, a study released in May 1996 showed that vitamin E supplements slowed age-related changes in the brain and immune system in mice.

"Eventually, these age-related changes will occur, but vitamin E slowed them," says Marguerite M. Kay,

M.D., who led the study at the University of Arizona.

MENTAL ABILITY
THE BRAIN
The older you get, the more slowly your brain works, says K. Warner Schaie, Ph.D., of Pennsylvania State University. With age, your ability to do more than one thing at a time also decreases. But, Schaie says, "it doesn't matter if you take a bit more time. The information, the vocabulary, the ability to use words all continue pretty well into old age."

Men versus women: As they age, men lose brain tissue from the area that affects planning and inhibition at almost three times the rate of women, according to Ruben C. Gur, Ph.D., of the University of Pennsylvania Medical Center. And, Gur notes, men's bodies compensate for the shrinkage by running their metabolisms at a higher rate. When brain (or any) cells are pushed too hard by a racing metabolism, they can die. Gur speculates this may be one reason men die sooner than women. Women, on the other hand, start with smaller brains but lose brain tissue more slowly, Gur found. They also tend to maintain a lower metabolic rate.

What you can do: "Use it or lose it" applies to the brain as well as to other muscles. Schaie and Gur agree that trying new activities, staying active and involved, and doing things you love are ways to stave off the slowing brain function that comes with age.

PERSONALITY
Were you a crotchety young man? Then you'll probably be a crotchety old man. Were you adventurous as a young woman? That sense of adventure will follow you to old age. "Personality doesn't change," says Barbara Waxman, a gerontologist in Kentfield, California.

Men versus women: Women tend to make more friends and remain more emotionally tied to them than men. That's significant because in a study of older people, "those with more social ties were less likely to be dead nine years later," finds Toni Antonucci, Ph.D., of the University of Michigan. "People who are productive and who receive and give social support live longer," says Yale University's Martha L. Bruce, Ph.D.

What you can do: Maintain social contacts—and make new ones. "Some people stop doing the things they enjoy when they retire—such as lunching with colleagues—and that's worrisome," Bruce says.

Regardless of whether you're a man or woman, you'll age. Men may look better with the passing years, but they don't live as long. Although women live longer, their lives are not necessarily healthier; they suffer more from chronic conditions such as arthritis and osteoporosis. In either case, one day, you'll look in the mirror and see an image staring back that you recognize only vaguely.

"Our outer layer does change," says gerontologist Waxman, "but our spirits don't. In the end, it's a question of melding the two. You've got to manage the spirit to stay vital."

ANDREA ATKINS, *a freelance writer who lives in Rye, New York, writes frequently on health and related subjects.*

The Latest Research
Meanwhile, Back in the Labs....
Can we learn to slow aging's inevitable advance? If we don't, it won't be for lack of trying. Researchers around the world are working in areas that range from diet to genes to hormones in an effort to slow the clock.

Cut the calories consumed by a laboratory rat, mouse or worm and it will live not only longer, but better. In hundreds of experiments, animals whose daily calories were cut by 35 percent aged better than those that ate what they wanted.

Research of this kind led University of Southern California's Caleb Finch, Ph.D., to conclude recently that caloric restriction could extend the average human life expectancy to 120 years. So scientists at the National Institute on Aging (NIA) began restricting the diets of monkeys. They wanted to see if the effect holds for a species more closely related to humans.

"The kinds of biological changes we saw in rats and mice also occur with monkeys," says NIA's George Roth, Ph.D., head of the monkey study. Sure, the monkeys are aging more slowly, but they *are* hungry, Roth acknowledges. Are they happy? A behavioral study now under way will answer that question. But more important, that study seeks to identify the mechanism that slows down aging when food is withheld. If the researchers can find that, Roth notes, then perhaps they can develop a drug that would mimic the effect of caloric restriction without necessarily cutting calories.

Researchers have also identified several genes in worms and fruit flies that, when mutated, increase life span. But they caution that the relationship to genes that control aging in humans remains unclear. Scientists may be somewhat closer to an answer with the identification of a gene responsible for a disease with symptoms of premature aging. But they're still a long way away from finding the genes that control aging.

And the use of hormones? Mitchell Harman, M.D., Ph.D., an endocrinologist with the NIA, says that work on human growth hormone is in its infancy. "We'll see the results of some large studies in the next few years, which will give us more information, but we'll need to experiment a lot more before we know what's going to work."

But, says Harman, the point of hormone research is not to help people live longer. "We're not trying to add years to life," he adds. "We're more interested in enabling people to feel better and not lose the capacity to work and play."—A.A.

Hormone Therapy: When and for How Long?

THE STORY

As women approach menopause, the decision of whether to take hormone replacement therapy (HRT) looms large. Sorting out the pros and cons of HRT makes the choice particularly confusing. While hormones can ease the sometimes troubling but temporary symptoms of menopause, such as hot flashes and night sweats, the bigger question is whether long-term HRT prevents or leads to common diseases.

Estrogen, the main component of HRT, is known to protect against osteoporosis and probably heart disease, but it raises the risk of endometrial cancer and possibly breast cancer. Progesterone, the other central player, is used as part of many hormone therapies because it can protect against endometrial cancer. But its influence on breast cancer is unclear.

Aside from the question of which hormones to take, there's also the consideration of when to start — and how long to take them.

Two studies published last month provide some new clues about the questions of timing. The first, in the February 19 *Journal of the American Medical Association*, measured the bone densities of 740 women ages 60 to 98. Most of the women — nearly 70 percent — had taken hormones for some period of time after menopause, though only 30 percent were still using hormones at the time of the study.

Not surprisingly, the women who started taking estrogen at menopause (usually between ages 48 and 53) and continued taking it into their later years had the highest bone density. But women who didn't start taking hormones until they turned 60 had bones that were nearly as dense as those of women who'd started on estrogen about a decade earlier, at menopause.

When women stopped the hormones, however, the benefits faded. The women who began estrogen therapy around menopause and stopped after 10 years were only slightly better off in their 70s than women who had never used the hormone.

In this study, most of the women were taking estrogen alone, with just one third taking progesterone in combination with the estrogen.

This so-called combination therapy is usually prescribed for women who still have a uterus, because taking estrogen alone increases the risk of endometrial cancer. Estrogen-only therapy causes the endometrium (the uterine lining) to build up, which means there's a chance that any abnormal cells in the endometrium may be overstimulated, possibly leading to cancer. Progesterone can prevent that process by prompting the uterine lining to slough off periodically — just like it does when a woman menstruates.

But progesterone's protective effect may depend on how it's taken, according to a report in the February 15 *Lancet*. Researchers interviewed 832 women with endometrial cancer and more than 1,000 women without the disease about their hormone use. They found that women whose regimen included progesterone fewer than 10 days a month had three times the risk of endometrial cancer of women who had never taken hormones. Among women who took estrogen alone, the risk was four times as high.

Women who took progesterone between 10 and 21 days per month had only a slightly increased risk of endometrial cancer compared with women who never took hormones. But if they stayed on that combination regimen for more than five years, their risk of the cancer was about two and a half times as high as women who never took hormones.

At first blush, the conclusions of these two studies may appear to confound the HRT issue even further, since the first seems to imply that women who take hormones the longest are the best off, while the second suggests a risk in taking them for more than five years. *HealthNews* associate editor Carolyn Runowicz, MD, offers help in interpreting the new findings.

— *The Editors*

THE PHYSICIAN'S PERSPECTIVE

Carolyn Runowicz, MD
Associate Editor

There are two main messages women should take away from these studies. The first is a familiar one: When making the decision about taking hormones, you need to carefully consider your own propensity for cancer, heart disease, and

---

TYPES OF HORMONE REPLACEMENT THERAPY

Estrogen alone – Via pill or skin patch

Cyclical therapy – Estrogen taken daily via pill or patch plus separate progesterone pill for a certain number of days per month

Continuous therapy – Estrogen plus low-dose progesterone in one or two pills taken every day

---

osteoporosis based on family history; your current symptoms; and your lifestyle. Unfortunately, that's not always how it happens. Many doctors automatically hand out prescriptions for hormones when women reach menopause — even if the woman isn't troubled by menopausal symptoms. Studies suggest that up to 60 percent of all postmenopausal women get prescriptions for hormones but only 25 percent actually fill them. And a quarter of those women stop taking the drugs within five years. In some cases, that might be appropriate; in other cases, it's not. Sometimes, women continue taking — or not taking — hormones simply out of habit. But both your symptoms and your lifestyle may change over the course of a decade.

That's the reasoning behind my second message: Women should reevaluate their hormone decision every five to ten years. For example, if you started taking hormones around menopause to treat bothersome hot flashes, you might consider tapering off the drugs if you aren't at high risk for osteoporosis or heart disease.

For women who still have a uterus, that choice may be particularly appropriate, because, as the *Lancet* article suggests, even women who take combined therapy for more than five years may raise their risk of endometrial cancer. Although endometrial cancer is the most common gynecological cancer, the overall risk is quite low. For every 100,000 50-year-old women, endometrial cancer will strike 20.

Tripling the risk would increase that number to 60. Also, endometrial cancer is rarely fatal, because its early warning sign (abnormal bleeding or spotting) alerts women to the problem, and a hysterectomy prevents the cancer from spreading. Still, we shouldn't discount the emotional upheaval and life-altering effects of a diagnosis of cancer, even one that is highly curable.

What's more, several studies have documented a slightly (around 30 percent) increased risk of breast cancer in women who took estrogen for more than 15 years. For every 100,000 50-year-old women, 250 will get breast cancer. A 30 percent increase would raise the number of cases to 325. So even a small increase in breast cancer risk suggests a possibly greater threat to a woman's health than the endometrial cancer risk. There's also some evidence that progesterone may stimulate breast tissue to divide abnormally. So long-term hormone therapy may be less advisable in women with other risk factors for breast cancer, such as having a mother or sister with the disease.

On the other hand, if you sailed through the "change of life" unfettered by the hormonal ups and downs that characterize this period, perhaps you didn't take any hormones. But if you're at risk of osteoporosis — that is, you have a family history of osteoporosis, have avoided high-calcium foods, and haven't exercised much, it's a good idea to get a bone density test. Your

BALANCING BENEFITS AND RISKS

ESTROGEN'S BENEFITS

▶ Relief from the classic symptoms of menopause: hot flashes, mood swings, vaginal dryness, thinning skin

▶ Proven reduced bone loss (osteoporosis) associated with menopause, including a probable reduction in hip fractures

▶ Probable reduced risk of heart disease by improving cholesterol levels and the flexibility of blood vessels

▶ Possible improved memory and better mental functioning of women with mild to moderate Alzheimer's disease

▶ Possible lowered risk of colon cancer

ESTROGEN'S RISKS

▶ An increased risk of endometrial cancer which may be countered by adding progesterone to a regimen of estrogen

▶ Symptoms similar to premenstrual ones (swelling, bloating, breast tenderness, mood swings, headaches)

▶ A menstrual discharge (when progesterone is taken with estrogen)

▶ Probable increased risk of breast cancer

▶ Stimulation of the growth of uterine fibroids and endometriosis

▶ Probable increased risk of gallstones and blood clots

▶ Possible weight gain

physician can order the test, which is painless, takes between 5 and 20 minutes depending on the number of sites (hip, spine, etc.) measured. The cost varies widely based on the type of machine used and is not always fully covered by insurance. If it reveals that your bones are weak, you should think about taking estrogen to strengthen them and decrease your risk of fracture. And, as the *JAMA* paper affirms, you don't risk any great bone loss by starting when you're older.

Fosamax, a drug that helps increase bone density and appears to prevent osteoporotic fractures, is another option for women who shouldn't or don't want to take estrogen. An FDA

panel recently recommended that the drug be approved for prevention, not just treatment, of osteoporosis.

What about heart disease? While it's true that heart disease is the number-one killer of older women, estrogen is only one way to prevent heart disease. Eating a low-fat, high-fiber diet and exercising to lower your cholesterol and blood pressure is vital — whether you take hormones or not.

Hormone replacement therapy is a personal decision, based on risk factors and symptoms. Remember, there isn't one right answer for all patients, and the answer may change with age and as your lifestyle changes.

Silent
SABOTAGE

The symptoms of this crippling,
sometimes fatal, bone disease often
go unnoticed. But there are changes
you can make—starting now—
to dramatically lower your risk.

JUDITH NEWMAN

I worry constantly about my health. Most nights you'll find me curled up with *The Merck Manual,* that bible for enlightened hypochondriacs, engrossed in yet another chapter of my ongoing medical drama; last night's installment, prompted by mild indigestion, was "Intestinal Threadworms: Could They Happen to You?"

Yet there's one body part I've never fretted about: my bones. They were there, they held me up, they were fine. During years of horseback riding I'd broken many and they'd all healed beautifully, with nothing but the occasional rainy-day ache to remind me of past mishaps. But, curious about a new medical technology, I went to Mount Sinai Hospital in New York City and got a dual-energy X-ray absorptiometry (DXA) scan, which measures bone density—and hence bone strength. This constituted one of my favorite activities: a visit to a place where serious-looking people would listen to me complain about assorted ills while administering a painless test. The DXA scan uses a tiny dose of radiation, emitted through a beam so focused the technician can sit in the room with you and chat while she monitors the procedure on a computer. I lie on a table, and the beam is passed through my hip, wrist, and spine.

The whole thing takes about 15 minutes, and I leave, whistling. Imagine my surprise when, a week later, Gail Rosselot, N.P., director of Mount Sinai's Osteoporosis Prevention and Detection Program, informs me that my hip density is 81 percent of what's considered normal for women my age (35). Nothing to fret about, though: Just take 1200 milligrams (mg) of calcium supplements a day, and come back in a year to see how things are going, she advises.

Immediately, I began popping calcium tablets like M&Ms.

In truth, I have every reason to be glad I took the test. It brought home a point I might not have learned otherwise: Bones are worth thinking about—even in your 30s and 40s. Especially in your 30s and 40s. Because osteoporosis, one of the most devastating and common diseases for women—80 percent of the 25 million Americans diagnosed with osteoporosis are female—is also one of the most preventable.

The trouble is, the disease—characterized by low bone mass, deterioration of bone tissue, and increased fragility and fracture risk—can go undetected for years. That's why specialists often call it the silent saboteur. But at some point a woman may begin to get subtle fractures of the spine, caused by an event as innocent as lifting a bag of groceries, which can cause excruciating pain and may result in the kind of back curvature we associate with old age. "And the bad news is that one fracture increases the risk of more fractures," says Ethel Siris, M.D., director of the Stabile Center for the Prevention and Treatment of Osteoporosis at Columbia-Presbyterian Medical Center in New York City.

We don't think of osteoporosis as life-threatening, but in fact, complications from fractures are a leading cause of death among older women. One in six women has a hip fracture during her lifetime, and many more have osteoporosis-related vertebral fractures. "Go into a nursing home, and look who's there," says Dr. Siris. "Fifty percent of people who break their hips do not live at home again. They need assistance." Thirty percent are unable to walk one year later, and up to 5 to 20 percent die within that time period, she adds.

But a diagnosis does not spell doom. Even if you have significant bone loss after menopause, you may never lose enough bone to develop full-blown osteoporosis—and even if you have osteoporosis right now, you may never suffer a fracture, develop a dowager's hump, or exhibit any other outward signs of the disease. "When I tell a fifty-year-old woman who feels just fine that she has osteoporosis, she thinks 'Oh my God! Any day now, I'm going to be a bent-over little old lady

From *Good Housekeeping*, April 1997, pp. 94-97. © 1997 by Judith Newman. Reprinted by permission.

with a walker!' Well, of course that's not the case," says Dr. Siris. "Being told you have osteo is like being told you have high blood pressure. It simply means you're more at risk for certain problems." But thanks to advancements in understanding—and treating—osteoporosis, there are many things you can do to keep the situation under control.

WHO'S AT RISK

When it comes to taking care of yourself, the experiences of Judy Black, a senior vice president of TicketMaster in Washington, DC, would make most of us quake in our Nikes. A former phys-ed teacher, the trim mother of two in her mid-40s runs, skis, and has always watched her diet. "When I needed to lose a few pounds, food that was fattening but also calcium-rich—like cheese—was always the first to go," she says.

Three years ago, Black pulled a muscle and had a lot of pain in her hip. She went to an orthopedic surgeon, who suggested that she also get a bone scan. It revealed significant loss in bone density, enough to be labeled osteoporosis. Black told her mother, Elinor Bergman,

71, also a former gym teacher, to get a scan too. Four years earlier Bergman had broken her ankle, just by stepping off a bench. "There were four or five other breaks in the last decade too," Black explains. "We never thought much about them." Her mother's tests confirmed that she also had the disease. Finally, Black convinced her younger sister, Jane, who was then only 38 and had no symptoms, to be tested; she, too, had osteoporosis.

Black, her mother, and sister share the biggest risk factor for osteoporosis: being female. It's not known exactly why, but with the loss of estrogen during menopause also comes bone loss. Thus far, scientists have no way of predicting the rate of deterioration, although it's thought that the tendency to lose bone quickly or slowly is hereditary. And Asians and Caucasians are at greater risk than African-Americans.

There are other risk factors as well, including:

NOT GETTING ENOUGH DIETARY CALCIUM. Dairy products—milk, cheese, yogurt—are the richest sources of calcium in food, and those who avoid them and don't take supplements are almost definitely not getting enough calcium. Additionally, a diet that's high in protein and/or sodium increases the amount of calcium that is excreted in urine. Studies also show that drinking more than three cups of caffeinated coffee a day can have the same effect. Heavy alcohol consumption is also bone-thinning.

SMALL FRAME AND/OR EXCESSIVE THINNESS. It has long been known that slight, petite women are at greater risk than their bigger-boned, better-padded sisters—especially if they were chronic dieters, or have suffered from anorexia or bulimia. (Eating disorders and extreme exercise regimens often result in long periods of amenorrhea, or the absence of normal menstrual cycles. The ovaries shut down and stop producing estrogen; this lack of estrogen wreaks havoc on bone building.)

SMOKING. This impedes the ability to build bone, although scientists aren't exactly sure why.

CERTAIN MEDICATIONS. Long-term use of steroids, such as prednisone and cortisone, anticonvulsants, and synthetic thyroid hormones can increase the risk.

BUILDING STRONGER BONES

Perhaps because we associate the skeleton with death, we assume it is inert. In fact, bone tissue is constantly renewing and repairing itself in a cellular renovation project that's sort of like a never-ending episode of *This Old House*. Cells called osteoclasts relentlessly chew on the skeletal surface, dissolving minerals and forming tiny potholes. Then, osteoblasts (think of them as millions of little backhoes) roll in and fill in the potholes with new bone, which is comprised mainly of collagen and minerals. Until about the age of 30, our bone mass is constantly increasing. For the next 15 to 20 years, it remains more or less stable. Then, with the onset of menopause, we lose bone at a rate of 2 to 4 percent a year, with the rate of loss slowing somewhat in our 60s and 70s. Some loss is normal and expected. Even after you've reached menopause, you can still retard bone loss, but the best bet is making sure that before menopause, you start out with the greatest density possible. It's like going deep-sea diving: One tank of oxygen might suffice, but why not take two?

Fortunately, the measures necessary to shore up your bone-density levels before and during menopause are relatively easy, affordable, and widely available:

SHOULD YOU BE SCREENED?

Doctors say the test of choice to assess risk for osteoporosis is the dual-energy X-ray absorptiometry (DXA) scan. The test (which costs $150 to $300, depending on where you live) compares your bone density to the bone densities of other women your age and body size, and to the density of a prototypical healthy 30-year-old. Doctors diagnose osteoporosis based on how many standard deviations you are away from the norm for someone your age. Less than one standard deviation away is good. Between one and two and a half deviations away: below the threshold of osteoporosis, but a sign that it's time to make some lifestyle changes and supplement your calcium intake. If your scan is between two and two and a half, you may want to talk to your doctor about more frequent monitoring. (My scan was one and a half deviations away from the norm.) Two and a half deviations or more below normal bone density: You have osteoporosis. To find the DXA screening center nearest you, call the National Osteoporosis Foundation at 202-223-2226.

There are also two urine tests available that can measure bone loss. These tests cannot diagnose osteoporosis per se, but they can determine whether you are losing bone for any number of reasons. They are also useful in evaluating whether the osteoporosis treatment you've chosen is working.

Should the DXA scan be required like a mammogram or Pap smear? Susan Love, M.D., doesn't think so. "Low bone density is only one piece of the puzzle," she notes. "If mine is lower than it should be for my age, it doesn't necessarily mean I'm going to get into trouble, because I could be a very slow bone loser." She suggests that only those who are at high risk of developing the disease need be tested—around the time of menopause, and every few years thereafter. Keep in mind that the DXA scan may not be covered by your health insurer, so discuss with your doctor whether you are at enough risk to make it worth your while.

FOOD AND SUPPLEMENTS. Even those of us with balanced diets may not be getting the recommended 1000 to 1200 mg of calcium a day (the equivalent of four glasses of milk). In addition to dairy products, other foods that are rich in calcium are bok choy, kale, broccoli, collard greens, calcium-enriched tofu, canned sardines, and canned salmon when eaten with the bones.

It can be difficult to get calcium through foods alone, because substances in certain vegetables and grains can bind to the calcium and make much of it unavailable for absorption. That's why more and more doctors and nutritionists are recommending calcium supplements. It's not important whether the supplements come in the form of calcium carbonate or calcium citrate; just look on the bottle for the amount of elemental calcium per tablet. Antacids like Tums and Rolaids are a cheap source—six regular-strength tablets a day give you about 1200 mg.

For optimal absorption, supplements should be taken just before meals and be split up over the course of the day with no more than 500 mg taken at any one time. Until you adjust to them, calcium carbonate supplements can cause gas and constipation. For the latter problem, you might also want to add a little extra fiber to your diet. And don't overdo it: Excess calcium in your bloodstream can lead to nausea, weight loss, kidney stones, internal bleeding, and even reduced bone strength.

Taking vitamin D or magnesium supplements to absorb the calcium isn't necessary. "You do need magnesium to absorb calcium, but virtually everyone gets enough in their diets without supplementation," notes Dr. Siris. You probably get enough vitamin D, too, especially if you're out in the sun for 15 minutes or more a day. If you're not sure, virtually all multivitamins contain the recommended 400 mg a day of vitamin D.

WEIGHT-BEARING EXERCISE. Various studies have proven conclusively: If you increase muscle mass, you increase bone density. "When you build muscle by weight training, you're also stimulating the bone that the muscle is attached to," says Wayne Westcott, Ph.D., fitness research director at South

NEW DRUG TREATMENTS

In 1995, the Food and Drug Administration approved two drugs that not only slow bone loss, but actually also seem to increase bone density:

Diphosphate alendronate (Fosomax) Studies show this nonhormonal drug decreases the risk of spine and hip fractures by 50 percent. But Fosomax is not an easy drug to take. Ten to 12 percent of users experience stomach upset or heartburn. And it must be taken first thing in the morning with at least eight ounces of water, and then you can't lie down, eat, or drink anything (even that all-essential jolt of java) for at least 30 minutes. Taking it improperly can lead to severe irritation of the esophagus. That's why it's not recommended for anyone with upper gastrointestinal problems, such as esophageal disease or difficulty in swallowing.

For now, Fosomax has been approved as a treatment only for those who already have osteoporosis. But researchers are looking into the possibility that, at a smaller dosage level, it may work as a preventive measure.

Calcitonin (Miacalcin) Once available only by injection, it's now available as a nasal spray. Though it hasn't been shown to prevent fractures, it does slow bone loss—and unlike Fosomax, it can be taken at any time of the day.

There are several other drugs in the pipeline that should be available in the next few years. Two in the same family as Fosomax—risedronate and tuludrinate—may not have to be taken first thing in the morning or every day. Another, Calcitriol, is already an extremely popular osteoporosis treatment in Europe, but it hasn't been approved yet in the United States. Finally, raloxifene may be the most intriguing treatment of all because in animal studies, it seems to offer the benefits of estrogen without the problems. But what raloxifene does in humans still remains to be seen.

Shore YMCA in Quincy, MA. "No matter what your age, doing weight-bearing exercise for as little as twenty to thirty minutes two days a week can result in a significant improvement in your muscle mass—and thus in your bone density," says Westcott.

ESTROGEN REPLACEMENT THERAPY (ERT). Although there are now several drugs available to treat osteoporosis, ERT is the only approved treatment for preventing it. Taking estrogen during and after menopause seems to slow the rate of bone loss, and may even add bone density. It's been shown to reduce future osteoporotic fractures by 50 percent or more. But to be most effective, it must be continued indefinitely.

Not all women are candidates for treatment, though. Since ERT seems to raise the risk of endometrial and breast cancer, it's not recommended for women with a family history of those diseases. Other women may be advised to stop ERT after ten years.

At least one high-profile physician—

Susan Love, M.D., adjunct associate professor of surgery at the University of California, Los Angeles, and author of *Dr. Susan Love's Hormone Book*—isn't convinced that ERT is a good osteoporosis preventive for *anyone*. She says, "Studies suggest that women with naturally lower estrogen levels have worse bones and a smaller chance of getting breast cancer, while women with higher estrogen levels have better bones, but a greater chance of getting breast cancer. And the lesson here, to me, is simple: There's no free lunch."

MY PERSONAL OSTEOPOROSIS-PREVENTION regimen now includes calcium supplements, weight training, and massive broccoli consumption. But sadly, there's one thing all these measures cannot do: make me graceful. As I was setting down a 12-pound weight recently, I dropped it squarely on my right foot. It swelled impressively—a good excuse, I felt, to visit the local radiologist.

I didn't break a single bone. Maybe I'm doing something right.

The Mammography Muddle

The Consensus Conference on Breast Cancer Screening for Women ages 40–49, which was held recently by the National Institutes of Health (NIH), reminded us that the most urgent questions in medicine often do not have ready answers. The consensus panel, which was convened to determine whether women in their 40s should have regular mammograms, abstained, citing inconclusive data. Instead, the panel advised each woman to weigh the evidence and decide whether or not regular mammograms were appropriate for her. By making no clear recommendation, the panel placed the responsibility for obtaining and evaluating the relevant information on women and health-care providers.

The report also carried a mixed message to insurers. It recommended that health plans cover the cost of regular mammography for women in their 40s. However, by failing to endorse regular mammography screening, it made it possible for insurers to contend that the practice does not merit reimbursement. As a result, women in their 40s who want mammograms may have to bear the cost, which averages around $90.

The anatomy of "consensus"

The 3-day conference was held as a part of the NIH consensus development program, in which ad hoc meetings are called to weigh the available scientific information concerning controversial topics of importance to public health. For these meetings, a panel of health professionals who are knowledgeable in the field, along with a representative of the public, is selected to evaluate the evidence. In this case, the NIH seemingly bent over backward to choose an unbiased jury of physicians, researchers, and consumer advocates who had neither participated in studies of mammography nor published articles about the topic. The NIH gave the panelists lists of articles to read in advance and brought in 32 speakers to present data at the conference. After considering a day and a half of testimony, the panel was given 20 hours to deliver a verdict and draft a report.

As that report was read aloud, it became apparent that the consensus process, which had been intended to resolve a controversy, had itself become mired in controversy. Some participants took issue with the structure of the program; others charged that the panel members harbored biases; still others contended that panelists lacked the expertise to make an informed decision. Even the director of the National Cancer Institute, Dr. Richard Klausner, stepped into the fray, voicing concern that the panel had overlooked new information favoring mammography.

Yet, despite the discordant climate, there were several points of true consensus at the conference, which, if you are in your 40s, may help you to make your decision about mammography. They are summarized in the following paragraphs.

• *If a benefit is present, it is small.* The conference reviewed data from the eight randomized controlled trials that have been conducted in women aged 40 and older over the last 30 years. In each of these studies, one group of women has had regular mammograms and a comparable group has not. Both groups have been followed for several years, and breast cancer deaths in each group have been compared.

These studies have yielded varied results. For women ages 50–69, the early data, compiled after 5–7 years of follow-up, were unequivocal—regular mammography seemed to reduce the risk of dying from breast cancer. During the same follow-up period, however, only one study indicated a similar reduction for women in their 40s. But after 10–18 years, at least three studies have demonstrated a reduction in risk in the 40–49 age group.

Some statisticians have combined all the data to indicate that mammograms produce a significant reduction in risk. Others have conducted similar analyses and found no such advantage. While statisticians continue to debate the meaning of these results, one thing is certain: regular mammography does not confer a reduction in the risk of a breast cancer death that is as dramatic for women in their 40s as for women in their 50s and 60s.

• *The studies may not represent the "real world."* Some of the studies considered at the conference were initiated in the 1960s and 1970s when mammography was in its infancy. Since then, the equipment used, imaging techniques employed, and interpretation of images have improved markedly. This is particularly important in screening premenopausal women who are more likely to have dense breast tissue that makes tumors more difficult to detect. Today all mammography facilities must meet rigorous federal standards.

A large majority of the women in the studies were caucasian. The data may not apply to black, Asian, or Hispanic women.

• *Mammograms detect smaller tumors.* Tumors diagnosed by mammography average less than 2 centimeters in diameter, and are much smaller than those picked up during a manual breast examination. Studies indicate that approximately 25% are ductal carcinoma in situ (DCIS), a precancerous condition in which abnormal cells are confined to mammary ducts, and which is discussed below. Another 40% are invasive cancer that hasn't metastasized. Only about 35% of breast cancer detected by mammography is metastatic.

• *Annual screening may be best.* There is increasing evidence that the nature of a breast tumor is determined early in the course of the disease. Because tumors that are destined to become invasive appear to progress more rapidly in premenopausal women, the risk of "interval cancers," which arise and metastasize between screenings, is higher in 40–49-year-olds. Thus opinion now favors mammography annually, rather than every other year, for women in this age group who decide to have it.

• *Risk of negative biopsy is higher.* Women in their 40s also have the highest rate of follow-up procedures after mammography, including ultrasound, needle aspiration, and surgical biopsy, as well as the highest rate of negative findings from these tests. By some estimates, the average 40-year-old woman who has an annual mammogram has a 30% chance of undergoing at least one biopsy before she's 50.

• *DCIS poses a dilemma.* The incidence of DCIS has risen precipitously since the advent of mammography because it previously went undetected until it became invasive disease. Many if not most, DCIS lesions will never become invasive tumors; yet DCIS, once diagnosed, rarely goes untreated. Women in their 40s have the highest rate of surgery for DCIS, and as many as 40% of women with DCIS still undergo mastectomy.

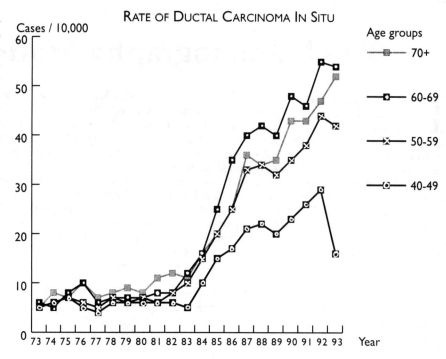

RATE OF DUCTAL CARCINOMA IN SITU

Cases / 10,000

Age groups
——■—— 70+
——□—— 60-69
——✕—— 50-59
——◉—— 40-49

Year

• *Mammography is less informative in this age group.* Because women in their 40s are more likely to have denser breast tissue than those in older age groups, they are also more likely to have mammograms that are difficult to read. That's because mammary tissue is seen as a white field against which tumors, which also appear to be white, must be detected. After menopause, women begin to have a lower ratio of mammary tissue to fat, which is gray on a mammogram and affords a sharper contrast to tumors. However, as with most physical characteristics, breast density varies widely from woman to woman; some may not have dense breasts in youth, while others retain density late in life. Unfortunately, clinical breast exams do not give an indication of breast density.

• *Radiation isn't risky.* Recent estimates provided by the National Cancer Institute indicate that at the current low levels of radiation in mammography, the risk of radiation-induced cancer is negligible for women 40 and older.

• *Your individual risk factors are important.* Breast cancer is the single most common cause of death among women in their 40s. Even so, the risk is still quite low: the average 40-year-old woman has a 0.3% chance of dying from breast cancer before age 50. The likelihood of being diagnosed with breast cancer during that decade is around 2%. Of course, certain factors—a history of breast cancer on either side of one's family, never having had a child, having one's first child after age 30, onset of menstruation before age 12,

and late menopause—may raise that risk. Nonetheless, 60–70% of breast cancers occur in women with no known risk factors.

• *Psychological concerns count.* For some women, having regular mammograms provides a sense of security; for others the test is a source of great anxiety. You undoubtedly know which group you're in. Although the psychological ramifications of mammography haven't been widely studied and are rarely discussed, your feelings are an important component of your decision.

What to do

We are in a state of changing knowledge and technology. Mammography is an imperfect screening tool, but it's the best one available at present. While the risk of unnecessary biopsy, and perhaps even unnecessary treatment for DCIS, is ever-present, so is the promise of detecting a small tumor in the early stages, when it requires less aggressive treatment and the prognosis is good.

This conundrum doesn't disappear on our 50th birthdays; we just enter a new statistical category in which the benefits of regular mammography clearly outweigh the disadvantages. Unfortunately, for women in their 40s, the decision isn't getting any easier yet.

FOR FURTHER INFORMATION

A copy of the NIH Consensus Development Conference: Breast Cancer Screening for Women Ages 40–49 can be ordered by calling 1-888-NIH-CONSENSUS. The latest draft is available on-line at http://consensus.nih.gov

---

Options for Hysterectomy

The decision to undergo hysterectomy isn't the only choice associated with the operation. After discussing the options with your clinician, you will probably have a few additional decisions to make; there are several approaches to hysterectomy.

If you are younger than 40 and have no evidence of ovarian disease, your ovaries and fallopian tubes will probably be left in place. You won't have periods, but your ovaries will continue to produce hormones. You'll still ovulate and the eggs will be absorbed by the body. Although no one knows exactly why, women who have had hysterectomies occasionally stop producing estrogen and enter menopause somewhat earlier than those who have an intact uterus.

If you are in your 40s, you should discuss with your surgeon whether your ovaries should be removed to eliminate the risk of ovarian cancer, which, though slight, increases with age. If your ovaries are taken, you will begin menopause, and your clinician will probably recommend estrogen replacement therapy to alleviate the symptoms of menopause, as well as to reduce the risk of osteoporosis.

If you are past menopause, your ovaries as well as your uterus are likely to be removed to eliminate the risk of ovarian cancer.

In any case, either a total hysterectomy or a supracervical hysterectomy may be performed. In a supracervical hysterectomy, the body of the uterus is removed and the neck of the cervix is sutured closed; the vagina is not noticeably altered, as illustrated on the next page, right. Some women prefer this approach, because the presence of the cervix enables them to have more pronounced vaginal contractions during orgasm. Because women who have had supracervical hysterectomies have a risk of cervical cancer similar to that of women with an intact uterus, they should follow the commonly recommended Pap screening schedule.

In a total hysterectomy, the surgeon closes the apex or "top" of the vagina. This creates a "blind" pouch. Intestines now fill the space once occupied by the uterus. Recent studies have indicated that regular Pap smears have little benefit for women who have had total hysterectomies and thus are no longer at risk for cervical cancer.

Surgical approaches

• *Abdominal hysterectomy.* This procedure is usually necessary when the uterus is substantially enlarged, there is extensive scar tissue in the abdomen, or cancer has been identified or is suspected. The surgeon makes either a vertical incision from the pubic line to below the navel or a horizontal incision at the pubic line from hipbone to hipbone. Because the surgeon must make a 4-6" incision through several layers of tissue and displace some abdominal organs, the operation requires general or regional anesthesia. Recovery may require 2-4 days in the hospital and 1-3 weeks at home. It can take up to three months before women who have had abdominal hysterectomies feel that they have recovered completely. They are usually advised to refrain from intercourse for six weeks.

• *Vaginal hysterectomy.* About one-third of hysterectomies are now performed through the vagina. In a standard vaginal hysterectomy, the surgeon makes a slit in the vaginal wall to gain access to the ligaments and tissues that anchor the uterus, ovaries, and fallopian tubes. After these tethers have been severed and the uterus freed, the organ is removed through the vagina. There is no visible surgical scar. Hospital stays are usually 1 to 2 days, and home convalescence is usually limited to two weeks. Women who have vaginal hysterectomies are asked to abstain from sexual intercourse for about 6 weeks.

In a laparoscopically-assisted vaginal hysterectomy (LAVH), the surgeon makes three or four small, half-inch incisions in the abdomen to enable the insertion of a fiber-optic viewing device or miniaturized video camera and surgical tools. The ligaments are severed laparoscopically, and the uterus is removed through the vagina. The procedure is more expensive than a vaginal hysterectomy because it takes longer to perform and requires more equipment and personnel. However, it enables surgeons to examine the abdomen for endometriosis and scar tissue, in much the same way open surgery does. It also makes it easier to remove the ovaries if necessary, and can facilitate vaginal hysterectomy in women who haven't had children. The recovery period is similar to that for standard vaginal hysterectomy.

Preparing for surgery

Several days before your operation, your surgeon will take a health history and you will have a standard physical examination including blood and urine tests. Although hospital policies vary, you may have an electrocardiogram and a chest x-ray.

During the pre-operative visit, your surgeon will explain the risks and ask you to sign a consent form indicating that you understand them. The most common complications of hysterectomy are reactions to anesthesia, infection, bleeding and blood clots. Rarer events include damage to the bowel, bladder or ureters — the vessels that carry urine from the kidneys. Your surgeon should give you an approximation of your particular risks, depending upon the type of hysterectomy you're having and your general state of health.

You will have to make some preparations for surgery. You may have to give yourself an enema or

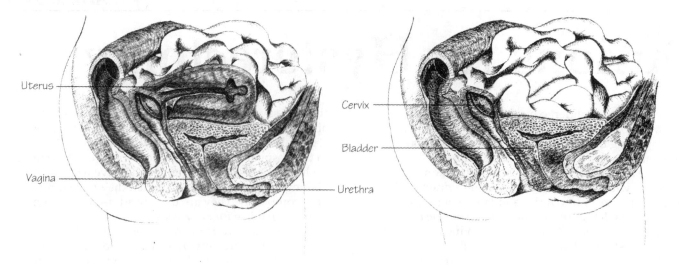

Before Hysterectomy   After Supracervical Hysterectomy

a laxative 1-2 days before surgery and restrict your diet to clear liquids the day before your operation. You may be asked not to eat or drink for 8-12 hours before you go to the operating room and may be prescribed antibiotics to take a few hours before your operation.

After hysterectomy

You will have a urinary catheter in place during surgery, and may still be wearing it when you wake up. You should be given liquids and foods as soon as you want them. You may be asked to cough periodically and may be given chest physiotherapy to prevent pulmonary complications. You'll also be monitored for signs of infection.

You will not be released from the hospital until the staff can be relatively certain that you can eat, drink, and move about on your own. Because you won't be able to drive, you'll want to make arrangements for transportation home in advance. You'll also need household help once you're home. While you may be up and about within a week or two, you may find that you tire easily for several months.

Recent surveys on the quality of life after hysterectomy have yielded surprisingly positive results. Although many women experience a sense of loss after the operation, such feelings are generally temporary; only women who suffered from depression before the procedure tended to be depressed afterward as well. In fact, most of the 800 participants in the Maine Women's Health Study and 1100 in a similar investigation by researchers from the University of Maryland, reported that the operation had improved their quality of life. In both of these studies, as in one conducted by the Centers for Disease Control several years earlier, the women polled also reported improved sexual satisfaction following hysterectomy.

These studies would seem to indicate that hysterectomy, though occasionally unnecessary, can also have substantial benefits. As with other things in life, preparation can make things go more smoothly. Hysterectomy is usually an elective procedure; you have time to evaluate alternative treatments, investigate the available surgical techniques, and get a second opinion if you have any qualms about the recommended surgical approach or the necessity for the operation. Most importantly, do whatever you need to do — be it adding iron to your diet or stopping smoking — to ensure that you're in the best shape possible should you decide to have the operation.

FOR FURTHER INFORMATION

National Women's Health Resource Center
2425 L Street NW, Washington, DC 20037
202-293-6045
http://www.womens-health.com/NWHRC.html

Hysterectomy Educational Resources and Services (HERS)
610-667-7757
Information on alternatives to and consequences of hysterectomy; telephone counseling; journal articles

National Women's Health Network
1325 G Street NW, Washington, DC 20005
202-347-1140
Information packets on hysterectomy

To obtain a free booklet,
"Understanding Hysterectomy," send SASE to:
The American College of Obstetricians and Gynecologists
Resource Center, 409 12th Street SW
Washington, DC 20024

Index

Credits/Acknowledgments

Cover design by Charles Vitelli

1. Women and Health
Facing overview—PhotoDisc, Inc. photo.

2. Nutrition and Fitness
Facing overview—Photo by Pamela Carley. 43—"Update '97" from *Mayo Clinic Health Letter*, June 1997, p. 3. © 1997 by the Mayo Foundation for Medical Education and Research, Rochester, MN 55905. Reprinted by permission.

3. Gynecological and Sexual Health
Facing overview—Illustration by Mike Eagle. 76—Photos by Richard Pierce.

4. Psychological Health
Facing overview—Photo by Louis P. Raucci.

5. Chronic Diseases
Facing overview—WHO photo by Jean Mohr.

6. Substance Abuse: New Trends for Women
Facing overview—Photo by Pamela Carley.

7. Violence in Women's Lives
Facing overview—New York Times Pictures photo by Bill Aller.

8. Special Issues for Older Women
Facing overview—Colonial Penn Group, Inc. photo.

ANNUAL EDITIONS ARTICLE REVIEW FORM

■ NAME: _____ DATE: _____

■ TITLE AND NUMBER OF ARTICLE: _____

■ BRIEFLY STATE THE MAIN IDEA OF THIS ARTICLE: _____

_____

■ LIST THREE IMPORTANT FACTS THAT THE AUTHOR USES TO SUPPORT THE MAIN IDEA:

_____

_____

_____

_____

■ WHAT INFORMATION OR IDEAS DISCUSSED IN THIS ARTICLE ARE ALSO DISCUSSED IN YOUR
TEXTBOOK OR OTHER READINGS THAT YOU HAVE DONE? LIST THE TEXTBOOK CHAPTERS AND
PAGE NUMBERS:

_____

_____

_____

_____

_____

■ LIST ANY EXAMPLES OF BIAS OR FAULTY REASONING THAT YOU FOUND IN THE ARTICLE:

_____

_____

_____

_____

■ LIST ANY NEW TERMS/CONCEPTS THAT WERE DISCUSSED IN THE ARTICLE, AND WRITE A SHORT
DEFINITION:

_____

_____

_____

_____

*Your instructor may require you to use this ANNUAL EDITIONS Article Review Form in any
number of ways: for articles that are assigned, for extra credit, as a tool to assist in developing
assigned papers, or simply for your own reference. Even if it is not required, we encourage
you to photocopy and use this page; you will find that reflecting on the articles will greatly
enhance the information from your text.

We Want Your Advice

ANNUAL EDITIONS revisions depend on two major opinion sources: one is our Advisory Board, listed in the front of this volume, which works with us in scanning the thousands of articles published in the public press each year; the other is you—the person actually using the book. Please help us and the users of the next edition by completing the prepaid article rating form on this page and returning it to us. Thank you for your help!

ANNUAL EDITIONS: WOMEN'S HEALTH 98/99
Article Rating Form

Here is an opportunity for you to have direct input into the next revision of this volume. We would like you to rate each of the 59 articles listed below, using the following scale:

1. **Excellent: should definitely be retained**
2. **Above average: should probably be retained**
3. **Below average: should probably be deleted**
4. **Poor: should definitely be deleted**

Your ratings will play a vital part in the next revision. So please mail this prepaid form to us just as soon as you complete it.
Thanks for your help!

Rating	Article	Rating	Article
	1. Women's Health Studies		30. The New Rite of Passage
	2. Women *Are* Different		31. Mending the Female Heart
	3. Work with Me, Doctor: How to Get Better Care		32. Heart Disease in Women: Special Symptoms, Special Risks
	4. Forgotten Women: How Minorities are Underserved by Our Health Care System		33. Consensus: No Long-Term Link between the Pill and Breast Cancer
	5. Fitting into Our Genes		34. Redesigning Women: Breast Cancer & Estrogen
	6. Give Your Body Time to Heal		35. The Cancer Nobody Talks About
	7. Say Good-Bye to Dieting		36. Mole Patrol
	8. Confessions of a Former Women's Magazine Writer		37. A Silent Epidemic
	9. Rebel against a Sedentary Life		38. Living with Lupus
	10. Diet Pills: Are Millions of Women Playing Russian Roulette with Their Health?		39. When Arthritis Strikes
	11. Dying to Win		40. Running on Empty
	12. Who *Isn't* on a Diet? In Search of Sensible Eating		41. What to Do for Urinary-Tract and Vaginal Infections
	13. The Diet Fix		42. What Does Being Female Have to Do with It?
	14. Weighty Matters in Women's Health		43. The Facts About . . . Women and Smoking
	15. The Smart Pap		44. Up in Smoke: Why Teen Girls Don't Quit
	16. Politically Incorrect Surgery		45. A Smoker's Tale
	17. Prevent Sexually Transmitted Diseases		46. Cigars, Women, and Cancer
	18. The Condom Report: What's New in Sheath Chic		47. Alcohol and Health: Mixed Messages for Women
	19. Rethinking Birth Control		48. Way Out West and Under the Influence
	20. Endometriosis: The Hidden Epidemic		49. Female Genital Mutilation: Balancing Intolerance of the Practice with Tolerance of Culture
	21. Overcoming Infertility		50. Domestic Violence: Why It's Every Woman's Issue . . . and What *You* Can Do
	22. The National Abortion Debate: Are Both Sides Asking the Wrong Questions?		51. A Woman's Killer Is Likely to Be Her Partner, A New Study in New York Finds
	23. Psychological Aftereffects of Abortion: The Rest of the Story		52. "I Was Raped"
	24. How Real Women Keep Stress at Bay		53. Dangerous Men: The Warning Signals You May Miss
	25. The Myth of the Miserable Working Woman		54. Our Mothers, Ourselves: Older Women's Health Care
	26. Stressed Out—and Sick from It: The Ultimate Prevention Guide		55. Who Age Better—Men or Women?
	27. Depression: Way beyond the Blues		56. Hormone Therapy: When and for How Long?
	28. Treating Eating Disorders		57. Silent Sabotage
	29. Childless by Choice		58. The Mammography Muddle
			59. Options for Hysterectomy

(Continued on next page)

ABOUT YOU

Name _____ Date _____

Are you a teacher? ❑ Or a student? ❑

Your school name _____

Department _____

Address _____

City _____ State _____ Zip _____

School telephone # _____

YOUR COMMENTS ARE IMPORTANT TO US !

Please fill in the following information:

For which course did you use this book? _____

Did you use a text with this *ANNUAL EDITION*? ❑ yes ❑ no

What was the title of the text? _____

What are your general reactions to the *Annual Editions* concept?

Have you read any particular articles recently that you think should be included in the next edition?

Are there any articles you feel should be replaced in the next edition? Why?

Are there any World Wide Web sites you feel should be included in the next edition? Please annotate.

May we contact you for editorial input?

May we quote your comments?